Mental Health Challenges during the COVID-19 Pandemic

Mental Health Challenges during the COVID-19 Pandemic

Editor

Alfonso Troisi

MDPI • Basel • Beijing • Wuhan • Barcelona • Belgrade • Manchester • Tokyo • Cluj • Tianjin

Editor
Alfonso Troisi
Department of Systems
Medicine
University of Rome Tor
Vergata
Rome
Italy

Editorial Office
MDPI
St. Alban-Anlage 66
4052 Basel, Switzerland

This is a reprint of articles from the Special Issue published online in the open access journal *Journal of Clinical Medicine* (ISSN 2077-0383) (available at: www.mdpi.com/journal/jcm/special_issues/Mental_Health_Pandemic).

For citation purposes, cite each article independently as indicated on the article page online and as indicated below:

LastName, A.A.; LastName, B.B.; LastName, C.C. Article Title. *Journal Name* **Year**, *Volume Number*, Page Range.

ISBN 978-3-0365-7195-9 (Hbk)
ISBN 978-3-0365-7194-2 (PDF)

Cover image courtesy of Maria Claudia Blanco
A depressed woman wearing a mask. Still from short film: "Au bord du délire" directed by Maria Claudia Blanco, La Fémis Production, FR, 2022

Contents

About the Editor . . . . **vii**

Preface to "Mental Health Challenges during the COVID-19 Pandemic" . . . . **ix**

Alfonso Troisi
Mental Health Challenges during the COVID-19 Pandemic
Reprinted from: *J. Clin. Med.* **2023**, *12*, 1213, doi:10.3390/jcm12031213 . . . . **1**

Alona Emodi-Perlman, Ilana Eli, Nir Uziel, Joanna Smardz, Anahat Khehra and Efrat Gilon et al.
Public Concerns during the COVID-19 Lockdown: A Multicultural Cross-Sectional Study among Internet Survey Respondents in Three Countries
Reprinted from: *J. Clin. Med.* **2021**, *10*, 1577, doi:10.3390/jcm10081577 . . . . **7**

Noelia Muñoz-Fernández and Ana Rodríguez-Meirinhos
Adolescents' Concerns, Routines, Peer Activities, Frustration, and Optimism in the Time of COVID-19 Confinement in Spain
Reprinted from: *J. Clin. Med.* **2021**, *10*, 798, doi:10.3390/jcm10040798 . . . . **19**

Dimitrios Kavvadas, Asimoula Kavvada, Sofia Karachrysafi, Vasileios Papaliagkas, Stavros Cheristanidis and Maria Chatzidimitriou et al.
Stress, Anxiety and Depression Prevalence among Greek University Students during COVID-19 Pandemic: A Two-Year Survey
Reprinted from: *J. Clin. Med.* **2022**, *11*, 4263, doi:10.3390/jcm11154263 . . . . **33**

Leilanie Apostol-Nicodemus, Ian Kim B. Tabios, Anna Guia O. Limpoco, Gabriele Dominique P. Domingo and Ourlad Alzeus G. Tantengco
Psychosocial Distress among Family Members of COVID-19 Patients Admitted to Hospital and Isolation Facilities in the Philippines: A Prospective Cohort Study
Reprinted from: *J. Clin. Med.* **2022**, *11*, 5236, doi:10.3390/jcm11175236 . . . . **49**

Beatriz Olaya, María Pérez-Moreno, Juan Bueno-Notivol, Patricia Gracia-García, Isabel Lasheras and Javier Santabárbara
Prevalence of Depression among Healthcare Workers during the COVID-19 Outbreak: A Systematic Review and Meta-Analysis
Reprinted from: *J. Clin. Med.* **2021**, *10*, 3406, doi:10.3390/jcm10153406 . . . . **63**

Raúl Soto-Cámara, Susana Navalpotro-Pascual, José Julio Jiménez-Alegre, Noemí García-Santa-Basilia, Henar Onrubia-Baticón and José M. Navalpotro-Pascual et al.
Influence of the Cumulative Incidence of COVID-19 Cases on the Mental Health of the Spanish Out-of-Hospital Professionals
Reprinted from: *J. Clin. Med.* **2022**, *11*, 2227, doi:10.3390/jcm11082227 . . . . **81**

Gaia Perego, Federica Cugnata, Chiara Brombin, Francesca Milano, Emanuele Preti and Rossella Di Pierro et al.
The "Healthcare Workers' Wellbeing [Benessere Operatori]" Project: A Longitudinal Evaluation of Psychological Responses of Italian Healthcare Workers during the COVID-19 Pandemic
Reprinted from: *J. Clin. Med.* **2022**, *11*, 2317, doi:10.3390/jcm11092317 . . . . **95**

Alfonso Troisi, Roberta Croce Nanni, Alessandra Riconi, Valeria Carola and David Di Cave
Fear of COVID-19 among Healthcare Workers: The Role of Neuroticism and Fearful Attachment
Reprinted from: *J. Clin. Med.* **2021**, *10*, 4358, doi:10.3390/jcm10194358 . . . . **113**

Marta Llorente-Alonso, Cristina García-Ael, Gabriela Topa, María Luisa Sanz-Muñoz, Irene Muñoz-Alcalde and Beatriz Cortés-Abejer
Can Psychological Empowerment Prevent Emotional Disorders in Presence of Fear of COVID-19 in Health Workers? A Cross-Sectional Validation Study
Reprinted from: *J. Clin. Med.* **2021**, *10*, 1614, doi:10.3390/jcm10081614 . . . . **121**

Camilla Gesi, Federico Grasso, Filippo Dragogna, Marco Vercesi, Silvia Paletta and Pierluigi Politi et al.
How Did COVID-19 Affect Suicidality? Data from a Multicentric Study in Lombardy
Reprinted from: *J. Clin. Med.* **2021**, *10*, 2410, doi:10.3390/jcm10112410 . . . . **137**

Flavia Marino, Paola Chilà, Chiara Failla, Roberta Minutoli, Noemi Vetrano and Claudia Luraschi et al.
Psychological Interventions for Children with Autism during the COVID-19 Pandemic through a Remote Behavioral Skills Training Program
Reprinted from: *J. Clin. Med.* **2022**, *11*, 1194, doi:10.3390/jcm11051194 . . . . **149**

Marina Letica-Crepulja, Aleksandra Stevanović, Diana Palaić, Iva Vidović and Tanja Frančišković
PTSD Symptoms and Coping with COVID-19 Pandemic among Treatment-Seeking Veterans: Prospective Cohort Study
Reprinted from: *J. Clin. Med.* **2022**, *11*, 2715, doi:10.3390/jcm11102715 . . . . **165**

Dariusz Wojciech Mazurkiewicz, Jolanta Strzelecka and Dorota Izabela Piechocka
Adverse Mental Health Sequelae of COVID-19 Pandemic in the Pregnant Population and Useful Implications for Clinical Practice
Reprinted from: *J. Clin. Med.* **2022**, *11*, 2072, doi:10.3390/jcm11082072 . . . . **177**

Vidya Rajagopalan, William T. Reynolds, Jeremy Zepeda, Jeraldine Lopez, Skorn Ponrartana and John Wood et al.
Impact of COVID-19 Related Maternal Stress on Fetal Brain Development: A Multimodal MRI Study
Reprinted from: *J. Clin. Med.* **2022**, *11*, 6635, doi:10.3390/jcm11226635 . . . . **195**

Hashir Ali Awan, Mufaddal Najmuddin Diwan, Alifiya Aamir, Muneeza Ali, Massimo Di Giannantonio and Irfan Ullah et al.
SARS-CoV-2 and the Brain: What Do We Know about the Causality of 'Cognitive COVID?
Reprinted from: *J. Clin. Med.* **2021**, *10*, 3441, doi:10.3390/jcm10153441 . . . . **209**

Niloufar Zia, Parsa Ravanfar, Sepideh Allahdadian and Mehdi Ghasemi
Impact of COVID-19 on Neuropsychiatric Disorders
Reprinted from: *J. Clin. Med.* **2022**, *11*, 5213, doi:10.3390/jcm11175213 . . . . **223**

About the Editor

Alfonso Troisi

Alfonso Troisi is a Professor of Psychiatry at the International Medical School of the University of Rome Tor Vergata. In addition, he is director of the outpatient treatment program for eating disorders at the Psychiatric Clinic of the Medical Center of the University of Rome Tor Vergata.

Alfonso Troisi has published over 200 papers and book chapters. He co-authored the book Darwinian Psychiatry (Oxford University Press, 1998) and authored the books The Painted Mind: Behavioral Science Reflected in Great Paintings (Oxford University Press, 2017) and Bariatric Psychology and Psychiatry (Springer, 2020). His Hirsch index is 40 based on the Scopus database and 55 based on the Google Scholar database. His name was included in the list of the World's Top Scientists published in October 2020 by the University of Stanford (PLoS Biol 18(10): e3000918). Among the 159,684 scientists in all disciplines, Alfonso Troisi's rank was 51,167. Among the limited number of psychiatrists included in the list (3,519), Alfonso Troisi's rank was 1,070.

The breadth of his current research covers: the analysis of nonverbal behavior in psychiatric patients, the relationship between adult attachment style and psychopathology, the role of social cognition deficits in psychoses, the impact of adverse early experiences on adult mental health and the psychiatric aspects of obesity. Professor Troisi was instrumental in promoting the development of the Darwinian approach for the study of mental disorders and in showing the clinical utility of concepts and methods derived from evolutionary disciplines including human ethology, behavioral ecology and evolutionary psychology. In line with his prolonged activity in this interdisciplinary endeavor, he has been nominated as a member of the Task Force for Evolutionary Psychiatry of the World Federation of Societies of Biological Psychiatry (WFSBP) and the Section on Evolutionary Psychiatry of the World Psychiatric Association (WPA).

Preface to "Mental Health Challenges during the COVID-19 Pandemic"

The papers included in this reprint were originally published in the Special Issue of the Journal of Clinical Medicine entitled, "Mental Health Challenges during the COVID-19 Pandemic". The Special Issue was launched in early 2021 and closed in late 2022, covering the most critical phase of the COVID-19 pandemic. The aim of the Special Issue was to provide readers with updated research findings on the psychological and psychiatric consequences of the pandemic. Review papers, clinical studies and theoretical models were equally considered for publication. The response from potential contributors went beyond my expectations, with there being many submissions and, ultimately, 17 papers accepted for publication.

The wide scope of the reprint reflects the complexity of the impact of the COVID-19 pandemic on mental health. The focus of the studies ranges from the psychological consequences of social distancing and the closure of schools to the neurological consequences of the viral infection, and from the stressful impact of an increased workload on frontline health workers to the unmet needs of special populations such as pregnant women, veterans and patients with neurodevelopmental disorders. Thanks to its richness in content and worldwide perspectives (contributors were from Canada, Croatia, Greece, India, Israel, Italy, Pakistan, the Philippines, Poland, Spain, and the USA), this reprint is a valuable source of information to researchers and clinicians interested in the mental health implications of the COVID-19 pandemic.

Finally, I wish to thank Phoebe Zhang, Assistant Editor at the MDPI Branch Office, for her excellent editorial support.

Alfonso Troisi
Editor

Journal of
Clinical Medicine

MDPI

Editorial

Mental Health Challenges during the COVID-19 Pandemic

Alfonso Troisi

International Medical School, University of Rome Tor Vergata, via Montpellier 1, 00133 Rome, Italy;
alfonso.troisi@uniroma2.it

The impact of the COVID-19 pandemic on mental health has unveiled the complexity of the relationship between psychiatry and the rest of medicine, as clearly shown by the collection of studies published in this Special Issue entitled "Mental Health Challenges during the COVID-19 Pandemic".

Mental health and well-being depend on the combination of many individual variables, including genetic background, physiological homeostasis, child rearing experiences, socio-economic conditions, lifestyle, and interpersonal relationships. Although these variables are partly interconnected, they belong to distinct levels of analysis and are the object of study of different disciplines. It is uncommon to observe a single medical condition causing adverse effects on mental health through its concurrent impact on many of the variables listed above. Yet, this is exactly what has been happening with the COVID-19 pandemic.

The papers by Muñoz-Fernández et al. [1] and Kavvadas et al. [2] show that home confinement and alteration of daily activities were associated with increased levels of negative affectivity in Spanish adolescents and Greek university students, respectively. These findings are in line with growing evidence showing the importance of rewarding interpersonal relationships for establishing and maintaining optimal levels of psychological well-being [3]. This explains why preventive measures that proved to be effective in terms of controlling the spread of the virus led to other problems, particularly relating to the mental health of younger people.

Reviewing research and clinical data on the neurological effects of the SARS-CoV-2 infection, the papers by Zia et al. [4] and Ali Awan et al. [5] focused on the other extreme of the continuum that extends from the social to the organic. COVID-19 may be associated with a variety of neurologic complications, and several plausible mechanisms exist to account for these observations. As the current understanding of COVID-19 continues to evolve, a synthesis of the literature on the neurological impact of this novel virus may help inform clinical management and highlight potentially important avenues of investigation. Interestingly, the pathogenesis of neurological damage can involve indirect mechanisms, as shown by Rajagopalan et al. [6], who found alterations in fetal brainstem structure associated with increased maternal perception of pandemic-related stress in pregnant women.

Pregnant women belong to those special populations that have been responding to the challenge of the COVID-19 pandemic in peculiar ways, as shown by the review paper by Mazurchiewicz et al. [7]. Other special populations were investigated by Letica-Crepulja et al. [8], who analyzed symptom levels and coping strategies during the COVID-19 pandemic among treatment-seeking veterans with pre-existing post-traumatic disorder (PTSD), and by Marino et al. [9], who assessed the efficacy of a web-based remote training program in the management of behavioral disorders of children with autism spectrum disorders. In effect, one of the few positive aspects imposed by the COVID-19 pandemic is that telehealth has been rapidly deployed to help meet critical mental health needs.

Not only individual but also group variables may modulate the impact of the COVID-19 on mental health. Cultural differences should not be neglected when developing public health strategies to mitigate the adverse effects of stress, social isolation, fear, and uncertainty. Emodi-Perlam et al. [10] conducted a cross-sectional online survey and found major

Citation: Troisi, A. Mental Health Challenges during the COVID-19 Pandemic. *J. Clin. Med.* **2023**, *12*, 1213. https://doi.org/10.3390/jcm12031213

Received: 6 January 2023
Accepted: 30 January 2023
Published: 3 February 2023

differences in personal worries about physical health, finances, and relations with relatives and friends of participants living in Canada, Israel, and Poland. These findings are consistent with one of the basic postulates of contemporary psychotraumatology: the individual response to stressors and traumatic events depends in part on the cultural context in which the person lives and the order and priority of ideological values [11].

The paper by Gesi et al. [12] reports on the number and characteristics of subjects accessing the emergency rooms for suicidal behavior in three Emergency Departments in Lombardy (Italy) before (2019) and during the first wave (2020) of the COVID-19 pandemic. The proportion of subjects accessing the Emergency Department for suicidality was significantly higher in 2020 than in 2019. Interestingly, during the pandemic, a greater proportion of subjects did not show any mental disorders and were psychotropic drug-free.

Five of the 16 papers published in this Special Issue focused on the mental health problems of healthcare workers (HCWs) working in COVID-19 healthcare facilities. HCWs face a high risk of contracting a potentially severe viral infection, as shown by mortality statistics. At the same time, compared to the general population, they have a better knowledge of infection risk factors and are consistently adopting preventive measures because of their professional duties. Thus, they are the ideal sample to study the interaction between emotional and rational psychological factors in modulating individual levels of fear of infection and its impact on mental health. Olaya et al. [13] carried out a systematic review and meta-analysis of the prevalence of depression among HCWs during the first wave of the COVID-19 pandemic. They found that almost half of the frontline HCWs showed increased levels of depression. The papers by Perego et al. [14] and Soto-Cámara et al. [15] identified several variables that act as risk factors for the development of depression and anxiety in HCWs (i.e., female gender, less work experience, lower levels of perceived social support, living with minors). Troisi et al. [16] found that personality was a significant predictor of fear of infection in HCWs working in a COVID-19 university hospital. Those participants who reported a more intense fear of infection had higher levels of neuroticism and fearful attachment. Considering that excessive fear of infection can put at risk HCWs' psychological well-being and occupational efficiency, these findings can be useful to identify vulnerable subgroups and to implement selective programs of prevention based on counseling and psychological support. In their paper, Llorente-Alonso et al. [17] discuss the utility of selective programs such as job crafting and psychological empowerment to reduce the emotional distress of HCWs fighting the COVID-19 pandemic.

The burden of taking care of COVID-19 patients falls not only on HCWs, but also on their family caregivers. Apostol-Nicodemus et al. [18] carried out a cohort prospective study to assess the psychosocial impact of the pandemic on Philippine families of adult COVID-19 patients in isolation. They found that 43.2% of the caregivers had anxiety symptoms and 16.2% had depressive symptoms two weeks after the discharge of their relatives with a COVID-19 infection.

Before the COVID-19 pandemic, it was difficult to imagine that the worldwide spread of a respiratory infectious disease could have so many implications for mental health. The papers published in this Special Issue help us to understand why this has been happening. By definition, psychiatry is an interdisciplinary field extending from the investigation of neural correlates to the analysis of social dynamics [19]. The challenge of facing a global infectious threat has confirmed the importance of psychiatry for the rest of medicine and the necessity of considering the relationship between physical and mental health in terms of bidirectional pathways.

In this regard, one specific aspect is worth discussing. The COVID-19 pandemic has revealed how primitive emotional reactions to the risk of being infected by a potentially severe contagious disease can impact prevention and treatment programs.

There is a substantial difference between the fear of infection and the fear of the degenerative diseases that rank at the top of the morbidity statistics in affluent countries. Cancer, Alzheimer's disease, heart disease, stroke, and diabetes are evolutionary novelties because their etiology and pathogenesis depend largely on risk factors and life habits that are typical of modern environments (e.g., extended longevity, high-calorie diet, sedentary lifestyle, obesity, smoking, drinking alcohol, pollution, etc.). Our ancestors living in the natural environment were not exposed to these risk factors and, therefore, they had an infinitesimal likelihood of getting cancer or developing senile dementia. Meanwhile, they had a very high likelihood of dying from an infection. From an evolutionary perspective, this means that infectious diseases have exerted strong selective pressures on human psychology and behavior.

Selection pressures have reinforced our defenses against infections by causing the evolution of a behavioral immune system that is separate from, and complementary to, the physiological immune system. The behavioral immune system includes a set of proactive mechanisms that inhibit contact with pathogens in the first place. These mechanisms offer a sort of psychological and behavioral prophylaxis against infection [20,21]. Like the physiological immune system, the behavioral immune system includes both detection and response mechanisms. When an external cue connoting infection risk (e.g., seeing another person with symptoms of infectious disease) is detected, it triggers a cascade of emotional and behavioral responses that minimize the infection risk (e.g., through social avoidance of people who appear to pose an infection risk). Fear of infection and pathogen disgust sensitivity are the two psychological mechanisms serving the adaptive function of the behavioral immune system [22].

Fear and disgust are deeply rooted in our emotional brain, and their activation can interfere with the implementation of public health strategies based on rational decisions. For example, one study reported a correlation between higher pathogen disgust sensitivity and negative attitudes toward COVID-19 vaccination [23]. A possible explanation for the negative impact of high pathogen disgust sensitivity on vaccination adherence is that vaccines are administered in ways that in and by themselves are cues to contamination, such as puncturing the skin or the inhalation or ingestion of a foreign substance [24].

One should consider that vaccination is an evolutionary novelty not directly linked with the cues that activate the behavioral immune system. Accordingly, the intention to vaccinate is a deliberate, conscious choice which might be only partially related to individual differences in germ aversion. In effect, when studies have focused on preventive measures other than vaccination, the functional utility of the behavioral immune system for combating the COVID-19 pandemic has emerged clearly. Shook et al. [25] found that germ aversion correlated with the frequency of preventive health behaviors such as social distancing, avoiding touching one's face, wearing a facemask, hand washing and disinfecting objects. Cox et al. [26] reported that heightened disgust proneness before the pandemic resulted in an increased use of protective behaviors during the pandemic. Makhanova and Shepherd [27] found that germ aversion was negatively associated with the number of face-to-face interactions and positively associated with anxiety about social proximity.

The study of the behavioral immune system is a paradigmatic model for understanding the complex relationship between psychiatry and the rest of medicine. For example, there is evidence that, when social distancing results in social isolation, the functionality of the physiological immune system is reduced [28]. By contrast, the activity of the physiological immune system is enhanced by visual exposure to symptoms of infectious disease in others [29]. In conclusion, a lesson we are learning from the COVID-19 pandemic is that public health strategies should routinely include psychiatry and allied disciplines within the theoretical framework developed for optimizing prevention and treatment programs.

Conflicts of Interest: The authors declare no conflict of interest.

References

1. Muñoz-Fernández, N.; Rodríguez-Meirinhos, A. Adolescents' Concerns, Routines, Peer Activities, Frustration, and Optimism in the Time of COVID-19 Confinement in Spain. *J. Clin. Med.* **2021**, *10*, 798. [CrossRef] [PubMed]
2. Kavvadas, D.; Kavvada, A.; Karachrysafi, S.; Papaliagkas, V.; Cheristanidis, S.; Chatzidimitriou, M.; Papamitsou, T. Stress, Anxiety and Depression Prevalence among Greek University Students during COVID-19 Pandemic: A Two-Year Survey. *J. Clin. Med.* **2022**, *11*, 4263. [CrossRef] [PubMed]
3. Troisi, A. Social stress and psychiatric disorders: Evolutionary reflections on debated questions. *Neurosci. Biobehav. Rev.* **2020**, *116*, 461–469. [CrossRef] [PubMed]
4. Zia, N.; Ravanfar, P.; Allahdadian, S.; Ghasemi, M. Impact of COVID-19 on Neuropsychiatric Disorders. *J. Clin. Med.* **2022**, *11*, 5213. [CrossRef] [PubMed]
5. Ali Awan, H.; Najmuddin Diwan, M.; Aamir, A.; Ali, M.; Di Giannantonio, M.; Ullah, I.; Shoib, S.; De Berardis, D. SARS-CoV-2 and the Brain: What Do We Know about the Causality of 'Cognitive COVID? *J. Clin. Med.* **2021**, *10*, 3441. [CrossRef]
6. Rajagopalan, V.; Reynolds, W.; Zepeda, J.; Lopez, J.; Ponrartana, S.; Wood, J.; Ceschin, R.; Panigrahy, A. Impact of COVID-19 Related Maternal Stress on Fetal Brain Development: A Multimodal MRI Study. *J. Clin. Med.* **2022**, *11*, 6635. [CrossRef] [PubMed]
7. Mazurkiewicz, D.; Strzelecka, J.; Piechocka, D. Adverse Mental Health Sequelae of COVID-19 Pandemic in the Pregnant Population and Useful Implications for Clinical Practice. *J. Clin. Med.* **2022**, *11*, 2072. [CrossRef]
8. Letica-Crepulja, M.; Stevanović, A.; Palaić, D.; Vidović, I.; Frančišković, T. PTSD Symptoms and Coping with COVID-19 Pandemic among Treatment-Seeking Veterans: Prospective Cohort Study. *J. Clin. Med.* **2022**, *11*, 2715. [CrossRef]
9. Marino, F.; Chilà, P.; Failla, C.; Minutoli, R.; Vetrano, N.; Luraschi, C.; Carrozza, C.; Leonardi, E.; Busà, M.; Genovese, S.; et al. Psychological Interventions for Children with Autism during the COVID-19 Pandemic through a Remote Behavioral Skills Training Program. *J. Clin. Med.* **2022**, *11*, 1194. [CrossRef]
10. Emodi-Perlman, A.; Eli, I.; Uziel, N.; Smardz, J.; Khehra, A.; Gilon, E.; Wieckiewicz, G.; Levin, L.; Wieckiewicz, M. Public Concerns during the COVID-19 Lockdown: A Multicultural Cross-Sectional Study among Internet Survey Respondents in Three Countries. *J. Clin. Med.* **2021**, *10*, 1577. [CrossRef]
11. Troisi, A. Psychotraumatology: What researchers and clinicians can learn from an evolutionary perspective. *Semin Cell Dev Biol.* **2018**, *77*, 153–160. [CrossRef]
12. Gesi, C.; Grasso, F.; Dragogna, F.; Vercesi, M.; Paletta, S.; Politi, P.; Mencacci, C.; Cerveri, G. How Did COVID-19 Affect Suicidality? Data from a Multicentric Study in Lombardy. *J. Clin. Med.* **2021**, *10*, 2410. [CrossRef]
13. Olaya, B.; Pérez-Moreno, M.; Bueno-Notivol, J.; Gracia-García, P.; Lasheras, I.; Santabárbara, J. Prevalence of Depression among Healthcare Workers during the COVID-19 Outbreak: A Systematic Review and Meta-Analysis. *J. Clin. Med.* **2021**, *10*, 3406. [CrossRef]
14. Perego, G.; Cugnata, F.; Brombin, C.; Milano, F.; Preti, E.; Di Pierro, R.; De Panfilis, C.; Madeddu, F.; Di Mattei, V. The "healthcare workers' wellbeing [Benessere Operatori]" project: A longitudinal evaluation of psychological responses of Italian healthcare workers during the COVID-19 pandemic. *J. Clin. Med.* **2022**, *11*, 2317. [CrossRef]
15. Soto-Cámara, R.; Navalpotro-Pascual, S.; Jiménez-Alegre, J.; García-Santa-Basilia, N.; Onrubia-Baticón, H.; Navalpotro-Pascual, J.; Thuissard, I.; Fernández-Domínguez, J.; Matellán-Hernández, M.; Pastor-Benito, E.; et al. On behalf of the IMPSYCOVID-19 Study Group Influence of the Cumulative Incidence of COVID-19 Cases on the Mental Health of the Spanish Out-of-Hospital Professionals. *J. Clin. Med.* **2022**, *11*, 2227. [CrossRef]
16. Troisi, A.; Nanni, R.; Riconi, A.; Carola, V.; Di Cave, D. Fear of COVID-19 among Healthcare Workers: The Role of Neuroticism and Fearful Attachment. *J. Clin. Med.* **2021**, *10*, 4358. [CrossRef] [PubMed]
17. Llorente-Alonso, M.; García-Ael, C.; Topa, G.; Sanz-Muñoz, M.; Muñoz-Alcalde, I.; Cortés-Abejer, B. Can Psychological Empowerment Prevent Emotional Disorders in Presence of Fear of COVID-19 in Health Workers? A Cross-Sectional Validation Study. *J. Clin. Med.* **2021**, *10*, 1614. [CrossRef]
18. Apostol-Nicodemus, L.; Tabios, I.; Limpoco, A.; Domingo, G.; Tantengco, O. Psychosocial Distress among Family Members of COVID-19 Patients Admitted to Hospital and Isolation Facilities in the Philippines: A Prospective Cohort Study. *J. Clin. Med.* **2022**, *11*, 5236. [CrossRef] [PubMed]
19. Troisi, A. Biological psychiatry is dead, long live biological psychiatry! *Clin. Neuropsychiatry* **2022**, *19*, 351–354. [CrossRef]
20. Schaller, M.; Murray, D.R.; Bangerter, A. Implications of the behavioural immune system for social behaviour and human health in the modern world. *Philos. Trans. R. Soc. London. Ser. B Biol. Sci.* **2015**, *370*, 20140105. [CrossRef] [PubMed]
21. Iwasa, K.; Yamada, Y.; Tanaka, T. Editorial: Behavioral Immune System: Its Psychological Bases and Functions. *Front. Psychol.* **2021**, *12*, 659975. [CrossRef] [PubMed]
22. Troisi, A. Fear of COVID-19: Insights from Evolutionary Behavioral Science. *Clin. Neuropsychiatry* **2020**, *17*, 72–75. [CrossRef] [PubMed]
23. Kempthorne, J.C.; Terrizzi, J.A., Jr. The behavioral immune system and conservatism as predictors of disease-avoidant attitudes during the COVID-19 pandemic. *Personal. Individ. Differ.* **2021**, *178*, 110857. [CrossRef] [PubMed]
24. Clay, R. The Behavioral Immune System and Attitudes About Vaccines: Contamination Aversion Predicts More Negative Vaccine Attitudes. *Soc. Psychol. Personal. Sci.* **2017**, *8*, 162–172. [CrossRef]
25. Shook, N.J.; Sevi, B.; Lee, J.; Oosterhoff, B.; Fitzgerald, H.N. Disease avoidance in the time of COVID-19: The behavioral immune system is associated with concern and preventative health behaviors. *PLoS ONE* **2020**, *15*, e0238015. [CrossRef]

26. Cox, R.C.; Jessup, S.C.; Luber, M.J.; Olatunji, B.O. Pre-pandemic disgust proneness predicts increased coronavirus anxiety and safety behaviors: Evidence for a diathesis-stress model. *J. Anxiety Disord.* **2020**, *76*, 102315. [CrossRef]
27. Makhanova, A.; Shepherd, M.A. Behavioral immune system linked to responses to the threat of COVID-19. *Personal. Individ. Differ.* **2020**, *167*, 110221. [CrossRef]
28. Hawkley, L.C.; Cacioppo, J.T. Loneliness matters: A theoretical and empirical review of consequences and mechanisms. *Ann. Behav. Med. A Publ. Soc. Behav. Med.* **2010**, *40*, 218–227. [CrossRef]
29. Schaller, M.; Miller, G.E.; Gervais, W.M.; Yager, S.; Chen, E. Mere visual perception of other people's disease symptoms facilitates a more aggressive immune response. *Psychol. Sci.* **2010**, *21*, 649–652. [CrossRef]

Journal of
Clinical Medicine

MDPI

Article

Public Concerns during the COVID-19 Lockdown: A Multicultural Cross-Sectional Study among Internet Survey Respondents in Three Countries

Alona Emodi-Perlman [1,†], Ilana Eli [1,†], Nir Uziel [1], Joanna Smardz [2], Anahat Khehra [3], Efrat Gilon [1], Gniewko Wieckiewicz [4], Liran Levin [3] and Mieszko Wieckiewicz [2,*]

1 Department of Oral Rehabilitation, The Maurice and Gabriella School of Dental Medicine, Tel Aviv University, Tel Aviv 6139001, Israel; dr.emodi@gmail.com (A.E.-P.); elilana@tauex.tau.ac.il (I.E.); niruziel@gmail.com (N.U.); gilon.efrat@gmail.com (E.G.)
2 Department of Experimental Dentistry, Wroclaw Medical University, 50-425 Wroclaw, Poland; joannasmardz1@gmail.com
3 Faculty of Medicine and Dentistry, University of Alberta, Edmonton, AB T6G 2R3, Canada; anahat@ualberta.ca (A.K.); liran@ualberta.ca (L.L.)
4 Chair and Clinical Department of Psychiatry, Medical University of Silesia, 40-055 Katowice, Poland; gniewkowieckiewicz@gmail.com
* Correspondence: m.wieckiewicz@onet.pl
† Authors with equal contribution.

Abstract: (1) Background: this study aimed to evaluate the worries, anxiety, and depression in the public during the initial coronavirus disease 2019 (COVID-19) pandemic lockdown in three culturally different groups of internet survey respondents: Middle Eastern (Israel), European (Poland), and North American (Canada). (2) Methods: a cross-sectional online survey was conducted in the mentioned countries during the lockdown periods. The survey included a demographic questionnaire, a questionnaire on personal concerns, and the Patient Health Questionnaire-4 (PHQ-4). A total of 2207 people successfully completed the survey. (3) Results: Polish respondents were the most concerned about being infected. Canadian respondents worried the most about their finances, relations with relatives and friends, and both physical and mental health. Polish respondents worried the least about their physical health, and Israeli respondents worried the least about their mental health and relations with relatives and friends. Canadian respondents obtained the highest score in the PHQ-4, while the scores of Israeli respondents were the lowest. (4) Conclusions: various factors should be considered while formulating appropriate solutions in emergency circumstances such as a pandemic. Understanding these factors will aid in the development of strategies to mitigate the adverse effects of stress, social isolation, and uncertainty on the well-being and mental health of culturally different societies.

Keywords: COVID-19; SARS-CoV-2; coronavirus pandemic; anxiety; depression; mental health

Citation: Emodi-Perlman, A.; Eli, I.; Uziel, N.; Smardz, J.; Khehra, A.; Gilon, E.; Wieckiewicz, G.; Levin, L.; Wieckiewicz, M. Public Concerns during the COVID-19 Lockdown: A Multicultural Cross-Sectional Study among Internet Survey Respondents in Three Countries. *J. Clin. Med.* **2021**, *10*, 1577. https://doi.org/10.3390/jcm10081577

Academic Editor: Mauro Giovanni Carta

Received: 4 February 2021
Accepted: 2 April 2021
Published: 8 April 2021

1. Introduction

Coronavirus disease 2019 (COVID-19) is a novel severe respiratory syndrome caused by a new betacoronavirus, severe acute respiratory syndrome coronavirus 2 (SARS-CoV-2) [1–5]. The COVID-19 pandemic has caught the world by surprise. Within a relatively short time, most countries were affected and responded with partial-to-total lockdowns to curb disease spread [6]. The daily lives of people were greatly affected in every aspect, including restrictions in socializing, working (up to full quarantine), and/or planning for the future.

Mid-March 2020, the rate of contraction and the rate of deaths by COVID-19 constantly rose. On 15 March 2020, the number of daily confirmed cases in Israel was 2 per million people. Within one month (on 15 April 2020), the number rose to 45.32 per million (relative change of +2169%). The total number of confirmed deaths from COVID-19 during that period (15 March till 15 April) rose from 1 to 139 (relative change of +13,800%) [7]. On 19 March 2020, the Israeli government declared an almost complete lockdown. All schools, kindergartens, and universities were shut down, and schooling was continued (partially) through the internet. Leaving home to a distance greater than 100 m was prohibited except in the cases of emergency, shopping for basic products, or work in vital posts (specifically defined by the government). Most adults were either put on a no-pay leave or were instructed to work from home. Personal contact with non-cohabitating family members and/or with friends was prohibited, even during traditional religious family gatherings such as Passover.

The situation in Poland on 15 March 2020 was that of 0.41 per million COVID-19 confirmed cases. Within one month, the number rose to 8.97 per million (relative change of +2100%). The total number of confirmed deaths from COVID-19 during that period rose from 3 to 286 (relative change of +9433%) [7]. An almost complete lockdown was implemented in the country in mid-March, with regulations similar to those in Israel except for no limitation on the distance from home.

In Canada, the number of daily confirmed cases on 15 March 2020 was 0.71 per million people. Within one month (on 15 April 2020), the number rose to 34.32 per million (relative change of +4725%). During that period of time, the total number of confirmed death cases due to COVID-19 rose from 1 to 1008 (relative change of +100,700%) [7]. In the Province of Alberta, a state of public health emergency was declared on 17 March 2020. Schools, shops, arenas, restaurants, places of worship, recreation centers, bars, etc. were closed. All the other provinces across Canada declared a similar state of public health emergency.

Undoubtedly, all communities experienced feelings of separation, apprehension, stress, anxiety, and even depression. Uncertainty regarding the length of the situation and its final consequences only added to the anguish.

A recent review on the psychological impact of quarantine reported that it had substantial negative psychological effects on people, contributing to posttraumatic stress symptoms, confusion, and anger. Stressors included longer durations of quarantine, infection fears, frustration, boredom, inadequate supplies, insufficient information, financial loss, and stigma [8].

A number of studies have been published about the emotional aspects of the COVID-19 pandemic. For instance, Germani et al. described the impact of this pandemic on young Italian adults [9]. In a study conducted in Denmark, the researchers reported that the psychological well-being of subjects was negatively affected by the situation [10]. In a study performed in China, more than half of the participants showed a significant psychological disturbance due to the pandemic, while in a study from the United States, nearly half of the participants were found to be anxious [11,12]. In a study conducted in India, Varshney et al. reported that the factors predicting higher psychological impact among the general public were younger age, female sex, and presence of known physical comorbidity [13]. The infection might also have a putative tropism toward the central nervous system (CNS) that may explain some of the symptoms seen in clinical practice, with possible late neuropsychiatric manifestations [14]. Clearly, the pandemic took its toll on societies worldwide. The effect may vary among cultures and societies. A previous study showed that the COVID-19 pandemic caused significant adverse effects on the psycho-emotional status of both Israeli and Polish populations, resulting in the intensification of their orofacial pain. However, the two populations varied in their reaction to the stress. For example, the odds of occurrence of orofacial pain symptoms among Polish subjects were on average over 3 times higher than that among Israeli subjects [15]. Understanding the factors that cause worries, anxiety, and depression among different communities will enable us to develop response strategies to mitigate the adverse effects of stress, social isolation, and uncertainty on well-being, and physical and mental health in culturally different societies.

The present study aimed to evaluate the worries, anxiety, and depression in the public during the initial pandemic lockdown in three culturally different groups of internet survey respondents: Middle Eastern (Israel), European (Poland), and North American (Canada).

2. Materials and Methods

A cross-sectional online survey was conducted using anonymous questionnaires. The final questionnaire was compiled from a tool commonly used with regard to anxiety and depression (Patient Health Questionnaie-4 (PHQ-4), as detailed below), and specific questions referring to demographics and concerns specific to the COVID-19. The latter were agreed upon and tested for content validity by a group of subject matter experts (SMEs). The group consisted of four researchers (A.E.-P., I.E., N.U., and E.G.) who work at the Tel Aviv University and have vast academic experience in population studies. Each SMEs proposed questions for the study, and following discussions, the final questions were agreed upon. The questionnaire was compiled in Hebrew and translated to Polish by the Polish group. One of the Israeli researchers (I.E.), who is native in the Polish language, verified the Polish translation by retranslating it to Hebrew and vice versa. The Israeli group translated the questionnaire to English. One of the members of the Canadian group (L.L.), who is native in Hebrew, verified the English translation as above.

SurveyGizmo (www.surveygizmo.com (accessed on 19 April 2020)) was used to collect data. The survey was anonymous. Therefore, due to the need to avoid respondents' identification, and according to the EU regulations, quality control measures could not be practiced.

In Israel, the survey was posted in Hebrew, which assured that only Hebrew-speaking Israeli responders participated. In Poland, the survey was posted in Polish, enabling the participation of only Polish-speaking participants. In Canada, the survey was posted in English, with most of the responders coming from the province of Alberta.

The surveys were posted at least 4 weeks after the implementation of the first lockdown in each of the countries while the pandemic was still progressing at a rapid pace (see below).

In Israel, the survey was posted on 16 April 2020. Since the beginning of the pandemic, the relative change in cumulative confirmed COVID-19 cases per million in Israel at that time was +1,294,700% [7]. The questionnaire was distributed through social media (WhatsApp groups and Facebook groups).

In Canada, collection of data started on 13 May 2020. The relative change in cumulative confirmed cases per million in Canada at that time was +7,356,700% [7]. The questionnaire was distributed through social media (Facebook, Instagram, Reddit, and WhatsApp groups).

In Poland, collection of data started on 29 April 2020. The relative change in the number of cumulative confirmed cases per million in Poland at that time was +1,263,900% [7]. The questionnaire was posted on Reddit (r/Polska subreddit).

All responses were obtained anonymously in all three countries.

The study was conducted in full accordance with the World Medical Association Declaration of Helsinki. In Israel, the Ethics Committee of the Tel Aviv University approved all the study procedures (ID: 0001332-1). In Poland, the study was approved by the Bioethical Committee of the Wroclaw Medical University (ID: KB-302/2020). In Canada, the Research Ethics Board at the University of Alberta approved the study (ID: Pro00100768). Informed consent was obtained from all the subjects as required.

2.1. Instruments

The following data were collected through questionnaires:

2.1.1. Demographic and General Information

This included the following:

a. Consent to participate in the study

b. Gender
c. Age—the age groups of participants were defined according to "young adults" (age of 18–35 years) and "adults" (36–56 years old) as accepted in the literature [16]. Subjects over 56 years old were defined as "older".

2.1.2. Personal Concerns Regarding the COVID-19 Pandemic

Subjects were requested to indicate the following:

a. Whether they were feeling at risk of contamination by the virus (yes/no)
b. To what extent does the pandemic make them worry about finances (5-score scale, ranging from 1—not at all to 5—very worried)
c. To what extent does the pandemic make them worry about their physical health, namely, do they worry that the pandemic might negatively affect their physical status, including decrease in stamina, possible aggravation of prior systemic conditions, etc. (scale as above)
d. To what extent does the pandemic make them worry about their mental health (scale as above)
e. To what extent does the pandemic make them worry about their relations with meaningful figures in their lives, such as spouse, children, relatives, friends, and colleagues (scale as above)

2.1.3. Information on Anxiety and Depression

Subjects responded to the Patient Health Questionnaire-4 (PHQ-4), a brief screening tool used for assessing anxiety and depression. The questionnaire is a four-item inventory and is rated on a 4-point Likert-type scale. It allows for a very brief and accurate measurement of depression and anxiety. The reliability and validity of PHQ-4 have been repeatedly established [17,18]. It has been incorporated as a part of various diagnostic protocols and has been translated to numerous languages, including Hebrew and Polish [19].

The total score of the PHQ-4 ranges from 0 to 12: the higher the score, the higher the chances of the presence of anxiety and depression. The recommended PHQ-4 cutoff scores are as follows: 0–2, normal; 3–5, mild; 6–8, moderate; and 9–12, severe [20]. In the present study, a total PHQ-4 score was used for comparisons among countries, genders, and age groups.

The questionnaire also enables separate assessments of anxiety and depression.

A score of $\geq$3 for the first two questions suggests anxiety. A score of $\geq$3 for the two last questions suggests depression. In the present study, scores of the first two questions (anxiety) and of the last two questions (depression) were used for comparisons among countries, gender, and age groups.

The questionnaire referred to the last 2 weeks, namely, to the lockdown period.

2.2. Statistical Analysis

Data were analyzed using the SPSS software.

A logistic regression analysis was carried out to evaluate subjects' feelings of being at risk of contamination by the virus. Variables that were entered into the equation were country, gender, age, and the interactions among them (age $\times$ country, country $\times$ gender, age $\times$ gender, and age $\times$ country $\times$ gender).

Four 3-way analyses of variance (ANOVA) were carried out to analyze subjects' worries regarding finances, physical health, mental health, and relations with others. The analyses evaluated the effects of country ($\times$3), gender ($\times$2), age ($\times$2), and possible interactions among them.

Three additional 3-way ANOVA were carried out to analyze subjects' total PHQ-4 score as well as the separate scores of anxiety and of depression. The analyses evaluated the effects of country ($\times$3), gender ($\times$2), age ($\times$2), and possible interactions among them.

3. Results

In Israel, a total of 867 subjects responded to the questionnaire during the study period, out of whom 80.7% ($n = 699$) completed the questionnaire in full.

In Poland, a total of 1096 subjects responded to the questionnaire during the study period, out of whom 99.63% completed the questionnaire in full ($n = 1092$).

In Canada, a total of 548 subjects responded to the questionnaire during the study period, out of whom 75.9% completed the questionnaire in full ($n = 416$). Among the responders, 93% were Canadians, mostly from the province of Alberta (78.4%).

3.1. *Demographics*

The distributions of gender and age of the study participants are presented in Table 1.

Table 1. Gender and age distributions.

Country		Israel		Poland		Canada	
		No.	%	No.	%	No.	%
Gender	Female	465	66.5%	638	58.3%	343	82.7%
	Male	234	33.5%	457	41.7%	72	17.3%
Age	18–35	203	29.6%	830	75.8%	337	82.8%
	35–56	283	41.3%	234	21.4%	56	13.8%
	>56	199	29.1%	31	2.8%	14	3.4%

Significant differences were observed among countries with respect to gender ($p < 0.000$) and age ($p < 0.0000$).

In all three countries, there was a higher proportion of female responders than males, with the number of female responders being the highest in Canada (83%) compared to Poland (58%) and Israel (66%).

In general, the Polish and Canadian participants were younger (76% and 83% in the "young adult" group, respectively) compared to Israeli participants, in which only 30% of participants were in this age group. Due to the small number of respondents in the "older" group (>56 years) in Poland and Canada (2.8% and 3.4%, respectively), this group was collapsed with the "adult" age group and only two age groups were analyzed: the "younger group" (18–35 years) and the "older group" (>35 years).

3.2. *Personal Concerns Regarding the COVID-19 Pandemic*

3.2.1. Feeling at Risk of Contamination

Significant differences were found among the respondents with regard to concerns of being at risk of contamination by the virus with respect to country, gender, and age group. Poles felt most at risk of contamination (46.8% positive response) compared to Canadians (21.9% positive response) and Israelis (20.7% positive response).

Logistic regression (with the variables country; gender; age group; and the interactions age × country, country × gender, age × gender, and age × country × gender) showed that, compared to Israelis, the odds of Poles feeling at risk of contamination were over three times as much (odds ratio 3.2, 95% CI 2.37–4.32, $p < 0.000$). In the case of Canadians, the odds of feeling at risk of contamination were almost twice that compared to the Israelis (odds ratio 1.91, 95% CI 1.09–3.35, $p < 0.05$).

Older responders felt in general more at risk than the younger responders (31.4% versus 19.9% positive response, odds ratio 1.87, 95% CI 1.49–2.34, $p < 0.000$).

Women felt in general more at risk than men (35.8% versus 30.7% positive response). The odds of Polish women feeling at risk of contamination was 1.86 compared to Israeli women (95% CI 1.44–2.38, $p < 0.000$).

3.2.2. Worry about Finances

Three-way ANOVA that compared subjects' levels of worry about finances showed the main effects of country ($F_{(2,2173)} = 8.53$, $p < 0.000$; Israel < Poland < Canada), gender ($F_{(1,2173)} = 4.74$, $p < 0.05$; male < female), and age ($F_{(1,2173)} = 6.33$, $p < 0.05$; younger < older).

Significant interactions among the variables country, age, and gender were also observed ($F_{(2,2173)} = 6.59$, $p < 0.005$). Parameter estimates of the 3rd-order interactions were as follows: (i) country (IL) × gender (F) × age (young)—B = 1.12, 95% CI 0.33–1.90, $p < 0.005$; (ii) country (PL) × gender (F) × age (young)—B = 1.41, 95% CI 0.64–2.17, $p < 0.000$ (*IL = Israel, PL = Poland, F = female*).

Generally, Poles worried the least (M = 2.38) while Canadians worried the most (M = 2.84). Females worried more than males, and younger subjects worried more than the older age groups. The group that worried the least about finances was Polish males (both age groups, M = 2.27), while the group that worried the most was Canadian younger males (M = 2.33).

3.2.3. Worry about Physical Health

Three-way ANOVA that compared subjects' worries about their physical health showed the main effects of country ($F_{(2,2167)} = 8.38$, $p < 0.000$; Poland < Israel < Canada) and gender ($F_{(1,2167)} = 4.44$, $p < 0.05$; male < female). The effect of age was borderline ($F_{(1,2167)} = 3.739$, $p = 0.05$).

A significant interaction between gender and age was also observed ($F_{(2,2167)} = 9.18$, $p < 0.005$). Parameter estimates of the 2nd-order interaction were B = −0.721, $p = 0.02$, 95% CI lower bound −1.317, upper bound −0.124.

Generally, Poles worried the least (M = 2.26) while Canadians worried the most (M = 2.61) about their physical health. Females worried more than males. The group that worried the most about their physical health were Canadian older males (M = 2.91), while Israeli adult males showed the least concern (2.10).

3.2.4. Worry about Mental Health

Three-way ANOVA that compared subjects' worries about their mental health showed the main effects of country ($F_{(2,2174)} = 44.62$, $p < 0.000$; Israel < Poland < Canada), gender ($F_{(1,2174)} = 33.61$, $p < 0.000$; male < female), and age ($F_{(1,2174)} = 15.75$, $p < 0.000$; older < younger). No interactions were detected among variables.

Generally, Canadians showed the highest concern about their mental health (M = 3.14) while Israelis showed the lowest concern regarding this aspect of the pandemic (M = 1.97). Females worried more than males and younger subjects, worried more than older subjects.

3.2.5. Worry regarding Relations with Meaningful Figures

Three-way ANOVA that compared subjects' worries about their relationships with meaningful figures in their lives showed the main effects of country ($F_{(2,2172)} = 6.75$, $p < 0.001$; Israel < Poland < Canada), gender ($F_{(1,2172)} = 11.73$, $p < 0.001$; male < female), and age ($F_{(1,2172)} = 24.48$, $p < 0.000$; older < younger). A significant interaction was observed between gender and age ($F_{(2,2172)} = 8.05$, $p < 0.000$). Parameter estimates of the 2nd-order interaction were B = −0.478, 95% CI lower bound −0.869, CI upper bound −0.086, $p < 0.05$.

Generally, the group that worried the most about their relations with relatives and friends was the Canadian subjects (M = 2.69) while Israelis was the group that worried the least (M = 1.94). Females worried more than males, while younger subjects worried more than older subjects. In the three countries, older females showed higher concern regarding relations with relatives and friends than their male counterparts (M = 2.10 versus 1.96).

3.3. Anxiety and Depression

3.3.1. Total PHQ-4 Score

Three-way ANOVA of the total PHQ-4 score showed the main effects of country ($F_{(2,2174)} = 27.103$, $p < 0.000$; Israel < Poland < Canada), gender ($F_{(1,2174)} = 38.85$, $p < 0.000$;

male < female), and age ($F_{(1,2174)}$ = 16.59, $p < 0.000$; older < younger). No interactions were observed among the variables.

All three countries scored within the "mild" category of the total PHQ-4 score. In general, Israeli respondents showed the lowest PHQ-4 scores (M = 2.91) and Canadian respondents showed the highest scores (M = 4.94). Females showed higher scores than males (M = 4.37 vs. 3.27), and younger subjects showed higher scores than the older age group (M = 4.43 vs. 3.24).

3.3.2. Anxiety (According to PHQ-4)

Three-way ANOVA analysis of the separate anxiety scores showed a basically similar pattern for the main effects of country ($F_{(2,2173)}$ = 16.418, $p < 0.000$; Israel < Poland < Canada), gender ($F_{(1,2173)}$ = 46.181, $p < 0.000$; male < female), and age ($F_{(1,2173)}$ = 10.843, $p < 0.000$; older < younger). No interactions were observed among variables.

None of the countries reached a definite score defined of "anxiety" (>3). Nevertheless, Israelis were the least anxious group (M = 1.46) while Canadians were the most anxious one (M = 2.65). Females were more anxious than males (M = 2.22 vs. 1.42), and younger subjects were more anxious than the older age group (M = 2.14 vs. 1.61).

3.3.3. Depression (According to PHQ-4)

A similar pattern was also revealed for the separate assessment of depression. Three-way ANOVA of the separate depression scores showed the main effects of country ($F_{(2,2174)}$) = 49.00, $p < 0.000$; Israel < Poland < Canada), gender ($F_{(1,2174)}$ = 29.94, $p < 0.000$; male < female), and age ($F_{(1,2174)}$ = 18.70, $p < 0.000$; older < younger). No interactions were observed among variables.

None of the countries reached a score definition of "depression" (>3). Nevertheless, Israelis were the least depressed group (M = 1.14) while Canadians were the most depressed one (M = 2.31). Females were more depressed than males (M = 2.01 vs. 1.54), and younger subjects were more depressed than the older age group (M = 2.12 vs. 1.40).

4. Discussion

In late December 2019, a new unfamiliar public health threat, the COVID-19 pandemic, began to spread around the world. With almost complete uncertainty concerning the method of virus spread and the modes of treatment, insufficient availability of local health services, and lack of a vaccine or efficient drugs for treatment, most countries adopted the policies of social distancing and partial-to-total lockdown. The new situation burdened people not only with immediate severe health threats but also with economic uncertainty and social isolation, causing further potential deleterious effects on their mental and physical health.

From recent studies indicating the direct and indirect influences of the pandemic, it is apparent that subjects around the world might react differently to the new stressful situation. In the present study, subjects from different regions—Middle Eastern, European, and North American—were compared in terms of their personal worries and emotional reactions. A summary of the main effects of the study is presented in Table 2.

Table 2. Summary of the study main effects.

Variable *	Country **	Gender	Age
Feeling at risk of contamination	IL < CA < PL	Male < female	Younger < older
Worry about finances	PL < IL < CA	Male < female	Younger < older
Worry about physical health	PL < IL < CA	Male < female	
Worry about mental health	IL < PL < CA	Male < female	Older < younger
Worry about relations	IL < PL < CA	Male < female	Older < younger
PHQ-4-total, Anxiety, Depression	IL < PL < CA	Male < female	Older < younger

* Variables as defined in the text; ** country: IL—Israel, PL—Poland, CA—Canada; PHQ-4—Patient Health Questionnaire-4.

The study showed that subjects' reactions to the situation varied significantly among the three countries. Except for worry about physical health, Canadians appeared to be the most worried. Israelis appeared to be consistently less worried than the Canadians, while the Poles showed mixed behavior.

Israelis are used to changing their routine way of life within a short period as they frequently face sudden emergencies. The country is under constant security threats from the outside (at the borders) and the inside (terror attacks). Every few years, an emergency arises requiring the citizens to react quickly (i.e., stay in shelters). In general, the armed forces are highly trusted to contain the situation and to bring back normalcy. During the initial stage of the COVID-19 pandemic, the country reacted quickly. Borders were closed, and the army was mobilized to help. Although the political system underwent continuous changes (despite several rounds of indecisive elections, there was great difficulty in creating a stable government), the pandemic situation was generally under control.

Unlike Israel, Canada has not faced any major emergencies for many decades. Although the country was affected by severe acute respiratory syndrome (SARS) in 2003, which led to partial quarantine, the effects were evident mainly in Ontario [21]. Based on the SARS experience, one could assume that Canadians were more prepared for the COVID-19 pandemic and, therefore, less worried about its different aspects compared to other countries such as Poland, which had no such experience. Interestingly, the results were found to be quite the opposite. The study showed that Canadians worried more than the two other groups regarding their finances, physical health, mental health, and relations with relatives and friends.

Apparently, the unexpected threat rocked the lives of the Canadian people to a greater extent than the other two countries. The results were in line with a previous publication regarding the impact of COVID-19 in Canada, which showed that 87% of the population were concerned about the impact on vulnerable people, 21% about their own health, 36% about family stress from confinement, and 34% about maintaining social ties [22].

During the initial stage of the pandemic in Poland, a public opinion study showed that most of Polish citizens were concerned about their own health and about the health of their relatives, especially those of old age [23]. A previously published survey also showed that up to 57% of Polish citizens had concerns about their finances due to the COVID-19 pandemic [24]. The present study confirmed these results to some extent as Polish participants showed the second highest concern about mental health and relations with relatives and friends.

Among the three studied countries, one of the most prominent differences was observed for the subjects' perceptions of being at risk of virus contamination. The odds of Poles and Canadian to worry about this issue were two to three fold higher than those of the Israelis. This may be explained by the advanced and generally good public health services available in Israel. In the country, all citizens have governmental health insurance and are entitled to all the necessary health services with no additional costs (besides a mandatory monthly fee). Hospitals are required to maintain high medical standards, and medical personnel are well-trained. Up until now, Israel has been efficiently carrying out vaccination processes against COVID-19, with high percentages of the adult population being already successfully vaccinated.

Although healthcare in Poland does not differ significantly from that in Israel and medical costs are reimbursed to some extent, access to some specialist procedures is limited. Due to the extended wait time for their implementation, there is distrust among Poles about their national healthcare system.

Apparently, the differences among countries with regard to subjects' worries about the situation are also reflected in their emotional status (anxiety and depression).

In a recent Canadian survey series, performed during the COVID-19 pandemic only half of the Canadians reported excellent and very good mental health [25]. In Poland, the ranges of depressive, anxiety, and stress symptoms were around 50% during the COVID-19 outbreak [26]. In Israel, more than one-third of the responders reported stress and anxiety due to the crisis [27].

The impact of COVID-19 lockdowns on the mental health of people suffering from psychiatric disorders may be even more substantial and may lead to an increase in general psychopathology, anxiety, fear, and stress related to the quarantine. Tele-psychiatry was implemented in some countries to address population concerns and worries. Acceptance of telemedicine by decision makers might allow for quick response in times where face-to-face visits are not accessible [28,29]. As the pandemic still prevails around the globe, such an approach should be seriously considered.

The differences between genders, in levels of worries, anxiety, and depression, are not surprising. As a global phenomenon, women seem to be hardest hit by unemployment due to the pandemic [30–33]. Regretfully, information regarding domestic and professional variables such as family responsibilities, education level, employment type, or annual income was not collected in the present study. According to the United Nation policy brief, the pandemic amplified and heightened all preexisting inequalities (such as gender inequality) and exposed vulnerabilities in social, political, and economic systems, which in turn amplify the impacts of the pandemic [34].

The effect of age on the personal concerns and emotional aspects of subjects reported in the present study was inconsistent. Findlay et al. showed that Canadian youth had a higher risk for poor mental health both before and during the COVID-19 pandemic, while Okruszek et al. showed that young Polish adults were more concerned about the collapse of healthcare than any other issue [35–37]. This confirms that, in the days of health threats and financial uncertainty, anxiety, depression, and worries about mental health and social relations affect young adults worldwide. It is noteworthy that the group of responders over the age of 56 years in the present study was especially small in both Canada and Poland and therefore could not be properly analyzed. Possibly, some of the subjects at that age are not active in the social media used to distribute the questionnaire.

The results showed complex interactions among some of the study variables. Men and women belonging to different age groups reacted differently in each of the examined countries. These interactions suggest that the reactions of different subgroups (gender/age) are affected by subtle factors that are specific for each country. Further research will be needed to better analyze these differences.

Personal concerns evoked by the pandemic not only adversely affect the emotional status of subjects but also can also take a toll on physiological phenomena [37–39]. A previous study showed that personal worries, depression, and anxiety during the COVID-19 pandemic can act as predictors of symptoms that cause aggravation of chronic pain, the effect of which varies between communities [15]. Researchers, clinicians, and politicians are in need of literature that can help them understand the impact of this crisis on people's emotional and mental health, which can be long lasting.

Study limitations: although an effort was made to perform the survey at similar times as far as the pandemic progression is concerned, the slightly later timing of gathering data in Canada might have biased the results in this country. Moreover, the study was carried out as an anonymous internet survey with no actual ability to control the participants. As a result, the study groups differ as far as gender and age are concerned and are not necessarily representative of the country's populations. As pointed above, there was a under representation of the older age group (>56), which might have shown a different pattern of behavior (such as being more worried about contamination and physical health but possibly less worried about financial issues than the younger groups).

5. Conclusions

Better understanding the factors that cause worries, anxiety, and depression among different communities will enable us to develop response strategies to mitigate the adverse effects of stress, social isolation, and uncertainty on well-being, and physical and mental health in culturally different societies.

Author Contributions: Study conception and design, A.E.-P. and I.E.; data collection, A.E.-P., I.E., G.W., N.U., A.K., L.L., and E.G.; data analysis and interpretation, A.E.-P. and I.E.; article drafting, A.E.-P., I.E., A.K., L.L., M.W., and J.S.; critical revision of the article, A.E.-P., I.E., and M.W. All authors have read and agreed to the published version of the manuscript.

Funding: This research received no external funding.

Institutional Review Board Statement: The study was conducted according to the guidelines of the Declaration of Helsinki and was approved by the following: in Israel, the Ethics Committee of the Tel Aviv University approved all the study procedures (ID: 0001332-1); in Poland, the Bioethical Committee of the Wroclaw Medical University approved the procedures (ID: KB-302/2020); in Canada, the Research Ethics Board at the University of Alberta approved the study (ID: Pro00100768).

Informed Consent Statement: Informed consent was obtained from all subjects involved in the study.

Data Availability Statement: The data presented in this study are available on reasonable request from the corresponding author.

Conflicts of Interest: The authors declare no conflict of interest.

References

1. Yang, X.; Yu, Y.; Xu, J.; Shu, H.; Xia, J.; Liu, H.; Wu, Y.; Zhang, L.; Yu, Z.; Fang, M.; et al. Clinical course and outcomes of critically ill patients with SARS-CoV-2 pneumonia in Wuhan, China: A single-centered, retrospective, observational study. *Lancet Respir. Med.* **2020**, *8*, 475–481. [CrossRef]
2. Zhou, P.; Yang, X.L.; Wang, X.G.; Hu, B.; Zhang, L.; Zhang, W.; Si, H.R.; Zhu, Y.; Li, B.; Huang, C.L.; et al. A pneumonia outbreak associated with a new coronavirus of probable bat origin. *Nature* **2020**, *579*, 270–273. [CrossRef]
3. Chen, Y.; Li, L. SARS-CoV-2: Virus dynamics and host response. *Lancet Infect. Dis.* **2020**, *20*, 515–516. [CrossRef]
4. Wu, Y.; Ho, W.; Huang, Y.; Jin, D.Y.; Li, S.; Liu, S.L.; Liu, X.; Qiu, J.; Sang, Y.; Wang, Q.; et al. SARS-CoV-2 is an appropriate name for the new coronavirus. *Lancet* **2020**, *395*, 949–950. [CrossRef]
5. Chu, D.K.; Akl, E.A.; Duda, S.; Solo, K.; Yaacoub, S.; Schünemann, H.J. COVID-19 systematic urgent review group effort (SURGE) study authors. Physical distancing, face masks, and eye protection to prevent person-to-person transmission of SARS-CoV-2 and COVID-19: A systematic review and meta-analysis. *Lancet* **2020**, *395*, 1973–1987. [CrossRef]
6. Hiremath, P.; Suhas Kowshik, C.S.; Manjunath, M.; Shettar, M. COVID 19: Impact of lock-down on mental health and tips to overcome. *Asian J. Psychiatr.* **2020**, *51*, 102088. [CrossRef]
7. University of Oxford, Oxford Martin School. Our World in Data. Available online: https://ourworldindata.org/covid (accessed on 15 December 2020).
8. Brooks, S.K.; Webster, R.K.; Smith, L.E.; Woodland, L.; Wessely, S.; Greenberg, N.; Rubin, G.J. The psychological impact of quarantine and how to reduce it: Rapid review of the evidence. *Lancet* **2020**, *395*, 912–920. [CrossRef]
9. Germani, A.; Buratta, L.; Delvecchio, E.; Mazzeschi, C. Emerging adults and COVID-19: The role of individualism-collectivism on perceived risks and psychological maladjustment. *Int. J. Environ. Res. Public Health* **2020**, *17*, 3497. [CrossRef] [PubMed]
10. Sønderskov, K.M.; Dinesen, P.T.; Santini, Z.I.; Østergaard, S.D. The depressive state of Denmark during the COVID-19 pandemic. *Acta Neuropsychiatr.* **2020**, *32*, 226–228. [CrossRef] [PubMed]
11. Wang, C.; Pan, R.; Wan, X.; Tan, Y.; Xu, L.; Ho, C.S.; Ho, R.C. Immediate psychological responses and associated factors during the initial stage of the 2019 Coronavirus disease (COVID-19) epidemic among the general population in China. *Int. J. Environ. Res. Public Health* **2020**, *17*, 1729. [CrossRef]
12. American Psychiatric Association. New Poll: COVID-19 Impacting Mental Well-Being: Americans Feeling Anxious, Especially for Loved Ones. Older Adults Are Less Anxious. Available online: https://www.psychiatry.org/newsroom/news-releases/new-poll-covid-19-impacting-mental-well-beingamericans-feeling-anxious-especially-for-loved-ones-older-adults-are-less-anxious (accessed on 25 March 2020).
13. Varshney, M.; Parel, J.T.; Raizada, N.; Sarin, S.K. Initial psychological impact of COVID-19 and its correlates in Indian community: An online (FEEL-COVID) survey. *PLoS ONE* **2020**, *15*, e0233874. [CrossRef]
14. De Berardis, D. How concerned should we be about neurotropism of SARS-Cov-2? A brief clinical consideration of the possible psychiatric implications. *CNS Spectr.* **2020**, *10*, 1–6.
15. Emodi-Perlman, A.; Eli, I.; Smardz, J.; Uziel, N.; Wieckiewicz, G.; Gilon, E.; Grychowska, N.; Wieckiewicz, M. Temporomandibular disorders and bruxism outbreak as a possible factor of orofacial pain worsening during the COVID-19 pandemic-concomitant research in two countries. *J. Clin. Med.* **2020**, *9*, 3250. [CrossRef] [PubMed]
16. Petry, N.M. A comparison of young, middle-aged, and older adult treatment-seeking pathological gamblers. *Gerontologist* **2002**, *42*, 92–99. [CrossRef]
17. Kroenke, K.; Spitzer, R.L.; Williams, J.B.; Löwe, B. An ultra-brief screening scale for anxiety and depression: The PHQ-4. *Psychosomatics* **2009**, *50*, 613–621. [CrossRef]

18. INfORM. Diagnostic Criteria for Temporomandibular Disorders. Available online: https://ubwp.buffalo.edu/rdc-tmdinternational/tmd-assessmentdiagnosis/dc-tmd/dc-tmd-translations (accessed on 15 December 2020).
19. Löwe, B.; Wahl, I.; Rose, M.; Spitzer, C.; Glaesmer, H.; Wingenfeld, K.; Schneider, A.; Brähler, E. A 4-item measure of depression and anxiety: Validation and standardization of the Patient Health Questionnaire-4 (PHQ-4) in the general population. *J. Affect. Disord.* **2010**, *122*, 86–95. [CrossRef] [PubMed]
20. Kroenke, K.; Spitzer, R.L.; Williams, J.B. The Patient Health Questionnaire-2: Validity of a two-item depression screener. *Med. Care* **2003**, *41*, 1284–1292. [CrossRef] [PubMed]
21. Public Health Agency of Canada. Learning from SARS: Renewal of Public Health in Canada—SARS in Canada: Anatomy of an Outbreak. Available online: https://www.canada.ca/en/public-health/services/reports-publications/learning-sars-renewal-public-health-canada/chapter-2-sars-canada-anatomy-outbreak.html (accessed on 15 May 2020).
22. STATCAN COVID-19. The Health and Behavioural Impacts of COVID 19 on Youth: Results from the Canadian Perspectives Survey Series 1. Available online: https://www150.statcan.gc.ca/n1/pub/45-28-0001/2020001/article/00020-eng.htm (accessed on 15 May 2020).
23. Statista. Health Concerns Due to the Coronavirus (COVID-19) Pandemic in Poland in March 2020. Available online: https://www.statista.com/statistics/1110597/poland-health-concerns-due-to-covid-19 (accessed on 12 May 2020).
24. Statista. Financial Concerns Due to the Coronavirus (COVID-19) in Poland in March 2020. Available online: https://www.statista.com/statistics/1110607/poland-financial-concerns-due-to-covid-19 (accessed on 12 May 2020).
25. STATCAN COVID-19. Data to Insights for a Better Canada Canadians Report Lower Self-Perceived Mental Health during the COVID-19 Pandemic. Available online: https://www150.statcan.gc.ca/n1/pub/45-28-0001/2020001/article/00003-eng.htm (accessed on 12 May 2020).
26. Larionov, P.; Mudło-Głagolska, K. Mental Health Risk Factors during COVID-19 Pandemic in the Polish Population. *PsyArXiv* **2020**. Available online: Psyarxiv.com/3ku8w (accessed on 12 December 2020).
27. Israel Central Bureau of Statistics. Civilian Resilience in Israel and the COVID-19 Pandemic: Analysis of a CBS Survey. Available online: https://www.inss.org.il/publication/coronavirus-survey (accessed on 17 May 2020).
28. Gamus, A.; Chodick, G. Telemedicine after COVID-19: The Israeli Perspective. *Isr. Med. Assoc. J.* **2020**, *22*, 467–469.
29. Gentile, A.; Torales, J.; O'Higgins, M.; Figueredo, P.; Castaldelli-Maia, M.J.; De Berardis, D.; Annamaria Petito, A.; Bellomo, A.; Ventriglio, A. Phone-based outpatients' follow-up in mental health centers during the COVID-19 quarantine. *Int. J. Soc. Psychiatry* **2020**, *9*. [CrossRef]
30. U.S. Bureau of Labor Statistics. Employment Situation Summary. Available online: https://www.bls.gov/news.release/empsit.nr0.htm (accessed on 12 July 2020).
31. STATCAN COVID-19. Gender Differences in Mental Health during the COVID-19 Pandemic. Available online: https://www150.statcan.gc.ca/n1/pub/45-28-0001/2020001/article/00047-eng.htm (accessed on 12 July 2020).
32. World Health Organization. Gender and Women's Mental Health. Available online: https://www.who.int/mental_health/prevention/genderwomen/en/ (accessed on 15 July 2020).
33. Qiu, J.; Shen, B.; Zhao, M.; Wang, Z.; Xie, B.; Xu, Y. A nationwide survey of psychological distress among Chinese people in the COVID-19 epidemic: Implications and policy recommendations. *Gen. Psychiatr.* **2020**, *33*, e100213. [CrossRef] [PubMed]
34. United Nation Policy Brief: The Impact of COVID-19 on Women. 9 April 2020. Available online: https://www.un.org/sexualviolenceinconflict/wp-content/uploads/2020/06/report/policy-brief-the-impact-of-covid-19-on-women/policy-brief-the-impact-of-covid-19-on-women-en-1.pdf (accessed on 28 March 2021).
35. Findlay, L.C.; Arim, R.; Kohen, D. Understanding the perceived mental health of Canadians during the COVID-19 pandemic. *Health Rep.* **2020**, *31*, 22–27. [CrossRef] [PubMed]
36. STATCAN. Depression and Suicidal Ideation among Canadians Aged 15 to 24. Available online: https://www150.statcan.gc.ca/n1/pub/82-003-x/2017001/article/14697-eng.htm (accessed on 16 July 2020).
37. Okruszek, Ł.; Aniszewska-Stańczuk, A.; Piejka, A.; Wiśniewska, M.; Żurek, K. Safe but lonely? Loneliness, mental health symptoms and COVID-19. *PsyArXiv* **2020**. Available online: Psyarxiv.com/9njps (accessed on 12 December 2020).
38. Talevi, D.; Socci, V.; Carai, M.; Carnaghi, G.; Faleri, S.; Trebbi, E.; di Bernardo, A.; Capelli, F.; Pacitti, F. Mental health outcomes of the CoViD-19 pandemic. *Riv. Psichiatr.* **2020**, *55*, 137–144. [CrossRef]
39. Gao, J.; Zheng, P.; Jia, Y.; Chen, H.; Mao, Y.; Chen, S.; Wang, Y.; Fu, H.; Dai, J. Mental health problems and social media exposure during COVID-19 outbreak. *PLoS ONE* **2020**, *15*, e0231924. [CrossRef]

Journal of
Clinical Medicine

MDPI

Article

Adolescents' Concerns, Routines, Peer Activities, Frustration, and Optimism in the Time of COVID-19 Confinement in Spain

Noelia Muñoz-Fernández [1] and Ana Rodríguez-Meirinhos [2,*]

[1] Department of Psychology, Universidad Loyola Andalucía, 41704 Seville, Spain; nmunoz@uloyola.es
[2] Department of Communication and Education, Universidad Loyola Andalucía, 41704 Seville, Spain
* Correspondence: arodriguezm@uloyola.es; Tel.: +34-9-5564-1600 (ext. 2633)

Abstract: The global outbreak of COVID-19 has brought changes in adolescents' daily routines, restrictions to in-person interactions, and serious concerns about the situation. The purpose of this study was to explore COVID-19-related concerns, daily routines, and online peer activities during the confinement period according to sex and age groups. Additionally, the relationship of these factors and optimism along with adolescents' frustration was examined. Participants included 1246 Spanish students aged 16–25 years old (M = 19.57; SD = 2.53; 70.8% girls). The results indicated that the top concern was their studies. COVID-19-related concerns, daily routines, and online peer activities varied by sex and age. Findings also revealed moderate to high levels of frustration, which were associated with adolescents' main concerns, online peer activities, maintaining routines, and optimism. The results are discussed in light of their implications in designing support programs and resources to reduce the psychological impact of COVID-19 on adolescent mental health.

Keywords: COVID-19; adolescents; concerns; activities; frustration

Citation: Muñoz-Fernández, N.; Rodríguez-Meirinhos, A. Adolescents' Concerns, Routines, Peer Activities, Frustration, and Optimism in the Time of COVID-19 Confinement in Spain. *J. Clin. Med.* **2021**, *10*, 798. https://doi.org/10.3390/jcm10040798

Academic Editor: Erik Roj Larsen

Received: 25 January 2021
Accepted: 12 February 2021
Published: 16 February 2021

1. Introduction

The novel coronavirus disease (COVID-19) has become a major public health concern and was declared a pandemic by the World Health Organization in March 2020. Since the first cases were confirmed, the epidemic has rapidly spread worldwide. To control the outbreak, the Spanish government, similar to the governments of other countries all over the world, ordered a nationwide restrictive confinement for three months, starting from mid-March. During this period, a high restriction of mobility was imposed. Citizens were not allowed to leave their house except for essential reasons (e.g., buying supplies in the supermarket or pharmacy, taking care of vulnerable people, or going to work if teleworking was not possible). Schools were closed and other educational, social, cultural, artistic, sporting, or similar activities were canceled.

Although adolescents and young people are at lower risk of critical COVID-19 symptoms [1], strict confinement orders entailed important changes in daily routines and social interactions. With schools closed, youths had to adapt quickly to new remote learning environments, while uncertainties about their studies and their near academic future emerged [2]. These difficulties have been particularly marked among higher education students, who were preparing for university entrance exams, taking semester assessments, or doing practical training that could not adequately be replaced by online instruction [3]. Other extracurricular (e.g., educational and sports) and out-of-home leisure activities (e.g., hanging out with friends and dating), which provide valuable resources for socialization [4] were canceled, leaving adolescents with limited opportunities for face-to-face social contact. Although online social networks and instant messaging apps may have compensated for these shortages [5], there is emerging evidence that COVID-19 confinement has increased the risk of social isolation and loneliness among youths [6]. However, changes in interpersonal relationships go beyond friendships, also affecting family interactions. Family dynamics have had to change according to the stay-at-home mandates, forcing families to spend all their time together [7]. As a consequence, adolescents may have experienced restrictions in their personal space, while parents have faced an increase in daily stressors (including demands of caregiving and parenting, teleworking, home-schooling, threat of contagion, or financial insecurity, among others).

Exposure to COVID-19 challenges is having a substantial cost on psychological wellbeing [8,9]. To date, a growing number of studies among children and youths have reported high rates of anxiety and stress, along with difficulties with concentrating and worrying [10–12]. Although research is still progressing, it seems that from the very beginning, concerns about the consequences of COVID-19 have been particularly salient among young people. In early reports at the first stage of the outbreak in China, college students acknowledged being fearful of what was happening [13]. As this epidemic spread worldwide, this finding has been confirmed by more recent studies with adolescents and university students. These studies have found moderate levels of concern about COVID-19 [14], which were significantly related with increased anxiety and depression [15–20]. However, these worries may not be experienced by all young people in the same way. Indeed, studies indicate that levels of anxiety and fear about COVID-19 increase with age [14] and are higher among females [12,17,18,21]. Given these findings, research aimed at identifying the particular concerns that young people are experiencing would help to define better how they are coping with this crisis. To date, research has focused more on analyzing the overall levels of fear of COVID-19, e.g., [14,17,22], rather than describing adolescents' reasons for these concerns. Among the few available sources of evidence, studies indicate that the main worries of adolescents revolve around the issues that currently cause more uncertainty: the health of those more vulnerable to COVID-19 and the economic situation [23,24]. Although less studied, school-related concerns may have also become magnified [12,25], especially when considering that the closure of schools during the pandemic is a global issue [2] and that education is of central importance for adolescents' future.

Another important, yet less studied, consequence of the confinement may be frustration [26]. As shown by previous research, feelings of frustration emerge in situations in which people feel pressured to comply with rules which are perceived as a threat to their freedom [27]. Although adolescents may have different motivations to adhere to imposed measures, the confinement situation has certainly involved a number of restrictions on individual choice and decision-making (i.e., limitations on non-essential movements, prohibition of gathering with friends, and the obligation of wearing a face mask), which may have resulted in elevated levels of frustration. However, in the context of this pandemic, individual experiences of feeling thwarted may have been not only a common but a harmful consequence of the lockdown. Accordingly, ample research has well established that the psychological costs of frustration are related to higher levels of stress, depression, or anxiety, among others (see [28] for a review).

While there is no doubt that COVID-19 is having negative consequences in different areas of young people's lives, research investigating the factors that help adolescents handle this stressful experience is very valuable [29]. Over the last months, social and health agencies have offered guidelines to support adolescents. However, empirical evidence on the factors that mitigate the risk of psychological distress is still lacking. Among these, experts have outlined the importance of establishing stay-at-home routines and doing a variety of activities (e.g., school-work, hobbies, and exercising) to reduce the psychological stress of the confinement [30], yet few studies have examined the role that these activities play in adolescent psychological functioning. On an interpersonal level, interactions with peers may also have an important influence on the way that adolescents experience this health crisis. In adolescence, peer relationships become especially salient as they contribute not only to satisfying the needs of intimacy and companionship but also to navigate the challenges of this developmental stage [31]. During the lockdown, youths stayed connected with their friends and classmates although face-to-face interactions moved to an online setting [32]. Technology and social media may have indeed helped to compensate for the lack of in-person interactions. Nonetheless, little is known about the specific online activities that youths have been engaging in with their peers, and the role of these activities in adolescent psychological outcomes during the lockdown. Finally, some authors have drawn attention to optimism as a factor that may favor better adaptive outcomes under challenging situations [31]. As such, recent studies demonstrated that keeping a more optimistic view of the situation was related to lower rates of anxiety and depressive symptoms during the COVID-19 pandemic [32,33].

The present study focused on the psychological impact of the COVID-19 lockdown in order to offer insights into the factors related to adolescents' feelings of frustration. Specifically, the first aim was to describe adolescents' main concerns about the impact of COVID-19. It was expected that school-related concerns [12,25], concerns about the health of those more vulnerable to COVID-19, and concerns about the economic situation [23,24] would be the most salient worries among young people. In addition, it was hypothesized that COVID-19-related concerns would be higher among females [12,17,18,21] and participants in higher age groups [14]. Second, this study explored the activities that, on a daily basis or with their peers, adolescents have been engaging in during the COVID-19 lockdown. Participants were expected to engage in several stay-at-home routines [30]. Besides, considering that social media by its nature may compensate for a lack of face-to-face social interactions [32], we hypothesized that youths may have been using technology to feel supported, loved, or cared for by their friends during the confinement period. Third, given that frustration experiences have significant costs on wellbeing and diminished functioning, this study also examined adolescents' feelings of frustration during the confinement period and their link with COVID-19-related concerns, daily routines, online activities with peers, and optimism. Additionally, sex and age differences were examined. Adolescents were expected to display moderate to high levels of frustration [26]. As literature addressing the role of adolescents' concerns and routines on frustration is still scant, the association between these variables was addressed in an exploratory fashion.

2. Materials and Methods

2.1. Participants and Procedure

The study sample consisted of 1246 students (70.8% girls) from Spain. The participant age range was 16–25 years (M = 19.57; SD = 2.53). Following Steinberg [34], participants in the 16 to 18 age group were considered middle adolescents, meanwhile, participants in the 19 to 25 age group were considered late adolescents. In this study, 42.3% ($n = 527$) were middle adolescents and 57.7% ($n = 719$) were late adolescents. The distribution of participants according to sex was similar between the younger (16–18 years old; 70.4% girls) and the older (19–25 years old; 71.07% girls) age groups, $\chi 2(1) = 0.07$, $p > 0.05$. In terms of geographic distribution, most participants (88.9%) came from the southern area of Spain (Andalucía), although students from all other regions of Spain were also represented in the sample. All respondents were students enrolled in compulsory secondary education or professional training (17.9%), post-secondary education (24%), or university (58.1%). During the confinement, participants were living in two-parent families (86.4%), single-parent families (7%), with other relatives (1.5%), with roommates and/or their partners (4.8%), or alone (0.3%).

Among the study sample, few participants (0.1%) and their relatives (3.1%) were diagnosed with COVID-19. Additionally, although testing for COVID-19 was not performed, other participants also indicated that they (7.1%) or their relatives (8.2%) had COVID-19-like symptoms. In terms of the socio-economic impact of the health crisis, more than half of the sample (52.4%) reported a significant reduction in their family's income as a result of COVID-19.

Data were collected through an online survey using the Qualtrics software platform during the fifth–sixth week of the state of emergency in Spain (from 17 April to 1 May 2020). Participants were recruited through snowball sampling. The authors first distributed the online questionnaire through colleagues and potentially eligible participants who met the inclusion criteria: students between 16–25 years old, of Spanish nationality, and who were living in Spain. Then, initial participants were asked to send the questionnaire to other potential informants that met the inclusion criteria. The survey link was also shared through social media (Facebook, Instagram, Twitter, and WhatsApp), in the newsletter of the authors' university, and with school institutions and local youth organizations. Of the 1582 students who actively consented to participate, 336 respondents were excluded from the study sample. Reasons for exclusion included the following: participants did not meet the inclusion criteria; the questionnaire was blank, or respondents only answered demographic questions; and the time spent to complete the questionnaire was less than 7 min, which is significantly faster (10th percentile) than the average (11 min).

The approval to conduct this study was obtained from the Ethics Committee of the Universidad Loyola Andalucía. Participation was voluntary and anonymity was guaranteed. Active informed consent was obtained prior to participation.

2.2. Measures

COVID-19-related concerns: An ad hoc five-item questionnaire was used to measure concerns about the impact of COVID-19 during the confinement. With the question "how much have you been worrying about . . . ?" participants indicated their concerns related to: their own health (i.e., "getting ill with COVID-19"); the health of others (i.e., "my relatives getting ill with COVID-19"); their family financial strain, currently (i.e., "your family financial situation in this moment") and in the future (i.e., "your family financial situation in few months"); and their education (i.e., "this situation could negatively affect your studies"). This measure was created considering the main results of previous studies about youth concerns [12,23]. Participants reported their level of concern with each statement on a scale ranging from 1 (nothing) to 5 (a lot). Cronbach's alpha for this study was 0.73.

Daily routines during the confinement: To assess routines during the confinement, participants were asked to indicate the frequency with which they engaged in a set of five activities on a daily basis. These activities included the following: "maintaining a routine (e.g., getting up, eating . . . at the same time)"; "doing physical or sports activities"; "doing intellectual activities (e.g., studying and reading)"; "doing leisure activities (e.g., playing games, watching a series, or listening to music)"; and "doing creative activities (e.g., writing and handcrafting)". A pilot study with nine adolescents was conducted to explore if this pool of items covered all the possible daily routines during the confinement. Participants agreed that no other daily routine should be included, so this measure was tested in the full sample. Items were answered on a frequency scale ranging from 1 (never) to 5 (many times).

Online peer activities during the confinement: Online activities that participants engaged in during the confinement to feel supported, loved, or cared for by their friends were measured with an ad hoc seven-item questionnaire. These activities included: "sharing personal pictures or videos of activities I do at home"; "sharing funny memes or videos"; "messaging on WhatsApp, Telegram, or others"; "making calls or video calls"; "playing online"; "doing challenges"; and "doing activities simultaneously with friends (e.g., watching series, doing homework, and playing sports)". Items were chosen based on a pilot study with nine participants who were asked about the online activities that they were doing during confinement. Items were answered on a frequency scale ranging from 1 (never) to 5 (many times). Cronbach's alpha for this study was 0.67.

Feelings of frustration: The general sense of frustration during the confinement was captured using a single item created for this study. Participants were asked "in the past two weeks, to what extent did you feel frustrated?" [35]. Response options were on a Likert scale from 1 (nothing) to 5 (very much).

Optimism: Dispositional optimism, deemed as the general expectation that good things will happen, was measured with the three-item optimism subscale of the Comprehensive Inventory of Thriving [36]. Respondents rated items (e.g., "I have a positive outlook on life") on a scale ranging from 1 (strongly disagree) to 5 (strongly agree). Cronbach's alpha for this study was 0.85.

2.3. Plan of Analysis

First, to examine adolescents' concerns about the impact of COVID-19, their daily routines during the COVID-19 lockdown, and the online peer activities used to help youths feel supported during the confinement, descriptive statistics were computed. Besides, three different two-way multivariate analyses of variance (MANOVAs) were conducted to examine mean differences in adolescents' concerns about COVID-19, their daily routines, and online peer activities based on sex, age groups, and the interaction between sex and age. Second, multiple regression analysis was calculated to examine the association of adolescents' concerns, their daily routines, online peer activities, and optimism with adolescents' experiences of frustration. We entered independent variables in the model using the stepwise method. Variables were organized in three blocks: sex and age groups were entered in Block 1; COVID-19-related concerns, online peer activities, and optimism were entered as predictors in Block 2; and finally, the five daily routines were entered in Block 3. The stepwise method used was iterative. The order in which predictors were entered into the model was based on a statistical criterion [37]. Thus, the number of models was not dependent on the number of blocks, but rather on the number of predictors that were significantly associated with the dependent variable. This method began by introducing the independent variable of Block 1 with the highest simple correlation with the outcome. If this predictor significantly improved the percentage of variance explained by the model, it was retained and another predictor was considered. The second predictor included was the next independent variable within the block that had the largest semi-partial correlation with the outcome or, in other words, the predictor that explained the largest part of the remaining variance in the model. If no other variable was identified, it moved on to the next block. The analysis concluded when no more variables from any of the three blocks could make a significant contribution to the predictive power of the model. Each time a variable was introduced, all the statistics of the model were recalculated, resulting in a new model. Collinearity was assessed by calculating tolerance and Variance Inflation Factors (VIF) for each independent variable introduced in the model. The partial eta square (ηp^2) and the coefficient R^2 were used as measures of effect size.

3. Results

3.1. Concerns about COVID-19 among Youths by Sex and Age

As shown in Table 1, among the top concerns were that a relative could get infected with COVID-19 and that the pandemic could impact studies. In contrast, participants were least concerned about their own health.

Table 1. Descriptive and MANOVA statistics for adolescents' concerns by sex and age groups.

Concerns about COVID-19	Total	Sex				Age Groups			
		Boys	Girls			16–18 Years	19–25 Years		
	M (SD)	M (SD)	M (SD)	F (1, 1067)	ηp^2	M (SD)	M (SD)	F (1, 1067)	ηp^2
Their own health	2.84 (1.25)	2.54 (1.23)	2.95 (1.24)	22.98 ***	0.02	2.89 (1.24)	2.80 (1.26)	2.06	0.00
Others health	4.29 (0.98)	4.04 (1.11)	4.39 (0.91)	29.41 ***	0.03	4.38 (0.92)	4.22 (1.02)	4.74 *	0.00
Current family financial situation	3.27 (1.35)	3.00 (1.32)	3.37 (1.35)	18.46 ***	0.03	3.28 (1.35)	3.25 (1.35)	0.00	0.00
Future family financial situation	3.55 (1.35)	3.25 (1.37)	3.66 (1.33)	20.31 ***	0.02	3.60 (1.33)	3.51 (1.37)	0.73	0.00
Their own education	4.25 (1.12)	3.89 (1.30)	4.40 (1.01)	47.49 ***	0.04	4.36 (1.02)	4.17 (1.19)	7.05 **	0.01

* $p < 0.05$, ** $p < 0.01$, *** $p \leq 0.001$. Abbreviations: MANOVA, Multivariate Analysis of Variance; M, Mean; F, F-Snedecor; SD, Standard Deviation; ηp^2, partial eta square.

Results from MANOVA with the five concerns about COVID-19 as dependent variables and sex and age groups as independent variables revealed significant multivariate effects for both sex, Wilks' $\lambda = 0.94$; $F(5, 1063) = 14.13$, $p \leq 0.001$, $\eta p^2 = 0.06$, and age, Wilks' $\lambda = 0.99$; $F(5, 1063) = 2.56$, $p = 0.026$, $\eta p^2 = 0.01$. Subsequent univariate ANOVAs on adolescents' concerns (see Table 1) indicated that girls showed significantly higher levels of concern for all issues than boys. Regarding age differences, the results also indicated that younger adolescents were significantly more worried about their studies and the health of their relatives than their older counterparts. Finally, the multivariate interaction between sex and age was not significant, Wilks' $\lambda = 0.99$; $F(5, 1063) = 0.77$, $p > 0.05$, $\eta p^2 = 0.00$.

3.2. Daily Routines of Youths during COVID-19 Confinement by Sex and Age

Regarding routines during the confinement, Table 2 displays descriptive statistics and mean comparisons based on participants' sex and age. In general, the results indicated that the most frequent activities were intellectual (e.g., studying and reading) and leisure (e.g., playing games, watching a series, and listening to music) activities. In contrast, the least frequent were creative activities (e.g., writing and handcrafting).

Table 2. Descriptive and MANOVA statistics for daily routines by sex and age groups.

Daily Routines	Total	Sex				Age Groups			
		Boys	Girls			16–18 Years	19–25 Years		
	M (SD)	*M (SD)*	*M (SD)*	*F (1, 1064)*	ηp^2	*M (SD)*	*M (SD)*	*F (1, 1064)*	ηp^2
Maintaining a routine	3.49 (1.25)	3.21 (1.25)	3.61 (1.24)	23.20 ***	0.02	3.38 (1.25)	3.58 (1.25)	8.03 **	0.01
Physical or sports activities	3.31 (1.32)	3.18 (1.37)	3.36 (1.29)	4.51 *	0.00	3.30 (1.29)	3.31 (1.33)	0.18	0.00
Intellectual activities	4.18 (1.00)	3.82 (1.14)	4.33 (0.90)	58.79 ***	0.05	4.22 (0.99)	4.16 (1.01)	0.02	0.00
Leisure activities	4.26 (0.93)	4.33 (0.91)	4.24 (0.93)	2.38	0.00	4.36 (0.90)	4.19 (0.94)	6.85 **	0.01
Creative activities	2.59 (1.34)	2.24 (1.36)	2.72 (1.31)	29.77 ***	0.03	2.61 (1.34)	2.56 (1.35)	0.01	0.00

* $p < 0.05$, ** $p < 0.01$, *** $p \leq 0.001$. Abbreviations: MANOVA, Multivariate Analysis of Variance; *M*, Mean; *F*, F-Snedecor; *SD*, Standard Deviation; ηp^2, partial eta square.

Next, a MANOVA, including sex and age as fixed factors and daily routines as dependent variables, yielded significant multivariate effects of sex, Wilks' $\lambda = 0.92$; $F(5, 1060) = 17.86$, $p \leq 0.001$, $\eta p^2 = 0.08$, and age, Wilks' $\lambda = 0.99$; $F(5, 1060) = 3.14$, $p = 0.008$, $\eta p^2 = 0.02$, on adolescents' daily routines during COVID-19 confinement. Next, univariate ANOVAs (see Table 2) indicated that girls and late adolescents were more likely to maintain daily routines during the confinement. Girls were more engaged in intellectual, creative, and sports activities on a daily basis. Similarly, younger adolescents reported doing leisure activities with greater frequency than older adolescents. No multivariate interaction effect between sex and age was found, Wilks' $\lambda = 0.99$; $F(5, 1060) = 1.03$, $p > 0.05$, partial $\eta^2 = 0.00$.

3.3. Online Peer Activities Used to Help Youths Feel Supported by Friends during COVID-19 Confinement by Sex and Age

Table 3 provides an overview of descriptive statistics for online peer activities during the confinement by adolescent sex and age. As shown, participants engaged in online activities to maintain relationships with friends quite regularly. Among the most frequent were activities aimed at maintaining communication (i.e., through messaging on WhatsApp, Telegram, or others, or making calls or video calls) and having companionship (i.e., doing leisure activities simultaneously with friends).

A MANOVA with sex and age as independent variables and online peer activities as dependent variables provided evidence of multivariate effects for both sex, Wilks' $\lambda = 0.82$; $F(7, 1189) = 36.99$, $p \leq 0.001$, $\eta p^2 = 0.18$, and age, Wilks' $\lambda = 0.97$; $F(7, 1189) = 5.25$, $p \leq 0.001$, $\eta p^2 = 0.03$. As shown in Table 3, separate univariate ANOVAs on the outcome variables revealed that girls used the internet more extensively than boys to maintain relationships with their friends. While boys played online games with peers more often than girls, girls shared more pictures or videos of themselves doing activities at home, used WhatsApp or Telegram more often to message their friends, did more challenges, and got involved in more simultaneous activities with their friends using the internet. Similarly, when comparing online activities across age groups, the results showed that the younger group of adolescents made more calls or video calls with their friends, were more engaged in challenges, and did more activities simultaneously with their peers. Finally, a multivariate interaction effect between sex and age was observed, Wilks' λ = 0.98; $F(7, 1189)$ = 3.04, p = 0.004, ηp^2 = 0.02. Subsequent univariate analyses indicated that the interaction between sex and age was significant for the activities of sharing videos or memes, $F(1, 1195)$ = 6.16, p = 0.013, ηp^2 = 0.01, making calls or video calls, $F(1, 1195)$ = 4.50, p = 0.034, ηp^2 = 0.01, and playing online games, $F(1, 1195)$ = 7.26, p = 0.007, ηp^2 = 0.01; with boys in the youngest age group doing these activities more frequently than boys in the older age group.

Table 3. Descriptive and MANOVA statistics for online peer activities by sex and age groups.

Online Peer Activities	Total	Sex				Age Groups			
		Boys	Girls			16–18 Years	19–25 Years		
	M (SD)	*M (SD)*	*M (SD)*	*F (1, 1195)*	ηp^2	*M (SD)*	*M (SD)*	*F (1, 1195)*	ηp^2
Sharing personal pictures or videos	3.14 (1.25)	2.72 (1.20)	3.31 (1.22)	60.92 ***	0.05	3.14 (1.26)	3.14 (1.23)	0.78	0.00
Sharing memes or funny videos	3.71 (1.23)	3.73 (1.24)	3.70 (1.23)	0.34	0.00	3.77 (1.24)	3.66 (1.22)	6.06 *	0.00
Messaging: WhatsApp, Telegram	4.57 (0.79)	4.36 (0.93)	4.66 (0.70)	31.10 ***	0.03	4.60 (0.77)	4.55 (0.80)	2.81	0.00
Making calls or video calls	3.88 (1.05)	3.80 (1.08)	3.91 (1.04)	3.08	0.00	3.98 (1.03)	3.81 (1.06)	13.04 ***	0.01
Playing online	2.88 (1.46)	3.52 (1.44)	2.62 (1.40)	108.02 ***	0.08	2.97 (1.46)	2.82 (1.46)	6.46 *	0.01
Doing challenges	2.05 (1.09)	1.84 (1.00)	2.14 (1.11)	21.94 ***	0.02	2.21 (1.11)	1.94 (1.06)	15.41 ***	0.01
Doing activities simultaneously with friends	4.12 (1.20)	3.88 (1.25)	4.22 (1.17)	21.21 ***	0.02	4.31 (1.04)	3.97 (1.29)	13.52 ***	0.01

* $p < 0.05$, *** $p \leq 0.001$. Abbreviations: MANOVA, Multivariate Analysis of Variance; *M*, Mean; *F*, F-Snedecor; *SD*, Standard Deviation; ηp^2, partial eta square.

3.4. Feelings of Frustration during the Confinement: The Role of Adolescents' Sex, Age, Concerns, Daily Routines, Online Peer Activities, and Optimism

The multiple regression (see Table 4) revealed that sex, optimism, COVID-19-related concerns, online peer activities, maintaining daily routines, and leisure activities contributed significantly to the regression model, $F(6, 1052)$ = 31.80, $p \leq 0.001$. Together the six independent variables accounted for 15.4% of the variance in frustration. Being female, experiencing more concerns about the impacts of COVID-19, and doing online peer activities more frequently were positively related to frustration. In contrast, higher levels of optimism, maintaining daily routines, and doing more leisure activities were negatively associated with frustration.

Regarding collinearity, tolerance values ranged from 0.88 to 0.92 and VIF values ranged from 1.08 to 1.13. These values indicate that the variables introduced in the model were not highly correlated and there was no collinearity among the independent variables.

As a follow up, correlations between adolescents' frustration and specific aspects of COVID-19-related concerns and online peer activities were computed. In relation to COVID-19-related concerns, frustration was positively associated with concerns about their relatives getting COVID-19 (r = 0.08, p = 0.010), their family financial strain, currently (r = 0.11, $p \leq 0.001$), and in the future (r = 0.13, $p \leq 0.001$) as well as about their own education (r = 0.20, $p \leq 0.001$). Regarding online peer activities, positive, although small correlations, were found between frustration and sharing personal pictures or videos (r = 0.07, p = 0.017), messaging friends on WhatsApp, Telegram, or others (r = 0.06, p = 0.038), and making calls or video calls (r = 0.08, p = 0.013).

Table 4. Results of the multiple linear regression on adolescents' frustration.

Model	Variables	*B*	*t*	ΔR^2
1	Sex	0.34	4.75 ***	0.02
2	Sex	0.30	4.50 ***	0.12
	Optimism	−0.32	−10.79 ***	
3	Sex	0.23	3.41 **	0.14
	Optimism	−0.32	−10.94 ***	
	COVID−19-related concerns	0.17	4.70 ***	
4	Sex	0.23	3.36 **	0.14
	Optimism	−0.33	−11.15 ***	
	COVID−19-related concerns	0.16	4.23 ***	
	Online peer activities	0.10	2.10 *	
5	Sex	0.27	3.87 ***	0.15
	Optimism	−0.31	−10.09 ***	
	COVID−19-related concerns	0.15	4.20 ***	
	Online peer activities	0.09	1.98 *	
	Maintaining daily routines	−0.08	−3.28 **	
6	Sex	0.26	3.82 ***	0.15
	Optimism	−0.30	−9.91 ***	
	COVID−19-related concerns	0.14	3.87 ***	
	Online peer activities	0.12	2.54 *	
	Maintaining daily routines	−0.09	−3.49 **	
	Leisure activities	−0.08	−2.50 *	

$N = 1059$; * $p < 0.05$, ** $p < 0.01$, *** $p \leq 0.001$. Abbreviations: *B*, Unstandardized beta coefficient; *t*, t-value; ΔR^2, increment in the fraction of the variation in frustration accounted for the independent variables of each model.

4. Discussion

This paper aimed to provide insight into the concerns that young people experienced during the COVID-19 confinement in Spain as well as to explore daily and online activities. Most previous studies have analyzed the psychological impact of COVID-19 in the general or university population, but there are still few studies focused on adolescents. Besides, considering that the progress of the pandemic is still uncertain, this study has also described the degree of frustration experienced by adolescents and tried to identify factors associated with it.

The first aim of this study was to explore adolescents' concerns about COVID-19. According to the hypotheses of this study, findings evidenced that adolescents were the most worried about the risk of their relatives getting sick and the least worried about their own risk of infection. Previous studies have also shown this result [14]. From a developmental perspective, the lesser degree of concern that adolescents showed about their own health may be explained from the hypothesis of the "personal fable". Previous studies suggest that a characteristic of adolescent thinking is their propensity to regard themselves as invulnerable. That is, they think that problems and difficulties are not going to happen to them. This cognitive feature is associated with greater involvement in risky behaviors [38]. In times of pandemic, breaking the social distancing guidelines or not following health and safety measures may be considered as new risk behaviors. As such, if adolescents are less concerned about their own health, they may become more involved in irresponsible behaviors that put everyone's health at risk [39,40]. For this reason, future studies may want to analyze the effectiveness of prevention campaigns aimed at fostering social responsibility. Perhaps personalizing the consequences of adolescents' risk behaviors on the health of their relatives (e.g., grandparents) may be a more effective way to achieve greater adherence to prevention measures. Beyond health concerns, the findings of this study also indicated that, consistent with research on university students [12], adolescents were very concerned about their studies. A review by Sahu [41] describes that some young people have had to adapt to online education with limited resources at home (e.g., teenagers have had to share computer equipment with different family members who need to telework and study). They have also faced an increase in the amount of schoolwork because of continuous evaluation in addition to uncertainty and pressure of highly monitored final evaluations. All of these factors may have been a source of stress for young people. Thus, these results were in line with the hypothesis of this study and underline that it is also crucial to take care of our education. Additionally, the results have contributed to understanding the role of sex and age on adolescents' experienced concerns. Regardless of the issue, girls were found to be more worried than boys. For age, although in general there were no differences, younger people were more concerned about the health of others and their studies. These results are in line with previous studies with young people and adults, which have reported increased levels of increased worry, fear, anxiety, and depression among girls [14,17,32]. Moreover, contrary to our expectations, the younger groups of participants were more worried than older adolescents. A previous study among Italian adolescents between 13 to 20 years old [14] has shown that older adolescents were moderately more concerned than younger adolescents. However, the study results are similar to previous studies with university and adult samples, which found higher levels of COVID-19 fear and concerns among younger participants [19,24]. Thus, the results highlight the relevance of understanding that the COVID-19 health crisis is not affecting all people equally, so it is necessary to redouble efforts to the most vulnerable.

The second aim of this study was to provide insights into the activities that young people have been participating in during the confinement on a daily basis and with their peers. Findings suggested that adolescents have spent time on intellectual and leisure activities. In contrast, creative and physical activities were undertaken less frequently. In view of these findings, it is important to implement resources aimed at reducing sedentary behaviors and sports activities should be promoted. In this regard, previous theoretical studies have warned that the possible increase in sedentary behavior together with the excessive time spent on technology may have affected the sleep patterns of children and adolescents, with consequent risk to their development and health [42]. Regarding online activities with peers, this study has also yielded interesting results. Before the pandemic, the analysis of the use of new technologies in peer relations was undertaken in the knowledge that young people tend to alternate face-to-face interactions with online interactions. However, the pandemic situation and the lack of in-person contact has provided a unique opportunity to analyze the contribution of the online world to interpersonal relationships. According to the expectations, the results of this study indicated that young people very often used new technologies to feel supported by their friends. The most frequent online activities were conversations via instant messaging applications and the use of new technologies to do activities simultaneously with peers. In contrast, challenges and online games were less frequently undertaken. Girls used the internet more often than boys, and younger people tried to see their friends more, even if it was through the screen, using challenges, or doing the same activities simultaneously with peers. All these interactions, which are related to spending time together, are traditionally known as companionship or intimacy [43]. In-person, higher levels of companionship are associated with better psychological and relational adjustment [44]. However, the role of these relationships on adolescents' wellbeing is less known when interactions are 100% online.

The third aim of this study was to examine the factors that related to adolescents' experiences of frustration during the lockdown. Although frustration itself is not an indicator of mental health, prior research has shown that it is a significant predictor of adolescents' psychological problems [28]. Findings revealed that optimism, followed by sex, COVID-19-related worries, online peer activities, daily routines, and leisure activities were significantly related to higher levels of frustration. Concerning daily routines, the results showed that keeping daily routines and doing leisure activities were related to lower levels of frustration. Possibly, routines during the confinement have been important to foster a sense of normality, providing structure in the uncertain. In further detail, subsequent analyses indicated that adolescents' more salient concerns about COVID-19 were associated with higher levels of frustration. Specifically, the findings showed that youths who were more worried about their education, the financial situation of their family, or the health of their relatives also reported more frustration. Another important finding concerns the online activities used to keep youths connected with their peers during the confinement. Although correlations were modest, results indicate that youths who spent more time sharing personal pictures or videos, messaging friends, and making calls or video calls experienced greater levels of frustration. This finding might seem counterintuitive because previous literature has shown that intimacy and companionship with peers are related to better psychological adjustment [44]. However, our results may be far from what is expected because the interaction with peers, due to the confinement, has been restricted to the online context. A previous study found that the balance between online and offline communication matters [45]. For example, among university student couples, closeness increased when online and offline communication was balanced (i.e., couples communicated by both means). In contrast, intimacy and closeness decreased when communication was only online. Thus, these results suggested that the online context was useful for socialization, especially when face-to-face interactions were restricted, but that the internet alone could not compensate or replace face-to-face interaction. Finally, it is important to note that higher levels of optimism were significantly related to lower rates of frustration. This result is consistent with research on the stress buffering effect of optimism [46]. Literature on the psychological impact of COVID-19 has also evidenced that optimism mediates the relationship between COVID-19-related stress and psychological problems, and is associated with lower levels of depression or anxiety, among others [47,48]. Perhaps adolescents with a more optimistic perspective reappraised the situation in a more positive way [49]. Thus, although further studies with adolescents are needed, the results seem to indicate that keeping an optimistic perspective is important in mitigating the psychological impacts of COVID-19.

Limitations

Despite the strengths of this study, some limitations should be outlined. First, the sample was mostly composed of young people from the southern area of Spain. Although the aim of the study was not to make comparisons between different areas of the country, future studies could benefit from a stratified sampling. Second, adolescents' frustration was assessed through a single-item questionnaire. The main reason was that online surveys should be short to facilitate participation. However, future studies could evaluate this construct through a validated multi-item instrument. Third, the cross-sectional design of this study did not allow for an analysis of the directionality of the relationships between the variables. Future longitudinal studies could explore the temporal association between the factors associated with adolescents' frustration. Finally, given that data were collected during the strict confinement period in Spain, this study assumed that participants were not having any actual face-to-face contact with their peers and that all their social routines were online. However, as they were not explicitly asked about the extent to which they followed the strict isolation measures imposed, it remains possible that a few individuals in the study had had actual contact with their friends.

5. Conclusions

The pandemic has led to moderate-to-high levels of frustration among adolescents. The results of this study have allowed us to delve deeper into the role that concerns, daily activities, online interactions with friends, and optimism play in the degree of frustration that young people have experienced. First, matters related to family health, family financial situation, and education were found to be associated with more frustration. Among these, the academic concern was the most relevant variable because of the magnitude of the association with adolescents' frustration. In this sense, it is necessary to develop an educational response that involves the different stakeholders (politicians, teachers, families, and students) to ensure that we take care of both students' physical and mental health. To this end, it is necessary to rethink the changes that should be implemented in order to prepare schools for a new COVID-19 outbreak. Second, findings have allowed us to make conclusions about the importance of adolescents maintaining a daily routine, and participating in physical, leisure, and creative activities. Special attention should be paid to creative activities because, despite being negatively related to frustration, they were the least frequent activity undertaken during confinement. Third, another relevant conclusion of this study was that optimism turned out to be the variable that showed a stronger negative association with adolescents' frustration. Thus, it seems that being able to reinterpret the situation positively represents a precious resource for adolescents in facing this health crisis. In summary, this work contributes to understanding the emotional impact that the COVID-19 crisis has on Spanish adolescents, exploring not only the factors that are related to more significant psychological effects but also to some variables that are associated with greater resilience.

Author Contributions: Conceptualization, N.M.-F. and A.R.-M.; Methodology, N.M.-F. and A.R.-M.; Formal analysis, N.M.-F. and A.R.-M.; Investigation, N.M.-F. and A.R.-M.; Resources, N.M.-F. and A.R.-M.; Data curation, N.M.-F. and A.R.-M.; Writing—original draft preparation, N.M.-F. and A.R.-M.; Writing—review and editing, N.M.-F. and A.R.-M.; Project Administration, N.M.-F. and A.R.-M. All authors have read and agreed to the published version of the manuscript.

Funding: This research received no external funding.

Institutional Review Board Statement: The study was conducted according to the guidelines of the Declaration of Helsinki, and approved by the Institutional Review Board of Universidad Loyola Andalucía (16 April 2020).

Informed Consent Statement: Informed consent was obtained from all subjects involved in the study.

Data Availability Statement: The datasets generated and analyzed during the current study are available from the corresponding author on reasonable request.

Conflicts of Interest: The authors declare no conflict of interest.

References

1. Mantovani, A.; Rinaldi, E.; Zusi, C.; Beatrice, G.; Saccomani, M.D.; Dalbeni, A. Coronavirus disease 2019 (COVID-19) in children and/or adolescents: A meta-analysis. *Pediatric Res.* **2020**. [CrossRef]
2. UNESCO. COVID-19 Educational Disruption and Response. Available online: https://en.unesco.org/covid19/educationresponse (accessed on 25 July 2020).
3. Lee, J. Mental health effects of school closures during COVID-19. *Lancet Child Adolesc. Health* **2020**, *4*, 421. [CrossRef]
4. Larson, R.W.; Eccles, J.S. *Organized Activities as Contexts of Development: Extracurricular Activities, after-School and Community Programs*; Lawrence Erlbaum Associates Publishers: Mahwah, NJ, USA, 2005.
5. DPhil, A.; Tomova, L.; Blakemore, S.J. The effects of social deprivation on adolescent development and mental health. *Lancet Child Adolesc. Health* **2020**, *4*, 634–640. [CrossRef]
6. Luchetti, M.; Lee, J.H.; Aschwanden, D.; Sesker, A.; Strickhouser, J.E.; Terracciano, A.; Sutin, A.R. The trajectory of loneliness in response to COVID-19. *Am. Psychol.* **2020**, *75*, 897–908. [CrossRef]
7. Prime, H.; Wade, M.; Browne, D.T. Risk and resilience in family during the COVID-19 pandemic. *Am. Psychol.* **2020**, *75*, 631–643. [CrossRef]
8. Fergert, J.; Vitielli, B.; Plener, P.; Clemens, V. Challenges and burden of the Coronavirus 2019 (COVID-19) pandemic for child and adolescent mental health: A narrative review to highlight clinical and research needs in the acute phase and the long return to normality. *Child Adolesc. Psychiatry Ment. Health* **2020**, *14*, 20. [CrossRef] [PubMed]
9. Wang, G.; Zhang, Y.; Zhao, J.; Zhang, J.; Jiang, J. Mitigate the effects of home confinement on children during the COVID-19 outbreak. *Lancet* **2020**, *395*, 945–947. [CrossRef]
10. Liang, L.; Ren, H.; Cao, R.; Hu, Y.; Qin, Z.; Li, C.; Mei, S. The effect of COVID-19 on youth mental health. *Psychiatr. Q.* **2020**, *91*, 841–852. [CrossRef]
11. Romero, E.; López-Romero, L.; Domínguez-Álvarez, B.; Villar, P.; Gómez-Fraguela, J.A. Testing the effects of COVID-19 confinement in Spanish children: The role of parents' distress, emotional problems and specific parenting. *Int. J. Environ. Res. Public Health* **2020**, *17*, 6975. [CrossRef] [PubMed]

12. Wang, C.; Zhao, H. The impact of COVID-19 on anxiety in Chinese university students. *Front. Psychol.* **2020**, *11*, 1168. [CrossRef]
13. Yang, H.; Bin, P.; Jingwei, A. Opinions from the epicenter: An online survey of university students in Wuhan amidst the COVID-19 outbreak. *J. Chin. Gov.* **2020**, *5*, 234–248. [CrossRef]
14. Buzzi, C.; Tucci, M.; Ciprandi, R.; Brambilla, I.; Caimmi, S.; Ciprandi, G.; Marseglia, G.L. The psycho-social effects of COVID-19 on Italian adolescents' attitudes and behaviors. *Ital. J. Pediatr.* **2020**, *46*, 69. [CrossRef]
15. Alvis, L.; Shook, N.; Oosterhoff, B. Adolescents' Prosocial Experiences During the COVID-19 Pandemic: Associations with Mental Health and Community Attachments. *PsyArXiv*. (preprint). [CrossRef]
16. Gao, J.; Zheng, P.; Jia, Y.; Chen, H.; Mao, Y.; Chen, S.; Wang, Y.; Fu, H.; Dai, J. Mental health problems and social media exposure during COVID-19 outbreak. *PLoS ONE* **2020**, *15*, e0231924. [CrossRef]
17. Gritsenko, V.; Skugarevsky, O.; Konstantinov, V.; Khamenka, N.; Marinova, T.; Reznik, A.; Isralowitz, R. COVID 19 fear, stress, anxiety, and substance use among Russian and Belarusian university students. *Int. J. Ment. Health Addict.* **2020**, *21*, 1–7. [CrossRef]
18. Pérez-Fuentes, M.C.; Molero, M.M.; Martos, A.; Gázquez Linares, J.J. Threat of COVID-19 and emotional state during quarantine: Positive and negative affect as mediators in a cross-sectional study of the Spanish population. *PLoS ONE* **2020**, *15*, e0235305. [CrossRef] [PubMed]
19. Reznik, A.; Gritsenko, V.; Konstantinov, V.; Khamenka, N.; Isralowitz, R. COVID-19 Fear in Eastern Europe: Validation of the Fear of COVID-19 Scale. *Int. J. Ment. Health Addict.* **2020**. [CrossRef] [PubMed]
20. Seçer, I.; Ulaş, S. An investigation of the effect of COVID-19 on OCD in youth in the context of emotional reactivity, experiential avoidance, depression and anxiety. *Int. J. Ment. Health Addict.* **2020**. [CrossRef] [PubMed]
21. Liu, N.; Zhang, F.; Wei, C.; Jia, Y.; Shang, Z.; Sun, L.; Wu, L.; Sun, Z.; Zhou, Y.; Wang, Y.; et al. Prevalence and predictors of PTSS during COVID-19 outbreak in China hardest-hit areas: Gender differences matter. *Psychiatry Res.* **2020**, *287*, 112921. [CrossRef]
22. Baloran, E.T. Knowledge, attitudes, anxiety, and coping strategies of students during COVID-19 pandemic. *J. Loss Trauma* **2020**, *25*, 635–642. [CrossRef]
23. Odriozola-González, P.; Planchuelo-Gómez, Á.; Irurtia, M.J.; de Luis-García, R. Psychological effects of the COVID-19 outbreak and lockdown among students and workers of a Spanish university. *Psychiatry Res.* **2020**, *290*, 113108. [CrossRef]
24. Sorokin, M.Y.; Kasyanov, E.D.; Rukavishnikov, G.V.; Makarevich, O.V.; Neznanov, N.G.; Lutova, N.B.; Mazo, G.E. Structure of anxiety associated with COVID-19 pandemic: The online survey results. *Bull. RSMU* **2020**, *3*, 70–76. [CrossRef]
25. Cohen, A.; Hoyt, L.; Dull, B. A Descriptive study of coronavirus disease 2019-related experiences and perspectives of a national sample of college students in spring 2020. *J. Adolesc. Health* **2020**, *67*, 369–375. [CrossRef]
26. Brooks, S.K.; Webster, R.K.; Smith, L.E.; Woodland, L.; Wessely, S.; Greenberg, N.; Rubin, G.J. The psychological impact of quarantine and how to reduce it: Rapid review of the evidence. *Lancet* **2020**, *395*, 912–920. [CrossRef]
27. Ryan, R.M.; Deci, E.L.; Vansteenkiste, M. Autonomy and autonomy disturbances in self-development and psychopathology: Research on motivation, attachment, and clinical process. In *Developmental Psychopathology*; Cichetti, D., Ed.; Wiley: New York, NY, USA, 2015; pp. 385–438.
28. Vansteenkiste, M.; Ryan, R.M. On psychological growth and vulnerability: Basic psychological need satisfaction and need frustration as a unifying principle. *J. Psychother. Integr.* **2013**, *23*, 263–280. [CrossRef]
29. Dvorsky, M.; Breaux, R.; Becker, S.P. Finding ordinary magic in extraordinary times: Child and adolescent resilience during the COVID-19 pandemic. *Eur. Child Adolesc. Psychiatry* **2020**. [CrossRef]
30. World Health Organization. Mental Health and Psychosocial Considerations during the COVID-19 Outbreak, 18 March 2020. Available online: https://apps.who.int/iris/bitstream/handle/10665/331490/WHO-2019-nCoV-MentalHealth-2020.1-eng.pdf (accessed on 23 December 2020).
31. Brown, B.B.; Larson, J. Peer relationships in adolescence. In *Handbook of Adolescent Psychology: Contextual Influences on Adolescent Development*; Lerner, R.M., Steinberg, L., Eds.; John Wiley & Sons Inc.: Hoboken, NJ, USA, 2009; pp. 74–103.
32. Zhou, S.-J.; Zhang, L.-G.; Wang, L.-L.; Guo, Z.-C.; Wang, J.-Q.; Chen, J.-C.; Liu, M.; Chen, C.; Chen, J.-X. Prevalence and socio demographic correlates of psychological health problems in Chinese adolescents during the outbreak of COVID 19. *Eur. Child Adolesc. Psychiatry* **2020**, *29*, 749–758. [CrossRef]
33. Xie, X.; Xue, Q.; Zhou, Y.; Zhu, K.; Liu, Q.; Zhang, J.; Song, R. Mental health status among children in home confinement during the coronavirus disease 2019 outbreak in Hubei Province, China. *JAMA Pediatr.* **2020**, *174*, 898–900. [CrossRef] [PubMed]
34. Steinberg, L. *Age of Opportunity: Lessons from the New Science of Adolescence*; Houghton Mifflin Harcourt: New York, NY, USA, 2014.
35. Ezpeleta, L.; Navarro, J.; de la Osa, N.; Trepat, E.; Penelo, E. Life conditions during COVID-19 lockdown and mental health in Spanish adolescents. *Int. J. Environ. Res.* **2020**, *17*, 7327. [CrossRef]
36. Su, R.; Tay, L.; Diener, E. The development and validation of the Comprehensive Inventory of Thriving (CIT) and the Brief Inventory of Thriving (BIT). *Appl. Psychol. Health Well Being* **2014**, *6*, 251–279. [CrossRef] [PubMed]
37. Field, A. Regression. In *Discovering Statistics using IBM SPSS Statistics*, 3rd ed.; Sage: London, UK, 2014; pp. 293–356.
38. Alberts, A.; Elkind, D.; Ginsberg, S. The personal fable and risk-taking in early adolescence. *J. Youth Adolesc.* **2007**, *36*, 71–76. [CrossRef]
39. Abbott, A.; Askelson, N.; Scherer, A.M.; Afifi, R.A. Critical reflections on COVID-19 communication efforts targeting adolescents and young adults. *J. Adolesc. Health* **2020**, *67*, 159–160. [CrossRef]
40. Oosterhoff, B.; Palmer, C. Psychological Correlates of News Monitoring, Social Distancing, Disinfecting, and Hoarding Behaviors among US Adolescents during the COVID-19 Pandemic. *PsyArXiv*. (preprint). [CrossRef]

41. Sahu, P. Closure of universities due to Coronavirus disease 2019 (COVID-19): Impact on education and mental health of students and academic staff. *Cureus* **2020**, *12*, e7541. [CrossRef]
42. Becker, S.P.; Gregory, A.M. Editorial Perspective: Perils and promise for child and adolescent sleep and associated psychopathology during the COVID-19 pandemic. *J. Child Psychol. Psychiatry* **2020**, *61*, 757–759. [CrossRef]
43. Furman, W.; Buhrmester, D. The Network of Relationships Inventory: Behavioral systems version. *Int. J. Behav. Dev.* **2009**, *33*, 470–478. [CrossRef] [PubMed]
44. Zimmer-Gembeck, M.J. The development of romantic relationships and adaptations in the system of peer relationships. *J. Adolesc. Health* **2002**, *31*, 216–225. [CrossRef]
45. Caughlin, J.P.; Sharabi, L.L. A communicative interdependence perspective of close relationships: The connections between mediated and unmediated interactions matter. *J. Commun.* **2013**, *63*, 873–893. [CrossRef]
46. Lai, J. Dispositional optimism buffers the impact of daily hassles on mental health in Chinese adolescents. *Personal. Individ. Differ.* **2009**, *47*, 247–249. [CrossRef]
47. Arslan, G.; Yildirim, M. Coronavirus stress, meaningful living, optimism, and depressive symptoms: A study of moderated mediation model. *PsyArXiv*. (preprint). [CrossRef]
48. Arslan, G.; Yildirim, M.; Tanhan, A.; Buluş, M.; Allen, K. Coronavirus stress, optimism-pessimism, psychological inflexibility, and psychological health: Psychometric properties of the coronavirus stress measure. *Int. J. Ment. Health Addict.* **2020**. [CrossRef] [PubMed]
49. Calvete, E.; Connor-Smith, J.K. Perceived social support, coping, and symptoms of distress in American and Spanish students. *Anxiety Stress Coping* **2006**, *19*, 47–65. [CrossRef]

Journal of
Clinical Medicine

MDPI

Article

Stress, Anxiety and Depression Prevalence among Greek University Students during COVID-19 Pandemic: A Two-Year Survey

Dimitrios Kavvadas [1,2,*], Asimoula Kavvada [1,3], Sofia Karachrysafi [1,2], Vasileios Papaliagkas [3], Stavros Cheristanidis [1,4], Maria Chatzidimitriou [3] and Theodora Papamitsou [1,2]

1 Post-Graduate Program "Health and Environmental Factors", School of Medicine, Faculty of Health, Aristotle University of Thessaloniki, 54124 Thessaloniki, Greece; akavvada@auth.gr (A.K.); sofia_karachrysafi@outlook.com (S.K.); stavrcher@auth.gr (S.C.); thpapami@auth.gr (T.P.)
2 Laboratory of Histology and Embryology, School of Medicine, Faculty of Health, Aristotle University of Thessaloniki, 54124 Thessaloniki, Greece
3 Department of Biomedical Sciences, School of Health Sciences, International Hellenic University, 57400 Thessaloniki, Greece; vpapal@auth.gr (V.P.); mchatzid952@gmail.com (M.C.)
4 Laboratory of Atmospheric Physics, Department of Physics, Aristotle University of Thessaloniki, University Campus, 54124 Thessaloniki, Greece
* Correspondence: kavvadas@auth.gr

Abstract: Background: The negative effect of COVID-19 pandemic on college students' mental health is well-demonstrated. The aim of this study is to assess the impact of the pandemic on the students of Aristotle University of Thessaloniki (Northern Greece), in terms of stress, anxiety, and depression, and to analyze the probable correlation of various social and phycological factors. Methods: The survey was conducted in the form of a questionnaire, which was first distributed in November 2020 and then re-launched in November 2021. The evaluation was carried out through the DASS21 screening tool. Associations regarding participants' characteristics and the three variables (stress, anxiety, and depression) were investigated with Pearson's chi-squared (X^2) test. Results: The first-year results (November 2020) revealed severe prevalence of stress, anxiety, and depression (37.4%, 27.2% and 47% respectively). The second-year results (November 2021) revealed a significant augmentation in all three variables, mainly for the extreme severe scales (47.3%, 41.1% and 55% respectively). Participants who were receiving psychiatric treatment exhibited higher levels of stress, anxiety, and depression, especially during the second year of the pandemic (p-Value < 0.00001). Female students' mental health was at higher risk, as elevated prevalence of negative symptoms was observed (p-Value < 0.00001). Conclusions: The community of Aristotle University of Thessaloniki has been greatly affected during the last 2 years. The inherent risks of the confinement measures on students' well-being and mental health are undeniable. Recurrent annual psychological evaluation in universities and colleges is strongly advised.

Keywords: mental health; college; students; DASS21; pandemic; gender

Citation: Kavvadas, D.; Kavvada, A.; Karachrysafi, S.; Papaliagkas, V.; Cheristanidis, S.; Chatzidimitriou, M.; Papamitsou, T. Stress, Anxiety and Depression Prevalence among Greek University Students during COVID-19 Pandemic: A Two-Year Survey. *J. Clin. Med.* **2022**, *11*, 4263. https://doi.org/10.3390/jcm11154263

Academic Editor: Alfonso Troisi

Received: 18 June 2022
Accepted: 20 July 2022
Published: 22 July 2022

1. Introduction

An unknown etiology outbreak of pneumonia turned into the pandemic of COVID-19 (Coronavirus disease-19) disease and spread rapidly throughout the planet [1,2]. The mortality was unexpectedly high, leading countries to take drastic measures [3].

Several studies focused on the correlation among demographic characteristics and psychological deterioration during the pandemic [4–6]. Remarkable efforts have been made on the evaluation of psychological and mental effects on university students. Evidence suggest an increase in stress, anxiety, and depression levels in several countries. In China, according to Ma et al., the probability of developing acute stress, depression, and anxiety disorder was 34.9%, 21.1%, and 11.0% respectively, based on a sample of 746,217 students during November 2020. In the United States, in a similar study conducted during 2020, 195 students were evaluated and 71% of the sample revealed increased stress and anxiety during the pandemic, in comparison to the pre-COVID period [7–9]. Post-traumatic stress disorder, accompanied by sleep disorders, has also been observed. These findings confirm that intense and constant concern can lead to a severe reduction of the academic performance and to psychological health distress. For instance, according to Son et al., over 90% of the sample of university students expressed concerns for their relatives' well-being and 89% had difficulties to concentrate. Almost 86% reported sleep disorders and deterioration of their social life. Moreover, 82% observed decreased performance in their academic courses. Similar reports were recorded by Tang et al., during the first year of the pandemic, on 2485 students from six Chinese universities [7,10]. An aggravating factor in the above is the loss of their jobs or the alteration to their employment routine [11]. Several studies suggest that younger age, poor health, extensive exposure to computer screens, and the constant fear for SARS-CoV-2 infection, pose significant risk factors for the students' mental health during the pandemic. There is a worldwide indication that female gender should be included in the risk factors. Chang et al. observed that female students were more likely to suffer from anxiety and depression during the COVID-19 period [9]. Browning et al. collected data from seven United States Universities during the first months of the pandemic. Their findings suggest that female gender is hampered by the already deteriorating mental health of American students during the pandemic [12]. Similar observations were made in a survey conducted in France, including 69,054 students during the first lockdown period of 2020 [13]. Other risk factors are financial hardship, distance learning, and uncertainty about the academic future due to the ongoing preventive measures and quarantine [14].

A comparative study revealed severe stress management imbalance during the pandemic, compared to 2018 [15]. Similarly to other studies, it was noticed that female students and students with disabilities and different sexual orientation respondents faced significant difficulties and their mental health was aggravated during the pandemic [15,16].

Studies were also carried out in Greece during the first year of the pandemic, presenting similar results. Kaparounaki et al. conducted a study on student mental health during the first months of the pandemic in Greece (April 2020). Among the 1000 participating students, increased stress and depression levels (42.5% and 74.3% respectively) were observed [17]. Patsali et al. collected data from April to May 2020. A total of 1104 female Greek students and 431 male Greek students participated in the study. The results showed that more than 65% of the respondents reported a significant increase in stress due to quarantine. Severe depression and feelings of despair were also reported. Female gender appeared as a potential risk factor of depression [18]. Moreover, a study on 1060 students (mostly females) from several Greek universities during the first months of the pandemic [19] was performed through the Depression Anxiety Stress Scale (DASS-21). Moderate to extreme severe depression was observed in 35.6% of the students, while 31.8% and 19.7% reported moderate to extreme severe stress and anxiety, respectively. The prevalence of negative emotions was particularly high compared to similar rates on Chinese students, but similar to Mediterranean countries like Italy and Spain [19].

The research hypothesis expected increased levels of stress, anxiety, and depression in the second distribution of the survey. In addition, it was assumed that demographic and individual characteristics of the participants (such as gender, cohabitation status, vaccination status, psychological or psychiatric treatment) were significantly correlated with the different levels of stress, anxiety, and depression. The hypothesis was derived from recent global data with evidence of continuous deterioration of university students' mental health during the pandemic [7–10,14].

2. Materials and Methods

2.1. Study Design

The study was conducted through an anonymous questionnaire, which assessed the psychological, social data of the participants and included the Depression Anxiety Stress Scale (DASS21). The survey was launched twice. The questionnaire was the same for both distributions.

The aim of this research was to assess the general mental health of the Aristotle University of Thessaloniki (AUTh) students during COVID-19 "peak" periods, in Greece. For this purpose, DASS21 screening test was used in order to evaluate stress, anxiety, and depression levels. Furthermore, the impact of physical, social, and phycological factors and their probable correlation to the students' current mental state were analyzed. According to the literature, a further gender analysis was considered to be essential.

2.2. Population and Samples

The study sample included students (BSc, MSc, PhD) of the university. The research was conducted at two time intervals. The first period of the survey took place in November 2020 (first major peak of the pandemic) and included 2322 participants, while the second was in November 2021 (second peak) with 3160 participations. Based on the official registration of the AUTh, as of November 2021 there were 51,577 active students [20]. Therefore, the collected students' samples represent approximately 5–6% of the students' population (2110 and 2916 for the first and the second year respectively) (Figure 1). The rest participants were excluded as they represented the academic and administrative staff of the university. It should be noted that more than 1500 respondents' entries were also excluded from the surveys due to incomplete completion of the questionnaire (Figure 1). The percentage of female active students was approximately 54% and of the male active students was 46%.

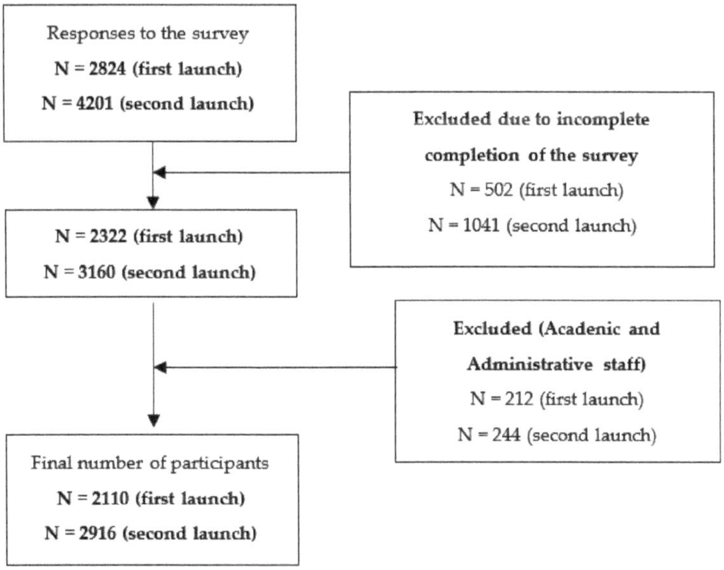

Figure 1. Participants' flow chart with inclusion and exclusion criteria.

2.3. Questionnaire Platform and Approvals

The hosting platform was the LimeSurvey AUTH (Aristotle University of Thessaloniki) under the supervision of the certified questionnaires authority of Aristotle University). Due to the legislation on personal data protection (GDPR), both the AUTh bioethics committee

(Bioethics Committee No. 1.254/20-10-20) as well as the AUTh Data Protection office, granted permission. The LimeSurvey AUTH platform gathered the responses and access was granted only to the head professor of the project (author T.P.) via a personalized link, which created a secure authorized profile.

2.4. Distribution and Content of the Questionnaire

The questionnaire was available from 15 November 2020 (08.00 A.M. Greece time) to 30 November 2020 (08.00 A.M.) (first launch) and from 15 November 2021 (08.00 A.M.) to 30 November 2021 (08.00 A.M.) (second launch). The survey was conducted in the form of an online questionnaire, which was distributed to participants via their institutional e-mail ("name"@auth.gr). All of the questions were closed-type questions and it was obligatory for participants to choose an answer, once they agreed to participate, in order to complete the survey.

The questionnaire was divided into three thematic sets (Table 1):

Table 1. The questionnaire used in both years' surveys.

A. Basic Information (Demographic, Psychological, COVID-19)		
1. Age range 2. Sex		
3. Marital Status 4. Health Professional (YES/NO) 5. Cohabitation 6. Changes in professional activity 7. Test for SARS-CoV-2 (YES/NO) 8. Known person diagnosed positive for COVID-19 (YES/NO) 9. Symptoms manifestation 10. Vaccination against COVID-19 (YES/NO) (only in the second launch, November 2021) 11. Concerns about an impending lockdown (0, 1, 2, 3) (only in the second launch, November 2021) 12. Psychological or psychiatric treatment in the past (YES/NO) 13. Psychological or psychiatric treatment at this time (YES/NO) 14. Psychotropic drugs intake (YES/NO) 15. Restriction due to quarantine had positive effects on relationships between people confined within the same house (YES/NO) 16. Restriction due to quarantine had negative effects on relationships between people confined within the same house (YES/NO) 17. Restriction due to quarantine had positive effects on social relations 18. Restriction due to quarantine had negative effects on social relations		
B. Information about the University Status		
19. Academic capacity (Students, Administrative staff, Academic staff) 20. Category of students (Undergraduate BSc or MD, MSc, PhD) 21. Year of study (for undergraduate students)		
C. DASS21 (Likert-4 Scale)		
22. I found it hard to wind down (s)	29. I felt that I was using a lot of nervous energy (s)	36. I felt I was close to panic (a)
23. I was aware of dryness of my mouth (a)	30. I was worried about situations in which I might panic and make a fool of myself (a)	37. I was unable to become enthusiastic about anything (d)
24. I couldn't seem to experience any positive feeling at all (d)	31. I felt that I had nothing to look forward to (d)	38. I felt I wasn't worth much as a person (d)
25. I experienced breathing difficulty (e.g., excessively rapid breathing, breathlessness in the absence of physical exertion) (a)	32. I found myself getting agitated (s)	39. I felt that I was rather touchy (s)
26. I found it difficult to work up the initiative to do things (d)	33. I found it difficult to relax (s)	40. I was aware of the action of my heart in the absence of physical exertion (e.g., sense of heart rate increase, heart missing a beat) (a)
27. I tended to over-react to situations (s)	34. I felt down-hearted and blue (d)	41. I felt scared without any good reason (a)
28. I experienced trembling (e.g., in the hands) (a)	35. I was intolerant of anything that kept me from getting on with what I was doing (s)	42. I felt that life was meaningless (d)

(a): evaluation of anxiety, (s): evaluation of stress, (d): evaluation of depression.

The first set was about the basic information and participant's profile, psychological evaluation, and experiences in relation to COVID-19 [16]. The aim was to extract information related to the basic characteristics of the respondents (questions 1–6) and their familiarization with COVID-19 (questions 7–10). Moreover, there was a short evaluation of their psychological state (questions 12–14) and their social well-being (questions 16–18).

The second section was about the university status (questions 19–21)

Both sets 1 and 2 were composed of well-established questions, similar to other published studies [16].

The third and most significant set of questions (questions 22–42) assessed the levels of anxiety, stress, and depression, as well as their physical manifestations, through the DASS21 [16,19].

The DASS21 (Depression, Anxiety, and Stress Scale) was introduced in 1995 by Lovibond and Lovibond [21]. It consists of three self-report scales designed for screening of depression, anxiety, and stress [16,19]. In 1998, a final version of the DASS that consisted of 21-item (DASS21) was described [22]. Each of the three DASS21 scales contain seven elements, divided into subscales with similar content. The Depression Scale assesses discomfort, despair, life devaluation, self-devaluation, lack of interest/engagement, and inaction. The stress scale assesses autonomic arousal, signs of stress through skeletal muscle movements, stress-induced anxiety, and the subjective experience of anxiety. The stress scale is sensitive to chronic non-specific stimulation. This scale evaluates the difficulty of relaxation, nervous agitation and upset/agitation, the case of an irritable/hyper-reactive characters, and impatience. Scores for depression, anxiety, and stress are calculated by summing the scores for the relevant data [21,22]. The DASS21 rating scale is used internationally to assess stress, anxiety, and depression levels. It is a recognized and accepted tool by psychologists and psychiatrists with a very good internal consistency [22]. It is, therefore, a valid Likert-4 scale (0. Not at all, 1. A little, 2. much, 3. Too much), which calculates the negative emotional states experienced by the participants during the period of time that the survey is available. The Greek version of the DASS-21 scale, based on Greek sources and official translations, was described by Lyrakos et al. [23]. This particular version was used in this survey. The results can be either normal, mild, moderate, severe, or extremely severe. For stress, a normal score is 0–7, 8–9 for mild stress, 10–12 for moderate, 13–16 for severe, and above 17 for extreme severe stress [21]. Similarly, 0–3 is the normal score for anxiety, 4–5 is the prevalence of the mild anxiety, 6–7 moderate, 8–9 severe and above 10 is the extreme severe anxiety [21]. Finally, a score of 0–4 is normal for depression, 5–6 is mild, 7–10 is moderate, 11–13 is severe, and above 14 is the score for extreme severe depression [21]. The scores for depression, anxiety, and stress are calculated by summing the scores for the relevant items [21].

The above questionnaire was distributed for the second time on November 2021. The second launch included the same questions with two extra questions (vaccine coverage and concerns for an impending lockdown).

During the 2-year study, all personal data protection measures were obtained for the participants, who were informed that they had the right to terminate their participation at any time. They were also informed about the purpose of the research, the population target of the university, and the DASS21 evaluation scale. It was stated to them that any processing of personal data would be done in accordance with the General Regulation of Personal Data Protection, taking the appropriate technical and organizational measures. Personal data were kept only for the period required for the lawful purposes for which they were collected ensuring their safe destruction, when the legally abovementioned period had elapsed or the purpose of their processing ceased to exist. Finally, they were informed that for the purposes of the investigation it was not required to verify their identity by those responsible for processing the data, with the result that the latter were not obliged to obtain or retain or process additional information to verify the identity of each participant. Consequently, the following rights did not exist: (a) the right of access to personal data, (b) the right of correction, (c) the right of deletion, (d) the right of restriction of processing, and (e) the right of data portability in accordance with the General Regulation Personal Data Protection. Contact details were provided for anyone seeking more information and clarifications.

2.5. Statistical Analysis

The Cronbach "alpha" factor was excellent in both years. More specifically, it was estimated at 0.946 for the DASS21 launched in 2020 and 0.954 for the DASS21 launched in 2021. As mentioned, the DASS-21 is based on a multi-dimensional and not a categorical perception of psychological distress [21,22]. The hypothesis on which the development of DASS21 was based (and which was confirmed by research data) is that the differences between depression, anxiety, and stress experienced by normal individuals and clinical populations, are gradually different [21]. The demographic characteristics of the participants and the answers to the first set of questions (psychological assessment, COVID-19, academic capacity) were studied with Pearson's chi-square test. Because of the large set of categorical variables, the multiple correspondence (correlations) analysis was performed for the second questionnaire (November, 2021) [24–28]. The aim was an in-depth psychological evaluation of the students after 2 consecutive years of the ongoing pandemic, during the second and largest peak of COVID-19 outbreak in Greece. The results of the 21 questions through which the score of anxiety, stress, and depression was obtained, are summarized within the multiple correspondence analysis in in three grades (Normal, Mild to Sever, Extreme Severe). The gradation was delineated based on the quadrants Q1 and Q3 of a continuous distribution of samples with a value range of 0–21, which consist of the sum of the DASS21 scores [29]. The multiple correspondence processing leads to the construction of the Burt tables, which are multiple coincidence tables. These tables were produced by the intersection of the classes of each variable [30]. The purpose of the multiple correspondence analysis is the calculation of the coordinates of the rows and columns on the factorial axes that are formed during the analysis of the data, in order to interpret the extracted information [24–28]. In this case the columns represented the levels of stress, anxiety, and depression, while the rows were the responses to the basic information received by the first part of the survey (demographic, psychological etc.) The statistical processing of the results was performed with the program SPSS version 24.0 (IBM, SPSS Inc., Chicago, IL, USA), Microsoft Excel (2019) version 16.43, and the the Méthodes d 'Analyses des Données (MAD) software [31].

3. Results

3.1. Two-Year Demographic Data

Female participants outnumbered males in both years (70% and 73%, first and second launch respectively). The cohabitation status changed in the second year, with a higher percentage stating to dwell in their houses without roommates (31%) or with one person (25%) (chi-square 281.2, p-value < 0.00001), compared to 2020 (15% and 21% respectively). Significant difference was also observed in the work status, with more employees reporting changes in their job routine during the first year (27.5%) (chi-square 23.8, p-value < 0.00001). During the second launch (November 2021), the majority of the participants reported to know an acquaintance who was diagnosed with COVID-19 (94.4%). This rate was significantly increased in comparison to the first launch (chi-square 81.5, p-value < 0.00001). Meanwhile, the cases of acquaintances who were diagnosed positive and were seriously ill or died were also significantly increased in 2021 (21%) (chi-square 99.0, p-value < 0.00001). Psychiatric care (chi-square 78.3, p-value < 0.00001) and psychotropic drugs intake (chi-square 14.3, p-value 0.00015) were also increased during the second year of the pandemic (14.5% and 3.9% respectively). Also, compared to the first year, the respondents felt that the relationship between people confined in the same house was significantly deteriorated (50%) (chi-square 12.4, p-value 0.00042).

The majority of students who had not been vaccinated by the time of the second launch were undergraduate and master students (25% and 19% respectively).

A statistically significant difference was observed regarding gender and the fear of an impending lockdown, due to the raised numbers of COVID-19 cases (p-value < 0.00001). The majority of females (60%) were more concerned compared to male participants (50%) (Supplementary Material; Tables S1–S14).

3.2. DASS-21 Results

The results of the DASS21 surveys are presented below (Table 2). In 2020, moderate to severe stress and extreme anxiety was observed in high rates. In the same year, 60% of the depression prevalence rates in students were distributed to the scales from mild (13%) to extremely severe (16.1%). In 2021, a significant increase was observed in all extreme severe scales (Table 2).

Table 2. DASS21 results of the Aristotle University of Thessaloniki students during the 2 years of the pandemic (2020–2021). The comparisons were performed with the chi-square test (*p*-Value significant at 0.05).

Students' Scores (%)	**Stress (%)**		**Anxiety (%)**		**Depression (%)**	
	2020	**2021**	**2020**	**2021**	**2020**	**2021**
Normal	1059 *(50.2)*	1188 *(40.7)*	1265 *(60.0)*	1295 *(44.4)*	844 *(40.0)*	1008 *(34.6)*
Mild	265 *(12.6)*	347 *(11.9)*	271 *(12.8)*	421 *(14.4)*	275 *(13.0)*	303 *(10.4)*
Moderate	316 *(15.0)*	476 *(16.3)*	194 *(9.2)*	298 *(10.2)*	433 *(20.5)*	590 *(20.2)*
Severe	294 *(13.9)*	502 *(17.2)*	116 *(5.5)*	243 *(8.3)*	219 *(10.4)*	382 *(13.1)*
Extreme severe	176 *(8.3)*	403 *(13.8)*	264 *(12.5)*	659 *(22.6)*	339 *(16.1)*	633 *(21.7)*
Total	2110 *(100.0)*	2916 *(100.0)*	2110 *(100.0)*	2916 *(100.0)*	2110 *(100.0)*	2916 *(100.0)*
p-Values	<0.00001		<0.00001		<0.00001	

In the second launch of the survey (November 2021), the extreme scale values for both female and male students were almost doubled (Tables 3 and 4).

Table 3. Chi-square statistical analysis between female students during the 2 years, based on the scores of the DASS21 scale (*p*-Value significant at 0.05).

Female Students	**Stress (%)**		**Anxiety (%)**		**Depression (%)**	
	2020	**2021**	**2020**	**2021**	**2020**	**2021**
Normal	718 (45.8)	736 (35.9)	890 (56.7)	817 (39.8)	584 (37.2)	662 (32.3)
Mild	207 (13.2)	252 (12.3)	203 (12.9)	288 (14.0)	194 (12.4)	197 (9.6)
Moderate	252 (16.1)	360 (17.6)	151 (9.6)	239 (11.7)	331 (21.2)	424 (20.7)
Severe	239 (15.2)	389 (18.9)	97 (6.4)	181 (8.8)	181 (11.5)	283 (13.8)
Extreme severe	152 (9.7)	314 (15.3)	227 (14.4)	526 (25.6)	278 (17.7)	485 (23.6)
p-Values	<0.00001		<0.00001		<0.00001	

Table 4. Chi-square statistical analysis between male students during the 2 years, based on the scores of the DASS21 scale (*p*-Value significant at 0.05).

Male Students	**Stress (%)**		**Anxiety (%)**		**Depression (%)**	
	2020	**2021**	**2020**	**2021**	**2020**	**2021**
Normal	341 (62.9)	452 (52.2)	375 (69.2)	482 (55.7)	260 (48.0)	341 (39.4)
Mild	58 (10.7)	95 (11.0)	68 (12.5)	129 (14.9)	81 (14.9)	107 (12.4)
Moderate	64 (11.7)	116 (13.4)	43 (7.9)	61 (7.0)	102 (18.8)	164 (19.0)
Severe	55 (10.1)	113 (13.1)	19 (3.5)	60 (6.9)	38 (7.0)	98 (11.3)
Extreme severe	24 (4.4)	89 (10.3)	37 (6.8)	133 (15.5)	61 (11.3)	155 (17.9)
p-Values	0.00008		<0.00001		0.00010	

A further study was performed on those who knew someone diagnosed with COVID-19 during the 2 years. The percentage of those who were familiar to someone who died of COVID-19 during the second year of the pandemic was doubled, in comparison to the first year (*p*-Value 0.0002).

In order for an in-depth analysis to be performed, the multiple correspondence analysis was implemented for the second-year responses (November 2021). DASS21 scores of our three variables stress, anxiety, and depression, were distributed in three grades: normal, mild to severe, and extremely severe (Table 5). From a total of 2916 students, 13 participants were removed. A total of 2903 students participated in the multiple correspondence analysis.

Table 5. The percentages of the three distribution grades for all participants.

	DASS21 Score	**Normal (%)**	**Mild to Severe (%)**	**Extreme Severe (%)**
Students (N = 2903)	Stress	651 (22.4)	1501 (51.7)	751 (25.9)
	Anxiety	1290 (44.4)	958 (33.0)	655 (22.6)
	Depression	1003 (34.6)	1269 (43.7)	631 (21.7)

3.3. *Multiple Correlations and Statistical Analyses*

The multiple statistical analysis was assessed on the prevalence of stress, anxiety, and depression (from November 2021), in association with the participants' demographic characteristics. Therefore, the Burt Tables were produced, alongside with the low-dimensional Euclidean spaces from which derived all the correlations (Table 6).

Table 6. The Burt table based on the variables and students' responses and statistical analysis. The variables are presented in odds ratios (ORs).

		Stress			**Anxiety**			**Depression**		
Burt Table/ Odds-Ratios		**Normal**	**Mild to Severe**	**Extreme Severe**	**Normal**	**Mild to Severe**	**Extreme Severe**	**Normal**	**Mild to Severe**	**Extreme Severe**
Age range	18–25	0.26	1.09	0.37	0.72	0.51	0.32	0.47	0.82	0.30
	26–35	0.30	1.08	0.34	0.96	0.46	0.24	0.62	0.72	0.25
	36–45	0.62	0.88	0.17	1.67	0.38	0.11	1.21	0.51	0.13
	≥46	0.71	0.82	0.16	2.07	0.31	0.10	1.41	0.46	0.11
	p-Values		<0.00001			<0.00001			<0.00001	
Gender	Male	0.45	0.97	0.24	1.24	0.42	0.18	0.65	0.74	0.22
	Female	0.23	1.12	0.40	0.66	0.53	0.34	0.48	0.79	0.30
	p-Values		<0.00001			<0.00001			0.00022	
Marital status	Unmarried	0.27	1.08	0.36	0.76	0.50	0.30	0.50	0.80	0.29
	Other	0.61	0.91	0.17	1.69	0.34	0.13	1.29	0.46	0.14
	p-Values		<0.00001			<0.00001			<0.00001	
Cohabitation status	I live alone	0.27	1.09	0.36	0.74	0.49	0.33	0.49	0.82	0.29
	With 1 person	0.28	1.08	0.35	0.77	0.50	0.30	0.50	0.76	0.30
	With 2 or more	0.31	1.05	0.34	0.87	0.49	0.26	0.58	0.76	0.26
	p-Values		0.79			0.12			0.26	
Vaccinated	Yes	0.28	1.07	0.36	0.77	0.49	0.31	0.52	0.78	0.29
	No	0.33	1.05	0.32	0.96	0.50	0.22	0.58	0.77	0.25
	p-Values		0.28			0.0093			0.36	

Table 6. *Cont.*

Burt Table/ Odds-Ratios		Stress			Anxiety			Depression		
		Normal	Mild to Severe	Extreme Severe	Normal	Mild to Severe	Extreme Severe	Normal	Mild to Severe	Extreme Severe
Concerns about an impending lockdown	None	0.57	0.78	0.25	1.22	0.41	0.19	0.76	0.63	0.22
	Little	0.38	1.15	0.23	1.10	0.46	0.19	0.69	0.75	0.19
	Much	0.23	1.25	0.35	0.69	0.55	0.30	0.48	0.85	0.28
	Very Much	0.18	0.91	0.59	0.53	0.48	0.49	0.35	0.77	0.44
	p-Values		<0.00001			<0.00001			<0.00001	
Psychological or psychiatric treatment in the past	Yes	0.15	1.08	0.54	0.47	0.55	0.48	0.29	0.86	0.45
	No	0.34	1.07	0.29	0.95	0.47	0.24	0.63	0.75	0.23
	p-Values		<0.00001			<0.00001			<0.00001	
Currently taking psychotropic drugs	Yes	0.14	0.66	0.93	0.27	0.54	0.77	0.23	0.61	0.77
	No	0.30	1.09	0.33	0.83	0.49	0.28	0.54	0.78	0.26
	p-Values		<0.00001			<0.00001			<0.00001	

p-Value significant at 0.05.

As shown (Table 6), there were significant differences on the anxiety, stress, and depression levels and several sociodemographic and psychological features of the students. Younger students, female, and unmarried participants presented significantly increased levels of our three variables, in comparison to older students, males, and married respondents (*p*-Value < 0.00001). Similarly, all three variables were elevated for students who claimed to have received psychological or psychiatric treatment and those who were receiving psychotropic drugs during the surveys' launch periods (*p*-Value < 0.00001). Vaccinated students' responses revealed an augmentation in anxiety levels, in comparison to the unvaccinated respondents (*p*-Value = 0.0093). Also, concerns for an impending lockdown affected the levels of stress, anxiety, and depression (*p*-Value < 0.00001) (Table 7).

Table 7. The severe extreme stress anxiety depression odds ratios (ORs).

Extreme Severe Scale	Stress	Anxiety	Depression
Age range: 18–25 vs. 26–35	1.1	1.33	1.2
Gender: Female vs. Male	1.7	1.9	1.4
Marital status: Unmarried vs. Other	2.1	2.3	2.1
Cohabitation status:			
I live alone vs. Live With 1 person	1.0	1.1	1.0
I live alone vs. With 2 or more	1.1	1.3	1.1
Vaccinated: Yes vs. No	1.1	1.4	1.2
Concerns about an impending lockdown:			
None vs. Little	1.1	1.0	1.1
None vs. Much	0.7	0.6	0.8
None vs. Very Much	0.4	0.4	0.5
Psychological or psychiatric treatment in the past: Yes vs. No	1.9	2.0	2.0
Currently taking psychotropic drugs: Yes vs. No	2.8	2.8	3.0

The same differences were also revealed on the gender-based analysis of our three variables regarding the psychological or psychiatric treatment, the psychotropic drugs intake, and the concerns on an impending lockdown (Tables 8 and 9). Female vaccinated students were significantly more anxious in comparison to the non-vaccinated (*p*-Value = 0.0079). Also, male students who lived alone presented higher anxiety levels in comparison to those who lived with one or more people (*p*-Value = 0.039).

Table 8. Gender-based Burt table of the male students and statistical analysis (p-Values significant at 0.05). The variables are presented in odds ratios (ORs).

Burt Table/ Odds Ratios		Male Students								
		Stress			Anxiety			Depression		
		Normal	Mild to Severe	Extreme Severe	Normal	Mild to Severe	Extreme Severe	Normal	Mild to Severe	Extreme Severe
Marital status	Unmarried	0.44	0.99	0.25	1.20	0.42	0.19	0.61	0.77	0.23
	Other	0.84	0.70	0.15	2.29	0.35	0.05	2.07	0.39	0.05
	p-Values		0.085			0.056			0.0002	
Cohabitation status	I live alone	0.45	0.92	0.26	1.15	0.40	0.22	0.61	0.74	0.24
	With 1 person	0.39	1.00	0.28	1.00	0.45	0.24	0.53	0.78	0.27
	With 2 or more	0.49	0.99	0.21	1.46	0.41	0.13	0.75	0.72	0.18
	p-Values		0.64			0.039			0.22	
Vaccinated	Yes	0.43	1.00	0.25	1.20	0.43	0.19	0.64	0.75	0.22
	No	0.54	0.85	0.23	1.45	0.37	0.16	0.71	0.69	0.21
	p-Values		0.46			0.57			0.83	
Concerns about an impending lockdown	None	0.79	0.70	0.17	1.57	0.36	0.14	0.82	0.62	0.20
	Little	0.61	0.80	0.21	1.65	0.38	0.12	0.81	0.76	0.14
	Much	0.33	1.44	0.19	1.06	0.52	0.17	0.60	0.81	0.21
	Very Much	0.26	0.93	0.45	0.87	0.38	0.35	0.43	0.72	0.39
	p-Values		<0.00001			0.00064			0.0004	
Psychological or psychiatric treatment in the past	Yes	0.21	1.09	0.43	0.65	0.56	0.33	0.26	1.07	0.38
	No	0.53	0.94	0.20	1.47	0.38	0.15	0.80	0.67	0.18
	p-Values		<0.00001			<0.00001			<0.00001	
Currently taking psychotropic drugs	Yes	0.26	0.61	0.71	0.38	0.53	0.61	0.26	0.45	0.93
	No	0.46	0.98	0.23	1.29	0.41	0.17	0.67	0.75	0.20
	p-Values		0.01			0.00072			0.00007	

Table 9. Gender-based Burt table of the female students and statistical analysis (*p*-Values significant at 0.05). The variables are presented in odds ratios (ORs).

Burt Table/ Odds Ratios		Female Students								
		Stress			Anxiety			Depression		
		Normal	Mild to Severe	Extreme Severe	Normal	Mild to Severe	Extreme Severe	Normal	Mild to Severe	Extreme Severe
Marital status	Unmarried	0.21	1.13	0.42	0.63	0.54	0.36	0.45	0.82	0.31
	Other	0.54	1.00	0.18	1.52	0.34	0.17	1.10	0.48	0.18
	p-Values		<0.00001			<0.0001			<0.00001	
Cohabitation status	I live alone	0.21	1.17	0.41	0.61	0.53	0.38	0.44	0.85	0.31
	With 1 person	0.24	1.11	0.39	0.69	0.52	0.33	0.49	0.75	0.32
	With 2 or more	0.24	1.08	0.40	0.69	0.53	0.32	0.51	0.77	0.29
	p-Values		0.83			0.60			0.68	
Vaccinated	Yes	0.22	1.11	0.41	0.63	0.52	0.37	0.47	0.79	0.31
	No	0.26	1.15	0.35	0.81	0.55	0.24	0.53	0.81	0.26
	p-Values		0.41			0.0079			0.34	
Concerns about an impending lockdown	None	0.45	0.84	0.31	1.04	0.45	0.22	0.73	0.65	0.23
	Little	0.29	1.36	0.24	0.91	0.51	0.23	0.63	0.75	0.22
	Much	0.19	1.19	0.41	0.60	0.57	0.36	0.44	0.87	0.30
	Very Much	0.15	0.91	0.65	0.43	0.52	0.55	0.32	0.79	0.46
	p-Values		<0.00001			<0.00001			<0.00001	
Psychological or psychiatric treatment in the past	Yes	0.13	1.07	0.58	0.42	0.55	0.54	0.30	0.81	0.48
	No	0.27	1.13	0.34	0.77	0.52	0.29	0.56	0.79	0.25
	p-Values		<0.00001			< 0.00001			<0.00001	
Currently taking psychotropic drugs	Yes	0.10	0.68	1.03	0.23	0.55	0.84	0.22	0.68	0.72
	No	0.24	1.14	0.38	0.69	0.53	0.33	0.49	0.80	0.29
	p-Values		0.00003			0.00002			0.00013	

4. Discussion

This study assessed the stress, anxiety, and depression levels of the Aristotle University of Thessaloniki community, through the DASS21, during the 2-year ongoing pandemic. Severe and extremely severe prevalence was revealed in alarmingly high rates. The deterioration of students' mental health was conspicuous in both years. These findings were similar to initial research projects carried out in other Greek universities [17,32,33]. Our study revealed a significant upward pace in students' stress, anxiety, and depression levels during the 2-year evaluation.

Setting a pre-pandemic background, studies before the COVID-19 outbreak in Greece revealed a mild depression prevalence, but the results were in most cases conflicting [34–40]. A survey launched in 2015 reported mild to normal depression, related to marital status and previous psychiatric evaluation [34]. During the years 2009–2011, a study assessed the changes in mental health in the general population of Greece, due to the beginning of the economic crisis. Depression levels were increased, while stress remained stable [35]. Moreover, the fact that students, particularly from Greece, are prone to alcohol consumption during their first years of college, could lead to psychological imbalance and negative feelings [36,37]. On the contrary, another pre-pandemic study assessed the effects of the Mediterranean diet on Greek university students and found reduced levels of depression and stress, due to the consumption of specific local products [38]. Regarding mental illness, a pre-pandemic large study in the AUTh found that students claim to be familiar with mental illness, but through unreliable sources [39]. This finding reinforced fear of stigma, especially during the COVID-19 pandemic. Consequently, their imbalanced psychology, the fear of stigma, and further burden due to the daily changes of routine, posed severe danger to the mental wellness of AUTh students [40].

In the current research, approximately 22–26% of the students were integrated to the severe and extreme severe scales of the three study variables (stress, anxiety, and depression). The present 2-year analysis of the AUTh community revealed similarities with the international studies. According to Carr et al., a large percentage of a UK university community was on the verge of depression and severe anxiety disorder, with analogous proportions (30% of the students) [41]. Van Niekerk et al., launched a resemblant extensive survey during the two quarantine periods (2020 and 2021) in an Eastern Cape university and suggested that the risk of mental health deterioration should not be underestimated [42]. In the United Arab Emirates, half of the participants were at psychological distress, with those suffering of mental illness being at highest risk [43]. In China, an early COVID-19 study revealed increased levels of fear, which were associated with the prevalence of depression in students who were close to graduation [9]. Symptoms of depression and anxiety were also found in students during lockdown periods in China, 1 year after the onset of the pandemic [44,45]. Similarly, in Malaysia, a significant prevalence of anxiety in students was observed during the first year of the pandemic [14]. However, their extreme scores were significantly lower than the ones found in the AUTh students. A study conducted in seven united states of America revealed that students with low quality of life and health, of low income, and of young age were at psychological distress due to the pandemic [12]. However, the case of Sweden was different [46]. The DASS21 survey was launched in Swedish students during the first 3 months of the pandemic and no significant increase in stress, anxiety, and depression levels was revealed. On the contrary, Swedish students' mental state was improved, especially during the summer months of the first year of the pandemic [46].

Furthermore, the increased levels of stress and anxiety were correlated with female gender, between the AUTh students. More than the half of the AUth female participants suffered from mild to severe stress. The numbers of female participants that scored on the extreme stress, anxiety, and depression scales was high (above the expected scores on both launches) (Table 3). The male sample was also affected by the pandemic but not at such extreme scales. Stress and depression were above the expected values for male students during the second launch (Table 4). The higher risk of psychological distress in females was confirmed by our findings, in accordance to other studies [12,13,33]. The present study confirmed that the ongoing pandemic has significantly affected the female population of the AUTh, especially after 2 years of consecutive measures and restrictions.

Several students declared to have received psychological or psychiatric care in the past. There was a significant correlation of the increased psychiatric treatment and the elevated stress, anxiety, or depression levels of the AUTh community. These findings were also in line with evidence from pre-pandemic studies [34]. A balanced social environment and resilience of character are essential for preserving the mental well-being during the home-confinement periods [47].

The Aristotle University of Thessaloniki has established a 24-h-communication line for members who seek counseling and psychological support. Records so far were in alignment with the evidence presented in this study. The cases of the AUTh community members who seek consultation and psychological support has quintupled. Two hundred and fifty members of the university community are currently supported by two psychologists (support center of AUTh) [48]. Therefore, re-evaluation through similar studies by the end of the next years is vital.

Strengths and Limitations

In the present study, the DASS21 was used independently of any other psychometric scales. This way, the researchers tried to increase the chances of higher participation rates, by constructing a short and coherent questionnaire that could independently screen for stress, anxiety, and depression our sample. Limitations were the lack of evaluation on routine habits (e.g., alcohol consumption, food, etc.), the lack of detailed psychiatric background evaluation of the students, and the lack of specialized questions on the respondents' physical and mental health. The authors made an effort to avoid long questionnaires in order to minimize the risk of losing participations. Regarding the female students' significantly higher participation in the survey, it should be noted that the AUTh reports a female population of 54%. The responses here were about 70%, which is much higher. Even though expected based on the literature, the higher female participation should be considered in the interpretation of our findings.

The strengths of this study are the repetition of the analysis, the multiple correlations analysis, and the number of participants.

5. Conclusions

The community of Aristotle University of Thessaloniki has been greatly affected by COVID-19, with students presenting high levels of stress, anxiety, and depression during the pandemic. The deterioration of the mental health of AUTh students was in line with international and Greek research data. The analysis of the demographic and social variables indicated a statistically significant correlation between elevated stress, anxiety, and depression levels and gender, age, and psychiatric treatment. Vaccination against COVID-19 was not associated with any significant difference on stress, anxiety, and depression levels. The majority of the female participants were worried about the future and concerned for an impending quarantine confinement. The continuous implementation of restrictive measures poses significant risks to the mental health of students. It is necessary to continue the evaluation in universities and colleges every year, even after the de-escalation of the pandemic.

Supplementary Materials: The following supporting information can be downloaded at: https://www.mdpi.com/article/10.3390/jcm11154263/s1, Table S1: Demographic characteristics of the participants during the first and second year of completing the questionnaire. Table S2: Questions about COVID-19 during the 2 years, Table S3: Participants' mental health characteristics and social burden due to the pandemic, Table S4: University status of participants, Table S5: Vaccination against COVID-19 infection (second-year participants only), Table S6: Concern about impending lockdown (second year participants), Table S7: Study of gender correlation and basic questions during the first year of completing the questionnaire (2020), Table S8: Gender-based student scores during the first year of the survey (2020), Table S9: Study of gender correlation and basic questions during the second year of completing the questionnaire (2021), Table S10: Gender-based student scores during the second year of the survey (2021), Table S11: Do you know anyone who has been diagnosed with COVID-19? (2020), Table S12: Do you know anyone who has been diagnosed with COVID-19? (2021), Table S13: Correlation of the question "Do you know anyone who has been diagnosed with COVID-19 infection?" with the DASS21 score during the 1st year of the survey, Table S14. Correlation of the question "Do you know anyone who has been diagnosed with COVID-19 infection?" with the score DASS21 during the second year of the research.

Author Contributions: Conceptualization, D.K. and S.C.; methodology, D.K., T.P., S.C. and S.K.; validation, A.K., S.K. and V.P.; formal analysis, D.K. and A.K.; investigation, A.K. and D.K.; resources, D.K. and T.P.; data curation, D.K.; writing—original draft preparation, D.K. and A.K.; writing—review and editing, A.K., V.P. and M.C. visualization, D.K. and A.K.; supervision, V.P., M.C. and T.P.; project administration, D.K.; funding acquisition, T.P. All authors have read and agreed to the published version of the manuscript.

Funding: This research received no external funding.

Institutional Review Board Statement: The study was conducted in accordance with the Declaration of Helsinki and approved by the Bioethics Committee of Aristotle University of Thessaloniki (1.254/20-10-20).

Informed Consent Statement: Informed consent was obtained from all subjects involved in the study.

Data Availability Statement: Not applicable.

Acknowledgments: We would like to acknowledge the valuable contribution of Dimitrios Karapistolis for the consultation on the multiple correlations' analysis and the permission to use his own developed statistical software "MAD". We would also like to acknowledge the valuable contribution of Konstantinos Stavrou (BSc English Literature) for the language revisions and Georgios Intzes for handling the data codification processes and assisting with the methodology.

Conflicts of Interest: The authors declare no conflict of interest.

References

1. Li, Q.; Guan, X.; Wu, P.; Wang, X.; Zhou, L.; Tong, Y.; Ren, R.; Leung, K.S.M.; Lau, E.H.Y.; Wong, J.Y.; et al. Early Transmission Dynamics in Wuhan, China, of Novel Coronavirus–Infected Pneumonia. *N. Engl. J. Med.* **2020**, *382*, 1199–1207. [CrossRef] [PubMed]
2. WHO Statement on Novel Coronavirus in Thailand. Available online: https://www.who.int/news-room/detail/13-01-2020-who-statement-on-novel-coronavirus-in-thailand (accessed on 3 February 2022).
3. Rello, J.; Belliato, M.; Dimopoulos, M.A.; Giamarellos-Bourboulis, E.J.; Jaksic, V.; Martin-Loeches, I.; Mporas, I.; Pelosi, P.; Poulakou, G.; Pournaras, S.; et al. Update in COVID-19 in the intensive care unit from the 2020 HELLENIC Athens International symposium. *Anaesth. Crit. Care Pain Med.* **2020**, *39*, 723–730. [CrossRef] [PubMed]
4. Konstantopoulou, G.; Iliou, T.; Karaivazoglou, K.; Iconomou, G.; Assimakopoulos, K.; Alexopoulos, P. Associations between (sub) clinical stress- and anxiety symptoms in mentally healthy individuals and in major depression: A cross-sectional clinical study. *BMC Psychiatry* **2020**, *20*, 428. [CrossRef] [PubMed]
5. Tsapou, K.; Psarra, E.; Konstantinou, J.; Kavvadas, D.; Cheristanidis, S.; Sidiropoulos, E.; Papazisis, G. The socio-psychological impact of the COVID-19 pandemic on Greek society: A survey of Greek adults. *Arch. Hell. Med.* **2022**, *39*, 89–97.
6. Kavvadas, D.; Papamitsou, T.; Cheristanidis, S.; Kounnou, V. Emotional crisis during the pandemic: A mini-analysis in children and adolescents. *Arch. Hell. Med.* **2021**, *38*, 237–239.
7. Son, C.; Hegde, S.; Smith, A.; Wang, X.; Sasangohar, F. Effects of COVID-19 on College Students' Mental Health in the United States: Interview Survey Study. *J. Med. Internet Res.* **2020**, *22*, e21279. [CrossRef]
8. Ma, Z.; Zhao, J.; Li, Y.; Chen, D.; Wang, T.; Zhang, Z.; Chen, Z.; Yu, Q.; Jiang, J.; Fan, F.; et al. Mental health problems and correlates among 746 217 college students during the coronavirus disease 2019 outbreak in China. *Epidemiol. Psychiatr. Sci.* **2020**, *29*, e181. [CrossRef]
9. Chang, J.; Yuan, Y.; Wang, D. Mental health status and its influencing factors among college students during the epidemic of COVID-19. *Nan Fang Yi Ke Da Xue Xue Bao* **2020**, *40*, 171–176. [CrossRef]
10. Tang, W.; Hu, T.; Hu, B.; Jin, C.; Wang, G.; Xie, C.; Chen, S.; Xu, J. Prevalence and correlates of PTSD and depressive symptoms one month after the outbreak of the COVID-19 epidemic in a sample of home-quarantined Chinese university students. *J. Affect. Disord.* **2020**, *274*, 1–7. [CrossRef]
11. Kecojevic, A.; Basch, C.H.; Sullivan, M.; Davi, N.K. The impact of the COVID-19 epidemic on mental health of undergraduate students in New Jersey, cross-sectional study. *PLoS ONE* **2020**, *15*, e0239696. [CrossRef]

12. Browning, M.H.E.M.; Larson, L.R.; Sharaievska, I.; Rigolon, A.; McAnirlin, O.; Mullenbach, L.; Cloutier, S.; Vu, T.M.; Thomsen, J.; Reigner, N.; et al. Psychological impacts from COVID-19 among university students: Risk factors across seven states in the United States. *PLoS ONE* **2021**, *16*, e0245327. [CrossRef] [PubMed]
13. Wathelet, M.; Duhem, S.; Vaiva, G.; Baubet, T.; Habran, E.; Veerapa, E.; Debien, C.; Molenda, S.; Horn, M.; Grandgenèvre, P.; et al. Factors Associated with Mental Health Disorders among University Students in France Confined during the COVID-19 Pandemic. *JAMA Netw. Open* **2020**, *3*, e2025591. [CrossRef] [PubMed]
14. Sundarasen, S.; Chinna, K.; Kamaludin, K.; Nurunnabi, M.; Baloch, G.M.; Khoshaim, H.B.; Hossain, S.F.A.; Sukayt, A. Psychological Impact of COVID-19 and Lockdown among University Students in Malaysia: Implications and Policy Recommendations. *Int. J. Environ. Res. Public Health* **2020**, *17*, 6206. [CrossRef] [PubMed]
15. Liu, Y.; Frazier, P.A.; Porta, C.M.; Lust, K. Mental health of US undergraduate and graduate students before and during the COVID-19 pandemic: Differences across sociodemographic groups. *Psychiatry Res.* **2022**, *309*, 114428. [CrossRef] [PubMed]
16. Odriozola-González, P.; Planchuelo-Gómez, Á.; Irurtia, M.J.; de Luis-García, R. Psychological effects of the COVID-19 outbreak and lockdown among students and workers of a Spanish university. *Psychiatry Res.* **2020**, *290*, 113108. [CrossRef] [PubMed]
17. Kaparounaki, C.K.; Patsali, M.E.; Mousa, D.V.; Papadopoulou, E.K.; Papadopoulou, K.K.; Fountoulakis, K.N. University students' mental health amidst the COVID-19 quarantine in Greece. *Psychiatry Res.* **2020**, *290*, 113111. [CrossRef] [PubMed]
18. Patsali, M.E.; Mousa, D.V.; Papadopoulou, E.K.; Papadopoulou, K.K.; Kaparounaki, C.K.; Diakogiannis, I.; Fountoulakis, K.N. University students' changes in mental health status and determinants of behavior during the COVID-19 lockdown in Greece. *Psychiatry Res.* **2020**, *292*, 113298. [CrossRef]
19. Kornilaki, A. The psychological consequences of COVID-19 pandemic on University students in Greece. The role of daily activities during the quarantine. *Psychol. J. Hell. Psychol. Soc.* **2022**, *26*, 144–164. [CrossRef]
20. Report on COVID-19 Cases in Aristotle University of Thessaloniki. Available online: https://www.amna.gr/macedonia/article/618766/Meiosi-tou-arithmou-krousmaton-COVID-19-sto-APTh (accessed on 18 May 2022).
21. Lovibond, S.H.; Lovibond, P.F. *Manual for the Depression Anxiety & Stress Scales*, 2nd ed.; Sydney Psychology Foundation: Sydney, Australia, 1995.
22. Gloster, A.T.; Rhoades, H.M.; Novy, D.; Klotsche, J.; Senior, A.; Kunik, M.; Wilson, N.; Stanley, M.A. Psychometric properties of the Depression Anxiety and Stress Scale-21 in older primary care patients. *J. Affect. Disord.* **2008**, *110*, 248–259. [CrossRef]
23. Lyrakos, G.N.; Arvaniti, C.; Smyrnioti, M.; Kostopanagiotou, G. Translation and validation study of the depression anxiety stress scale in the greek general population and in a psychiatric patient's sample. *Eur. Psychiatry* **2011**, *26*, 1731. [CrossRef]
24. Karapistolis, D. *Multivariate Statistical Analysis*, 1st ed.; A. Altintzis: Thessaloniki, Greece, 2011.
25. Benzecri, J.P. *Correspondence Analysis Handbook*, 1st ed.; Dekker P.: New York, NY, USA, 1992.
26. Jérôme, P. *Multiple Factor Analysis by Example Using R*; The R Series; Chapman & Hall/CRC: London, UK, 2014; p. 272.
27. Greenacre, M. *Correspondence Analysis in Practice*, 2nd ed.; Chapman & Hall/CRC: London, UK, 2007.
28. Drosos, G. Statistical Analysis of Linguistic Information Data. Ph.D. Thesis, Aristotle University of Thessaloniki, Thessaloniki, Greece, 2005.
29. Hogg, R.; McKean, J.; Craig, A. *Introduction to Mathematical Statistics*, 8th ed.; Pearson Education, Inc.: Boston, MA, USA, 2019.
30. Lestari, K.; Pasaribu, U.; Indratno, S.; Garminia, H. The comparative analysis of dependence for three-way contingency table using Burt matrix and Tucker3 in correspondence analysis. *J. Phys. Conf. Ser.* **2019**, *1245*, 012056. [CrossRef]
31. Karapistolis, D. MAD software. In *Workbooks of Data Analysis*; Athanasios Altintzis: Thessaloniki, Greece, 2002; Volume II, p. 133.
32. Sazakli, E.; Leotsinidis, M.; Bakola, M.; Kitsou, K.S.; Katsifara, A.; Konstantopoulou, A.; Jelastopulu, E. Prevalence and associated factors of anxiety and depression in students at a Greek university during COVID-19 lockdown. *J. Public Health Res.* **2021**, *10*, 2089. [CrossRef]
33. Karakasi, M.V.; Sismanidou, R.; Spourita, E.; Dimtsis, A.; Karakasi, A.I.; Bakirtzis, C.; Pavlidis, P. The emotional burden of the SARS-CoV-2 pandemic on medical students in Greece. *Psychiatrike* **2021**, *32*, 328–332. [CrossRef] [PubMed]
34. Kontoangelos, K.; Tsiori, S.; Koundi, K.; Pappa, X.; Sakkas, P.; Papageorgiou, C.C. Greek college students and psychopathology: New insights. *Int. J. Environ. Res. Public Health* **2015**, *12*, 4709–4725. [CrossRef] [PubMed]
35. Economou, M.; Peppou, L.; Fousketaki, S.; Theleritis, C.; Patelakis, A.; Alexiou, T.; Madianos, M.; Stefanis, C. Economic crisis and mental health: Effects on the prevalence of common mental disorders. *Psychiatrike* **2013**, *24*, 247–261. [PubMed]
36. Dazzio, R.E.; Daley, S.S.; Budesheim, T.L.; Klanecky Earl, A.K. The interaction between Greek affiliation and religiosity on problem drinking in college students. *J. Am. Coll. Health* **2021**, *2021*, 1–8. [CrossRef] [PubMed]
37. Martinez, H.S.; Klanecky, A.K.; McChargue, D.E. Problem drinking among at-risk college students: The examination of Greek involvement, freshman status, and history of mental health problems. *J. Am. Coll. Health* **2018**, *66*, 579–587. [CrossRef]
38. Antonopoulou, M.; Mantzorou, M.; Serdari, A.; Earl, A.K.K. Evaluating Mediterranean diet adherence in university student populations: Does this dietary pattern affect students' academic performance and mental health? *Int. J. Health Plann. Manag.* **2020**, *35*, 5–21. [CrossRef]
39. Kaparounaki, C.K.; Koraka, C.A.; Kotsi, E.S.; Ntziovara, A.M.P.; Kyriakidis, G.C.; Fountoulakis, K.N. Greek university student's attitudes and beliefs concerning mental illness and its treatment. *Int. J. Soc. Psychiatry* **2019**, *65*, 515–526. [CrossRef]
40. Economou, M. Social Distance in COVID-19: Drawing the line between protective behavior and stigma manifestation. *Psychiatrike* **2021**, *32*, 183–186. [CrossRef]

41. Carr, E.; Davis, K.; Bergin-Cartwright, G.; Lavelle, G.; Leightley, D.; Oetzmann, C.; Polling, C.; Stevelink, S.A.M.; Wickersham, A.; Razavi, R.; et al. Mental health among UK university staff and postgraduate students in the early stages of the COVID-19 pandemic. *Occup. Environ. Med.* **2022**, *79*, 259–267. [CrossRef] [PubMed]
42. Van Niekerk, R.L.; van Gent, M.M. Mental health and well-being of university staff during the coronavirus disease 2019 levels 4 and 5 lockdown in an Eastern Cape university, South Africa. *S. Afr. J. Psychiatry* **2021**, *27*, 1589. [CrossRef] [PubMed]
43. Saravanan, C.; Mahmoud, I.; Elshami, W.; Taha, M.H. Knowledge, Anxiety, Fear, and Psychological Distress about COVID-19 among University Students in the United Arab Emirates. *Front. Psychiatry* **2020**, *11*, 582189. [CrossRef] [PubMed]
44. Luo, W.; Zhong, B.L.; Chiu, H.F.K. Prevalence of depressive symptoms among Chinese university students amid the COVID-19 pandemic: A systematic review and meta-analysis. *Epidemiol. Psychiatr. Sci.* **2021**, *30*, e31. [CrossRef]
45. Li, H.Y.; Cao, H.; Leung, D.Y.P.; Mak, Y.W. The Psychological Impacts of a COVID-19 Outbreak on College Students in China: A Longitudinal Study. *Int. J. Environ. Res. Public Health* **2020**, *17*, 3933. [CrossRef]
46. Johansson, F.; Côté, P.; Hogg-Johnson, S.; Rudman, A.; Holm, L.W.; Grotle, M.; Jensen, I.; Sundberg, T.; Edlund, K.; Skillgate, E. Depression, anxiety and stress among Swedish university students before and during six months of the COVID-19 pandemic: A cohort study. *Scand. J. Public Health* **2021**, *49*, 741–749. [CrossRef]
47. Vasileiou, D.; Moraitou, D.; Papaliagkas, V.; Pezirkianidis, C.; Stalikas, A.; Papantoniou, G.; Sofologi, M. The Relationships between Character Strengths and Subjective Wellbeing: Evidence from Greece under Lockdown during COVID-19 Pandemic. *Int. J. Environ. Res. Public Health* **2021**, *18*, 10868. [CrossRef]
48. Increased Number of Students Receive Psychological Support in Relation to the Pre-Pandemic Period. Available online: https://www.ertnews.gr/roi-idiseon/apth-pentaplasios-o-arithmos-ton-foititon-poy-lamvanei-psychologiki-ypostirixi-se-schesi-me-tin-pro-pandimias-periodo/ (accessed on 5 April 2022).

Journal of
Clinical Medicine

Article

Psychosocial Distress among Family Members of COVID-19 Patients Admitted to Hospital and Isolation Facilities in the Philippines: A Prospective Cohort Study

Leilanie Apostol-Nicodemus [1,*,†], Ian Kim B. Tabios [2,3,*,†], Anna Guia O. Limpoco [1], Gabriele Dominique P. Domingo [4] and Ourlad Alzeus G. Tantengco [3]

[1] Department of Family and Community Medicine, University of the Philippines—Philippine General Hospital, Taft Avenue, Manila 1000, Philippines
[2] Institute of Biology, College of Science, University of the Philippines Diliman, Quezon City 1101, Philippines
[3] College of Medicine, University of the Philippines Manila, Manila 1000, Philippines
[4] One Hospital Command Center, Pasay 1709, Philippines
* Correspondence: lsapostolnicodemus@up.edu.ph (L.A.-N.); ibtabios2@up.edu.ph (I.K.B.T.)
† These authors contributed equally to this work.

Abstract: This study determined the psychosocial impact of COVID-19 on families of adult COVID-19 patients in isolation facilities in Metro Manila, Philippines. This prospective cohort study was conducted in COVID-19 healthcare facilities. Data collection was undertaken 2 weeks and 8 weeks after discharge. Logistic regression was performed to determine the socioeconomic and clinical factors influencing anxiety, depression, and family function. Based on HADS-P, 43.2% of the participants had anxiety symptoms, and 16.2% had depression symptoms 2 weeks after the discharge of their relative with COVID-19 infection. The prevalence of anxiety and depression significantly decreased to 24.3% and 5.4%, respectively, 8 weeks after discharge. The percentage of participants with a perceived moderate family dysfunction was 9.5% in the 2nd week and 6.8% in the 8th week post discharge. Participants with perceived severe family dysfunction increased from none to 4.1%. The most inadequate family resources for the participants were economic, medical, and educational resources. Patient anxiety ($p = 0.010$) and perceived inadequate family resources ($p = 0.032$) were associated with anxiety symptoms among family members. Patient anxiety ($p = 0.013$) and low educational attainment ($p = 0.002$) were associated with anxiety symptoms among family members 8 weeks after discharge. On the other hand, patient depression ($p = 0.013$) was a factor related to depressive symptoms among family members 2 weeks after discharge. This study provided an in-depth understanding of the mental health status of family members caring for relatives with COVID-19 infection. This can be used to guide healthcare professionals caring for COVID-19 patients and their family members.

Keywords: anxiety; coronavirus; depression; family; mental health; pandemic

Citation: Apostol-Nicodemus, L.; Tabios, I.K.B.; Limpoco, A.G.O.; Domingo, G.D.P.; Tantengco, O.A.G. Psychosocial Distress among Family Members of COVID-19 Patients Admitted to Hospital and Isolation Facilities in the Philippines: A Prospective Cohort Study. *J. Clin. Med.* **2022**, *11*, 5236. https://doi.org/10.3390/jcm11175236

Academic Editor: Alfonso Troisi

Received: 8 July 2022
Accepted: 2 September 2022
Published: 5 September 2022

1. Introduction

COVID-19 is a global pandemic caused by SARS-CoV-2. The Philippines is one of the countries in Southeast Asia that suffered greatly from COVID-19. There have been surges in cases due to the new variants and changes in the health response. Throughout the pandemic, containment and mitigation measures such as physical distancing, home quarantine, and self-isolation remain at the forefront of the country's response [1,2]. Families have an essential role in implementing these measures to control COVID-19.

Families are the basic social unit of society [3,4]. Filipinos are known for their close-knit extended family structures. Family members are the first line of support during times of sickness [5]. During disease outbreaks, families experience emotional upheaval due to anxiety and fear of the possibility of contracting the disease [6–8]. This emotional distress is further exacerbated by strict infection control measures that inadvertently promote stigmatization, social isolation, and economic problems stemming from losing income due to the lack of job opportunities [5,9].

The COVID-19 pandemic has caused radical changes to the average Filipino's life, such as loss of income and decreased social interaction due to the mitigating interventions implemented by the government [10,11]. Further psychosocial distress is likely to impact those directly affected by COVID-19 by either contracting the disease or having to take care of a family member who has been infected with COVID-19. Furthermore, COVID-19 severely affects the elderly, who require more attention and care [12–14].

Previous studies showed that COVID-19 infection affects the mental health of the patients [15,16]. Patients infected with COVID-19 experienced severe psychological distress, including symptoms of anxiety and depression [15,16]. Lower education level and family history of psychiatric disorder were risk factors for anxiety, and home isolation was a risk factor for depression [15]. Aside from patients, there were few studies that showed that family members taking care of COVID-19 patients also experienced mental health impacts, including anxiety and depressive symptoms [17–19].

COVID-19 infection negatively affected family function. Family members experienced the highest dysfunction in the areas of growth and affection [20]. Family members were dissatisfied with the support they received from their families regarding their decisions to take on new activities and directions, and the way their family members expressed affection and responded to their emotions, such as anger or love [20]. Family members, particularly parents, also reported increased family conflicts due to the pandemic [21]. However, our knowledge of the psychosocial effects of COVID-19 on the families and caregivers of COVID-19 patients in the Philippines is still limited.

Therefore, understanding the impact of COVID-19 illness on families taking care of COVID-19 patients will contribute to guidelines and policies for responding to pandemics such as COVID-19 effectively. Hence, this study determined the psychosocial impact of COVID-19 on families of adult patients in isolation facilities in Metro Manila, Philippines. We showed the proportion of COVID-19 patient family members with psychological symptoms of anxiety and depression, their perceived family function and resources, and the factors associated with psychological symptoms and family dysfunction among study participants.

2. Materials and Methods

2.1. Ethical Consideration

This study was approved by the University of the Philippines Manila Research Ethics Board (UPMREB Code: 2020-280-01) and the Philippine Department of Health Single Joint Research Ethics Board (SJREB Code: 2020-100). Written informed consent was obtained from all participants (family members of COVID-19 patients) and the patients at the beginning of the study and during the subsequent follow-up interviews.

2.2. Study Design

The study employed a cohort study design using quantitative methodologies. The participants were interviewed during their family member's two-week home quarantine after discharge from the facility. A follow-up data collection was performed 8 weeks post discharge of the participants' family member who had COVID-19 using the same procedure.

2.3. Sampling Design

The study employed non-probabilistic sampling. Participants were chosen as convenient from the list of patients of selected COVID-19 healthcare facilities. The selection was based on the availability of contact details and ease of coordination.

2.4. Study Sites

The following COVID-19 designated healthcare facilities in Metro Manila were included in the study: (1) two community isolation units (CIUs) in Metro Manila, namely the PNP Kiangan Quarantine Facility in Camp Crame, Quezon City, and the University of the Philippines Diliman Silungan Molave Quarantine Facility in Diliman, Quezon City; and (2) one hospital facility, namely the COVID-19 areas of the Philippine General Hospital (PGH) in Ermita, Manila.

2.5. Study Population

The study involved family members taking care of adult patients diagnosed with COVID-19 at the study sites. The inclusion criteria included: (1) age greater than or equal to 18 years; (2) family member (as previously defined) of a COVID-19 patient admitted in a hospital or quarantine facility; (3) has lived in the same household as the patient for at least 12 months before the interview; (4) involved in the care of the patient; (5) agrees to participate in the study with a signed informed consent form. The exclusion criteria included: (1) with non-consenting family members of COVID-19 patients; (2) with pre-existing clinically diagnosed psychiatric disorder before COVID-19 admission; (3) unable to provide consent due to physical or mental illness, including cognitive impairment; (4) unable to participate fully and answer questions due to physical or mental illness. Family members were able to discontinue their study participation and cancel their consent.

2.6. Data Collection Procedure

Data collection was undertaken through telephone or online calls with family members at 2 weeks and 8 weeks after discharge of their relative with COVID-19 infection. The research assistant or field interviewer used a semi-structured questionnaire during the data collection (interviewer-administered). Handwritten notes and voice recordings of calls using a call recording application were made. Electronic data is being stored in a well-secured data cloud for storage. If the participant warranted initial psychosocial supportive care during the interview, the research assistant or field interviewer referred the patient to the principal investigator and co-investigators. The co-investigators then provided initial counseling to the participants through telephone, online voice, or video calls. If further management was necessary, the participant was referred to the Family Health Unit (FHU) clinic at the Outpatient Department of the Philippine General Hospital.

2.7. Data Collection Tools

In this study, quantitative data were obtained to determine the impact of the COVID-19 experience on families caring for COVID-19 patients. The questionnaire was pre-tested practically with 20 family members of COVID-19 patients who were not included in this study, to increase data quality before data collection began. The assessment tools used in the study have validated Filipino translation.

2.7.1. Hospital Anxiety and Depression Scale (HADS)

Psychological symptoms of anxiety and depression were assessed using the Hospital Anxiety and Depression Scale (HADS). It is a self-report instrument designed to detect symptoms related to anxiety and depression. Initially designed for hospitalized patients, HADS has been used and validated in community settings and primary care practice. In the Philippines, a Filipino translation (HADS-P) has been validated among Filipino patients. It has fourteen items and two subscales, anxiety and depression, and each item is scored on a four-point scale of 0 to 3. A score of $\geq$11 was interpreted as positive for the emotional illness being tested since similar studies which used HADS/HADS-P utilized the same cut-off [22–24]. This tool has been used and validated in previous studies using telephone interviews with a Cronbach alpha of 0.76 to 0.86 [25].

2.7.2. Family Assessment Tools

The following family assessment tools were used in the study: Filipino family APGAR (Adaptability, Partnership, Growth, Affection, and Resolve), and SCREEM (Social, Cultural, Religious, Economic, Education, and Medical) Family Resources Survey (SCREEM-RES). Filipino family APGAR, a translated and validated Filipino version of Smilkstein's family APGAR, was used to assess family functioning based on five parameters: Adaptability, Partnership, Growth, Affection, and Resolve. Each parameter is scored with a three-point scale ranging from 0 (hardly ever) to 2 (almost always). The total scores range from 0 to 10, with higher scores indicating higher satisfaction with family functioning. A score of 0–3 shows severe family dysfunction, 4–7 moderate family dysfunction, and 8–10 highly functional families [26].

The SCREEM Family Resources Survey (SCREEM-RES) is a validated and reliable tool to measure family resources used to cope with difficult situations. This instrument is a brief twelve-item questionnaire containing all the six original SCREEM domains and includes two items per domain. Participants were asked to choose one of the following responses: strongly disagree, disagree, agree, and strongly agree. The total SCREEM-RES scores were grouped using the following key: Severely Inadequate Family Resources = 0 to 12, Moderately Inadequate Family Resources = 13 to 24, Adequate Family Resources = 25 to 36. For each domain subscale, scores were grouped using the following key: Severely Inadequate Family Resources = 0 to 2, Moderately Inadequate Family Resources = 3 to 4, Adequate Family Resources = 5 to 6. This was previously validated in Filipino patients with a Cronbach's alpha of 0.80 for the entire scale [26].

2.8. Data Analysis

Data were analyzed using SPSS statistical software version 28.0 (IBM Corp). Statistical significance was set at $\alpha = 0.05$, and all tests were two-tailed. Collected data were summarized using descriptive statistics, tables, and graphs. Means, medians, standard deviations, and interquartile ranges were computed for continuous variables, whereas frequencies and percentages were obtained from categorical variables. The internal consistencies of the questionnaires were reported as Cronbach alpha coefficients. Statistical comparisons between continuous variables were performed with an independent Student t-test for normally distributed data, whereas a Mann–Whitney U test was used if otherwise. A χ^2 test or Fisher's exact test was done for categorical variables. To check for statistical differences in the proportions of mental and social outcomes between 2 and 8 weeks after discharge, a paired-samples proportion test using McNemar was used. Binary logistic regression analysis was performed to determine factors influencing anxiety, depression, and family dysfunction symptoms. Associations between the exposure and outcome variables are presented as odds ratios and 95% CIs, after adjustment for confounders defined as exposure variables with $p > 0.25$ based on univariate analysis.

3. Results

3.1. Sociodemographic Characteristics of the Participants

A total of 104 participants were recruited for the project and completed the first interview, and 74 participants completed the second interview. Baseline sociodemographic characteristics of the 74 participants who completed the first and second interviews are shown in Table 1.

Table 1. Baseline sociodemographic characteristics of the family members of patients who completed the two interviews (n = 74).

Characteristic	Participants
Age in years, mean (SD)	41.2 (11.8)
Age group, *n* (%)	
18 to 34 years old	23 (31.1)
35 to 49 years old	30 (40.5)
50 to 64 years old	19 (25.7)
65 years old and above	2 (2.7)
Sex assigned at birth, *n* (%)	
Female	49 (66.2)
Male	25 (33.8)
Health care facility, *n* (%)	
PGH COVID-19 Designated Referral Center	42 (56.8)
UP Diliman Silungan Molave Quarantine Facility	22 (29.7)
PNP Kiangan Quarantine Facility	10 (13.5)
COVID-19 severity of relative during admission, *n* (%)	
Critical and severe	24 (32.4)
Moderate	11 (14.9)
Mild	35 (47.3)
Asymptomatic	4 (5.4)
Civil status, *n* (%)	
Married	45 (60.8)
Cohabitation	9 (12.2)
Separated	1 (1.4)
Widow	1 (1.4)
Single	18 (24.3)
Relationship with the patient, *n* (%)	
Romantic partner	35 (47.3)
Parent	16 (21.6)
Sibling	17 (23.0)
Close relatives (cousin, niece, nephew, aunt, uncle, etc.)	6 (8.1)
Educational attainment, *n* (%)	
Post-graduate	2 (2.7)
College	48 (64.9)
Vocational	7 (9.5)
Secondary school	15 (20.3)
Primary school	2 (2.7)
Employment status, *n* (%)	
Regular, *n* (%)	30 (40.5)
Self-employed, *n* (%)	7 (9.5)
Contractual, *n* (%)	15 (20.3)
Unemployed, *n* (%)	22 (29.7)
Number of household members, median (IQR)	5 (4–6)
Number of household members, *n* (%)	
less than 5	32 (43.2)
5 or more	42 (56.8)
Diagnosed with at least one chronic disease, *n* (%)	33 (44.6)
Had previous hospital admission, *n* (%)	36 (48.6)
Had previous surgery, *n* (%)	33 (44.6)
Income classification based on PIDS 2018, *n* (%)	
Poor (monthly salary below ₱ 10,957.0)	15 (20.3)
Low income (monthly salary of ₱ 10,957.0 to 43,828.0)	31 (41.9)
Middle income (monthly salary of ₱ 43,828 to 219,140)	28 (37.8)
Knew someone who died due to COVID-19, *n* (%)	21 (28.4)
Knew someone else who had COVID-19, *n* (%)	42 (56.8)

Abbreviations: SD, standard deviation; IQR, interquartile range; PGH, Philippine General Hospital; PNP, Philippine National Police; UP, University of the Philippines; PIDS, Philippine Institute for Development Studies; ND, No Data.

3.2. Dynamics of Anxiety and Depression among Family Members of COVID-19 Patients

At the cut-off HADS-P anxiety score of 11, 43.2% of the participants had anxiety symptoms 2 weeks after discharge of their relative with COVID-19 infection. The prevalence of anxiety significantly decreased to 24.3% 8 weeks after discharge ($p = 0.002$). At the cut-off HADS-P depression score of 11, 16.2% of the participants had symptoms of depression 2 weeks after the discharge of their relatives with COVID-19 infection. The prevalence of depression significantly decreased to only 5.4% at 8 weeks post discharge ($p = 0.021$). Lastly, 13.5% of the participants had a mixed diagnosis of anxiety and depression at 2 weeks and 4.1% at 8 weeks post discharge ($p < 0.001$) (Table 2 and Table S1).

Table 2. The proportion of family members with symptoms of anxiety and depression at 2 and 8 weeks after discharge of their relatives with COVID-19 from the study sites ($n = 74$).

Mental Health Outcomes	2 Weeks after Discharge		8 Weeks after Discharge		*p* Value
	n	% (95% CI)	*n*	% (95% CI)	
Anxiety	32	43.2 (31.7–55.3)	18	24.3 (15.7–35.0)	0.002
Depression	12	16.2 (8.7–26.6)	4	5.4 (1.9–12.3)	0.021
Mixed diagnosis, *n* (%)	10	13.5 (6.7–23.5)	3	4.1 (1.2–10.4)	<0.001

Among participants with anxiety symptoms at 2 weeks post discharge, 53.1% had resolved symptoms, and 46.9% had persistent anxiety symptoms at the 8th-week post-discharge follow-up. Most participants without anxiety symptoms at the second-week follow-up remained asymptomatic during the 8th-week follow-up. However, 7.1% developed new-onset anxiety symptoms during the 8th-week follow-up (Table 3). Among participants with depression 2 weeks post discharge, 83.3% had resolved symptoms, and only 16.7% had persistent symptoms of depression during the 8th-week follow-up. Most of the participants (96.8%) without symptoms of depression during the 2nd-week follow-up remained asymptomatic, whereas 3.2% developed new-onset symptoms of depression during the 8th-week follow-up (Table 3).

Table 3. Dynamics of anxiety and depressive symptoms among family members at 2 and 8 weeks after discharge ($n = 74$).

Psychosocial Condition	Symptomatic at 2 Weeks			Asymptomatic at 2 Weeks		
	n	Resolved Symptoms at 8 Weeks *n* (%)	Remained Symptomatic at 8 Weeks *n* (%)	*n*	Remained Asymptomatic at 8 Weeks *n* (%)	Developed Symptoms at 8 Weeks *n* (%)
Anxiety	32	17 (53.1)	15 (46.9)	42	39 (92.9)	3 (7.1)
Depression	12	10 (83.3)	2 (16.7)	62	60 (96.8)	2 (3.2)

3.3. Perceived Family Dysfunction

The Family APGAR index was used to measure the general family function. The percentage of participants with a perceived moderate family dysfunction decreased from 9.5% at 2 weeks post discharge to 6.8% at 8 weeks post discharge, whereas those with perceived severe dysfunction increased from none to 4.1% from the 2nd week to 8th week post discharge (Tables 4 and S1). However, these observed changes did not reach statistical significance.

Analysis of the dynamics of perceived family dysfunction showed that among those with perceived dysfunction at 2 weeks, 57.1% retained the same view at 8 weeks after discharge. On the other hand, 7.5% of those without perceived dysfunction at 2 weeks developed perceived family dysfunction 8 weeks post discharge (Table 5).

Table 4. The proportion of family members with perceived family dysfunction at 2 and 8 weeks after discharge of their relatives with COVID-19 from the study sites (n = 74).

Social Outcome	2 Weeks after Discharge		8 Weeks after Discharge		p Value
	n	% (95% CI)	n	% (95% CI)	
Dysfunctional	7	9.5 (3.8–18.5)	8	10.8 (4.8–20.2)	0.655
Moderately	7	9.5 (3.8–18.5)	5	6.8 (2.6–14.2)	
Severely	0	0 (0.1–4.4)	3	4.1 (1.2–10.4)	

Table 5. Dynamics of perceived family dysfunction among adult patients and family members at 2 and 8 weeks after discharge of their relatives with COVID-19 from the study sites (n = 74).

Psychosocial Condition	With Dysfunction at 2 Weeks			Without Dysfunction at 2 Weeks		
	n (%)	Resolved at 8 Weeks n (%)	Remained with Dysfunction at 8 Weeks n (%)	n (%)	Remained at 8 Weeks n (%)	Developed Dysfunction at 8 Weeks n (%)
Family dysfunction	7 (9.5)	3 (4.1)	4 (5.4)	67 (90.5)	62 (83.78)	5 (6.8)

3.4. Perceived Inadequacy of Family Resources

Among the resources measured by the SCREEM-RES questionnaire, the most inadequate resources for the family member participants were the economic, medical, and educational resources. The prevalence of perceived economic resource inadequacy decreased at 8 weeks post discharge. However, medical inadequacy increased. The resources least perceived to be inadequate were social, cultural, and religion. Perceived inadequacy in these resources increased at 8 weeks compared with 2 weeks after discharge. There was no increase in the overall perceived inadequacy from 2 weeks to 8 weeks post discharge (Tables 6 and S1).

Table 6. The proportion of patients' family members with perceived inadequate family resources at 2 and 8 weeks after discharge of their relatives with COVID-19 infection from the study sites (n = 74).

Social Outcome	2 Weeks after Discharge		8 Weeks after Discharge		p Value
	n	% (95% CI)	n	% (95% CI)	
		Overall Resources			
Inadequate	25	33.8 (23.2–45.7)	28	36.5 (25.6–48.5)	0.827
Moderate	25	33.8 (23.2–45.7)	26	35.1 (25.0–46.4)	
Severe	0	0 (0.0–2.4)	2	2.7 (0.6–8.4)	
		Social Resources			
Inadequate	27	36.5 (25.6–48.5)	27	36.5 (25.6–48.5)	0.819
Moderate	27	36.5 (25.6–48.5)	26	35.1 (25.0–46.4)	
Severe	0	0 (0.0–2.4)	1	1.4 (1.0–6.1)	
		Cultural Resources			
Inadequate	31	42.3 (33.1–51.9)	38	51.4 (39.4–63.2)	0.072
Moderate	31	42.3 (33.1–51.9)	33	44.6 (33.7–55.9)	
Severe	0	0 (0.0–2.4)	5	6.8 (2.6–14.2)	
		Religion Resources			
Inadequate	30	40.5 (29.3–52.6)	28	37.8 (26.8–49.9)	0.467
Moderate	28	37.8 (26.8–49.9)	26	35.1 (25.0–46.4)	
Severe	2	2.7 (0.3–9.4)	2	2.7(0.6–8.4)	
		Economic Resources			
Inadequate	57	77.0 (65.8–86.0)	56	75.7 (64.3–84.9)	0.617
Moderate	45	60.8 (48.7–72.0)	44	59.5 (48.1–70.1)	
Severe	12	16.2 (8.7–26.6)	12	16.2 (9.2–25.8)	
		Educational Resources			
Inadequate	42	56.8 (44.7–68.2)	46	62.2 (50.1–72.2)	0.532
Moderate	38	51.4 (39.4–63.2)	42	56.8 (45.4–67.6)	
Severe	4	5.4 (1.5–13.3)	4	5.4 (1.9–12.3)	
		Medical Resources			
Inadequate	61	82.4 (71.8–90.3)	57	77.0 (65.8–86.0)	0.225
Moderate	44	59.5 (47.4–70.7)	39	52.7 (41.4–63.8)	
Severe	17	23.0 (14.0–34.2)	18	24.3 (15.7–35.0)	

Analysis of the dynamics of perceived inadequacy of family resources showed that most participants with perceived inadequacy at 2 weeks retained the same view 8 weeks after discharge (59.3%). Meanwhile, 25.5% of those without perceived inadequacy at 2 weeks developed it 8 weeks post discharge (Table 7).

Table 7. Dynamics of perceived inadequacy of family resources among patients and family members at 2 and 8 weeks after discharge (n = 74).

Psychosocial Condition	With Perceived Inadequate Family Resources at 2 Weeks			Without Perceived Inadequate Family Resources at 2 Weeks		
	n	Resolved at 8 Weeks *n* (%)	Remained with Inadequacy at 8 Weeks *n* (%)	*n*	Remained at 8 Weeks *n* (%)	Developed Perceived Inadequacy at 8 Weeks *n* (%)
Inadequate family resources	27	11 (14.9)	16 (21.6)	47	35 (47.3)	12 (16.2)

3.5. Factors Influencing Psychological Impact of COVID-19 Experience

At 2 weeks after discharge, patient anxiety (p = 0.010) and perceived inadequate family resources (p = 0.032) were associated with anxiety symptoms among family members. Patient anxiety (p = 0.013) and low educational attainment (p = 0.002) were associated with anxiety symptoms among family members 8 weeks after discharge. On the other hand, patient depression (p = 0.013) was a factor related to depressive symptoms among family members 2 weeks after discharge (Table 8). Using multivariate logistic regression analysis, no identified factors were associated with depressive symptoms among family members at 8 weeks after discharge.

Table 8. Factors associated with psychological symptoms in patients' family members identified by multivariate logistic regression analysis.

Explanatory Variable	Adjusted Odds Ratio (95% CI)	*p* Value
Condition: Anxiety in Family Members at 2 Weeks after Facility Discharge [1]		
Patient anxiety at 8 weeks after facility discharge		
With anxiety	34.3 (2.3–500.5)	0.010
No anxiety	1	
Family resources at 8 weeks after facility discharge		
Inadequate	6.5 (1.2–35.7)	0.032
Adequate	1	
Condition: Anxiety in Family Members at 8 Weeks after Facility Discharge [2]		
Patient anxiety at 2 weeks after facility discharge		
With anxiety	5.9 (1.5–23.8)	0.013
No anxiety	1	
Highest educational attainment		
Lower than high school	0.1 (0.0–0.4)	0.002
College or higher	1	
Condition: Depression in Family Members at 2 Weeks after Facility Discharge [3]		
Patient depression at 2 weeks after facility discharge		
With depression	18.0 (1.8–176.4)	0.013
No depression	1	

[1] Adjusted for number of household members, diagnosed with chronic disease, employment status, perceived family functioning at 2 and 8 weeks after facility discharge, social resources at 2 weeks after facility discharge, overall family resources at 8 weeks after facility discharge, presence of patient anxiety at 2 and 8 weeks after facility discharge; [2] adjusted for highest educational attainment, perceived family functioning at 2 weeks after facility discharge, patient anxiety and depression at 2 weeks after facility discharge; [3] adjusted for marital status, number of household members, presence of chronic disease, knew somebody who died due to COVID-19, perceived family functioning at 2 weeks after facility discharge, medical resources at 2 weeks after facility discharge, patient anxiety and depression at 2 and 8 weeks after facility discharge.

4. Discussion

This prospective cohort study revealed a high prevalence of psychosocial symptoms among participants at 2 and 8 weeks after the discharge of their family member admitted for COVID-19 infection. Overall, family function and family resources contributed to anxiety and depression among patients and families post COVID. The study explored the impact of COVID-19 on the psychological symptoms of anxiety and depression and its associated sociodemographic, economic, and clinical factors. Anxiety was high in family members at 2 weeks and 8 weeks post COVID infection. Similarly, common mental health conditions such as anxiety, depression, post-traumatic stress disorder, and overall lower quality of life occur for up to 3 months or 12 weeks post COVID-19 infection.

The unpredictability of COVID-19 infection contributes to anxiety and depression among family members of patients with COVID-19. It impairs work, family engagements, and health [27]. Families may experience high stress, anxiety, and financial burden from missing work and unemployment concerns [28]. Moreover, family members' anxiety also stemmed from their inability to feel connected to the patient and informed about care [29]. During the pandemic, family members were not allowed to stay and visit their relatives who were admitted to the hospital for COVID-19. Family members struggled to feel informed about the care they could not witness and had difficulty understanding information. A previous study showed that visits to COVID-19 patients in the ICU reduced anxiety among family members [19]. Another study showed that the family members of COVID-19 patients experienced mental health symptoms 12 months after ICU admission of their relatives for COVID-19 infection. Family members also experienced disruption of quality of life and work-related problems [17].

In this study, risk factors identified for anxiety among family members were patient depression and a low level of educational attainment. Similar findings have been made in other studies on family members of COVID-19 patients [18,29]. COVID-19 has resulted in massive unemployment worldwide. Several studies have already shown that the unemployment rate increased negative mental health outcomes during the COVID-19 pandemic [30–32]. It exacerbated pre-existing mental health disorders and created new disorders for others [32]. Collectively, these data showed that the government and the health care system should support patients' families financially.

The family function measurements taken using APGAR scores showed that the participants' perceived family dysfunction increased during the period from 2 weeks to 8 weeks after the discharge of their family member. This suggests that family dysfunction exacerbated by admission of a family member to a health facility due to COVID-19 could have long-term effects. Previous studies showed that social and family relationships were disrupted for patients and their caregivers [33]. The stresses created by the COVID-19 pandemic have put families and their interrelationships under tremendous pressure [34]. A previous study in Portugal showed that almost 20% of the participants perceived their families to have severe dysfunction or moderate dysfunction [20]. Family dysfunction is a predisposing factor for developing the emotional problems of anxiety and depression during the COVID-19 pandemic [35].

Interestingly, despite the decrease in the prevalence of anxiety and depression in the participants during the period from 2 weeks to 8 weeks after discharge, perceived severe family dysfunction still increased. We surmised that family-level dysfunction manifests later than personal-level conditions, such as anxiety and depression. The family members and the patient need to adapt to the consequences of COVID-19 infection [36], such as long COVID-19 symptoms, financial responsibility accrued from hospitalization, loss of productivity due to inability to go to work, and unemployment. Caregiver fatigue may occur later, hence, the appearance of severe family dysfunction later after the patient's discharge. Previous studies showed that the COVID-19 pandemic changed the structure and routine of the family, especially for those who suffered from the disease [21,37,38]. The disruptions in the usual routine resulted in physical and mental health problems and family matters [37]. Family members, particularly parents, also reported increased family conflicts due to the pandemic [21].

The perceived inadequate family resources did not decrease 8 weeks post COVID-19 discharge. The economic burden did not decrease during the period from 2 weeks to 8 weeks post discharge. Financial factors may contribute to severe family dysfunction, as shown by the APGAR score. COVID-19 has generated a considerable economic and financial burden on patients. Aside from the high cost of hospitalization, long-term health effects of COVID-19 such as kidney disease and long COVID-19 symptoms may induce chronic medical needs that expose patients and their families to long-term financial risk [39,40]. A previous study conducted in the Philippine General Hospital showed that the average out-of-pocket payment for COVID-19 patients less than 60 years old ranged from Php 25,899 to Php 44,428.63 ($538 to $924.44), whereas for patients older than 60 this ranged from Php 4005.60 to Php 32,920.20 ($83.35 to $684.98) [41]. Despite the financial help from national health insurance in the Philippines, the patients still need to pay out of pocket. This puts a financial burden on the patients and their families, especially since the daily minimum wage of an average worker in the National Capital Region of the Philippines only ranges from Php 533 to Php 570 ($9.54 to $10.20) [42].

The participants perceived a significant lack of access to medical resources at 8 weeks post discharge. The persistent perception of the participants of having inadequate access to medical resources is not surprising. The pandemic has brought disruption and barriers to accessing medical care. The availability of healthcare services related to COVID-19 disease and other chronic diseases has deteriorated due to the diversion of health services for urgent COVID-19 cases [43,44]. This lack of access to medical care was more pronounced among those belonging to the lower socioeconomic strata [45,46].

This study also showed that inadequate family resources and low educational attainment were associated with anxiety in the participants. Previous studies showed that low educational levels were significantly associated with both anxiety and depression [47,48]. On the other hand, higher educational attainment is protective against developing a spectrum of psychiatric disorders [48]. Higher educational attainment is also associated with higher income [49] and being more capable of shouldering medical expenses from COVID-19 hospitalization. The material advantage is protective of the negative effect of COVID-19 on the mental health of individuals, as shown in a previous study [50].

This study supports the need for more holistic COVID-19 practice guidelines to include psychosocial interventions among family caregivers. We emphasize the need to have family assessments in routine medical history taking. The use of validated tools for early detection and screening of mental disorders such as the Patient Health Questionnaire (PHQ) and Depression, Anxiety, and Stress Scale (DASS) is recommended. In addition, the Family APGAR and SCREEM-RES are good family assessment tools to check functional family relationships and family resource adequacy. Healthcare professionals should involve family members during active treatment and post-COVID-19 care of hospitalized patients and those in the quarantine facilities as part of treatment protocols. A multi-disciplinary approach to the active and follow-up care of COVID-19 patients and their family caregiver is needed. The care team must include health professionals who can provide psychological, social support, and home care.

This study has several limitations. The study only recruited family members of patients from selected COVID-19 healthcare facilities within Metro Manila, the epicenter of the pandemic in the Philippines. Experiences in areas outside Metro Manila and other metropolitan cities, where healthcare facilities have significantly different situations, may vary substantially from those recorded in the study. Second, the structural distance inherent in telephone interviews affected the engagement and retention of samples of the study because of the absence of an interpersonal relationship commonly established in face-to-face interviews. Lastly, symptoms of anxiety and depression were detected using a screening tool, and the presence of either anxiety or depression disorders was not confirmed with a diagnostic tool commonly used in psychiatry, such as DSM-5.

5. Conclusions

This study provided a valuable in-depth understanding of the mental health status of family members caring for relatives with COVID-19 infection. This study described the prevalence of and factors associated with psychological distress, particularly symptoms of anxiety and depression, in family members of patients with COVID-19 admitted to hospital and quarantine facilities. They experienced symptoms of anxiety and depression even after the discharge of their relative with COVID-19 infection. They also perceived moderate to severe family dysfunction and inadequacy of economic, medical, and educational resources in the family. These symptoms and perceptions persisted for 2 to 8 weeks after the discharge of their relative with COVID-19 infection. Depressive symptoms in a relative with COVID-19 infection tend to influence the occurrence of anxiety among family members. Our findings can be used to guide healthcare professionals caring for COVID-19 patients and their family members. COVID-19 infection generates a secondary public health crisis through stress-related disorders among family members of COVID-19 patients. Therefore, relevant interventions are recommended.

Supplementary Materials: The following supporting information can be downloaded at: https://www.mdpi.com/article/10.3390/jcm11175236/s1, Table S1: Instrument scores of patients' family members at 2 and 8 weeks after discharge of their relatives with COVID-19 from the study sites ($n = 74$).

Author Contributions: Conceptualization, L.A.-N., I.K.B.T., A.G.O.L. and G.D.P.D.; methodology, L.A.-N., I.K.B.T., A.G.O.L. and G.D.P.D.; Formal analysis, L.A.-N., I.K.B.T., A.G.O.L., G.D.P.D. and O.A.G.T.; Investigation, L.A.-N., I.K.B.T., A.G.O.L. and G.D.P.D.; data curation, L.A.-N., I.K.B.T., A.G.O.L., G.D.P.D. and O.A.G.T.; writing—original draft preparation: L.A.-N., I.K.B.T., A.G.O.L., G.D.P.D. and O.A.G.T.; writing—review and editing, I.K.B.T. and O.A.G.T.; supervision: L.A.-N.; funding acquisition, L.A.-N. and I.K.B.T. All authors have read and agreed to the published version of the manuscript.

Funding: This study was funded by the Department of Health AHEAD Program 2018.

Institutional Review Board Statement: This study was approved by the University of the Philippines Manila Research Ethics Board (UPMREB Code: 2020-280-01) and the Philippine Department of Health Single Joint Research Ethics Board (SJREB Code: 2020-100).

Informed Consent Statement: Written informed consent has been obtained from the participants to publish this paper.

Data Availability Statement: The data that supports the findings of this study are available in the Supplementary Material of this article.

Acknowledgments: We would like to thank DOH, DOST-PCHRD, and the University of the Philippines Manila for supporting the study. We would also like to express our utmost gratitude to the officials and staff of the Philippine General Hospital, UP Diliman Silungan Molave Quarantine Facility, and PNP Kiangan Quarantine Facility who helped us in the participant identification, recruitment, and interviews.

Conflicts of Interest: The authors declare no conflict of interest. The funders had no role in the design of the study; in the collection, analyses, or interpretation of data; in the writing of the manuscript; or in the decision to publish the results.

References

1. Amit, A.M.L.; Pepito, V.C.F.; Dayrit, M.M. Early Response to COVID-19 in the Philippines. *West. Pacific Surveill. Response J. WPSAR* **2021**, *12*, 56–60. [CrossRef]
2. S Talabis, D.A.; Babierra, A.L.H.; Buhat, C.A.; Lutero, D.S.; Quindala, K.M.; Rabajante, J.F. Local Government Responses for COVID-19 Management in the Philippines. *BMC Public Health* **2021**, *21*, 1711. [CrossRef]
3. Akhmedov, B.T. The Family as the Basic Unit of Society. *Int. J. Multicult. Multirelig. Underst.* **2021**, *8*, 201. [CrossRef]
4. Ebrahim, G.J. (Ed.) The Family as a Child-Rearing Unit of Society. In *Child Health in a Changing Environment*; Macmillan Education UK: London, UK, 1982; pp. 68–97, ISBN 978-1-349-17031-9.

5. Rahimi, T.; Dastyar, N.; Rafati, F. Experiences of Family Caregivers of Patients with COVID-19. *BMC Fam. Pract.* **2021**, *22*, 137. [CrossRef]
6. Wister, A.; Li, L.; Mitchell, B.; Wolfson, C.; McMillan, J.; Griffith, L.E.; Kirkland, S.; Raina, P. Levels of Depression and Anxiety Among Informal Caregivers during the COVID-19 Pandemic: A Study Based on the Canadian Longitudinal Study on Aging. *J. Gerontol. Ser. B* **2022**, *77*, 1740–1757. [CrossRef]
7. Irani, E.; Niyomyart, A.; Hickman, R.L. Family Caregivers' Experiences and Changes in Caregiving Tasks during the COVID-19 Pandemic. *Clin. Nurs. Res.* **2021**, *30*, 1088–1097. [CrossRef]
8. Cohen, S.A.; Kunicki, Z.J.; Drohan, M.M.; Greaney, M.L. Exploring Changes in Caregiver Burden and Caregiving Intensity Due to COVID-19. *Gerontol. Geriatr. Med.* **2021**, *7*, 2333721421999279. [CrossRef]
9. Wittenberg, E.; Saada, A.; Prosser, L.A. How Illness Affects Family Members: A Qualitative Interview Survey. *Patient* **2013**, *6*, 257–268. [CrossRef]
10. Tee, M.L.; Tee, C.A.; Anlacan, J.P.; Aligam, K.J.G.; Reyes, P.W.C.; Kuruchittham, V.; Ho, R.C. Psychological Impact of COVID-19 Pandemic in the Philippines. *J. Affect. Disord.* **2020**, *277*, 379–391. [CrossRef]
11. Aruta, J.J.B.R.; Callueng, C.; Antazo, B.G.; Ballada, C.J.A. The Mediating Role of Psychological Distress on the Link between Socio-Ecological Factors and Quality of Life of Filipino Adults during COVID-19 Crisis. *J. Community Psychol.* **2022**, *50*, 712–726. [CrossRef]
12. Agrupis, K.A.; Smith, C.; Suzuki, S.; Villanueva, A.M.; Ariyoshi, K.; Solante, R.; Telan, E.F.; Estrada, K.A.; Uichanco, A.C.; Sagurit, J.; et al. Epidemiological and Clinical Characteristics of the First 500 Confirmed COVID-19 Inpatients in a Tertiary Infectious Disease Referral Hospital in Manila, Philippines. *Trop. Med. Health* **2021**, *49*, 48. [CrossRef]
13. Malundo, A.F.G.; Abad, C.L.R.; Salamat, M.S.S.; Sandejas, J.C.M.; Planta, J.E.G.; Poblete, J.B.; Morales, S.J.L.; Gabunada, R.R.W.; Evasan, A.L.M.; Cañal, J.P.A.; et al. Clinical Characteristics of Patients with Asymptomatic and Symptomatic COVID-19 Admitted to a Tertiary Referral Centre in the Philippines. *IJID Reg.* **2022**, *2*, 204–211. [CrossRef]
14. Salva, E.P.; Villarama, J.B.; Lopez, E.B.; Sayo, A.R.; Villanueva, A.M.G.; Edwards, T.; Han, S.M.; Suzuki, S.; Seposo, X.; Ariyoshi, K.; et al. Epidemiological and Clinical Characteristics of Patients with Suspected COVID-19 Admitted in Metro Manila, Philippines. *Trop. Med. Health* **2020**, *48*, 51. [CrossRef]
15. Mohamed, A.E.; Yousef, A.M. Depressive, Anxiety, and Post-Traumatic Stress Symptoms Affecting Hospitalized and Home-Isolated COVID-19 Patients: A Comparative Cross-Sectional Study. *Middle East Curr. Psychiatry* **2021**, *28*, 28. [CrossRef]
16. Moayed, M.S.; Vahedian-Azimi, A.; Mirmomeni, G.; Rahimi-Bashar, F.; Goharimoghadam, K.; Pourhoseingholi, M.A.; Abbasi-Farajzadeh, M.; Hekmat, M.; Sathyapalan, T.; Guest, P.C.; et al. Depression, Anxiety, and Stress Among Patients with COVID-19: A Cross-Sectional Study. *Adv. Exp. Med. Biol.* **2021**, *1321*, 229–236. [CrossRef]
17. Heesakkers, H.; van der Hoeven, J.G.; Corsten, S.; Janssen, I.; Ewalds, E.; Burgers-Bonthuis, D.; Rettig, T.C.D.; Jacobs, C.; van Santen, S.; Slooter, A.J.C.; et al. Mental Health Symptoms in Family Members of COVID-19 ICU Survivors 3 and 12 Months after ICU Admission: A Multicentre Prospective Cohort Study. *Intensive Care Med.* **2022**, *48*, 322–331. [CrossRef]
18. Khaleghparast, S.; Ghanbari, B.; Maleki, M.; Zamani, F.; Peighambari, M.-M.; Karbalaie Niya, M.H.; Mazloomzadeh, S.; Safarnezhad Tameshkel, F.; Manshouri, S. Anxiety, Knowledge and Lived Experiences of Families with COVID-19 Patients: A Mixed-Method Multi-Center Study in Iran. *Iran. J. Med. Sci.* **2022**, *47*, 131–138. [CrossRef]
19. Bartoli, D.; Trotta, F.; Pucciarelli, G.; Simeone, S.; Miccolis, R.; Cappitella, C.; Rotoli, D.; Rocco, M. The Lived Experiences of Family Members Who Visit Their Relatives in COVID-19 Intensive Care Unit for the First Time: A Phenomenological Study. *Heart Lung* **2022**, *54*, 49–55. [CrossRef]
20. Fernandes, C.S.; Magalhães, B.; Silva, S.; Edra, B. Perception of Family Functionality during Social Confinement by Coronavirus Disease 2019. *J. Nurs. Health* **2020**, *10*, 1–14. [CrossRef]
21. Gadermann, A.C.; Thomson, K.C.; Richardson, C.G.; Gagné, M.; McAuliffe, C.; Hirani, S.; Jenkins, E. Examining the Impacts of the COVID-19 Pandemic on Family Mental Health in Canada: Findings from a National Cross-Sectional Study. *BMJ Open* **2021**, *11*, e042871. [CrossRef] [PubMed]
22. Snaith, R.P. The Hospital Anxiety And Depression Scale. *Health Qual. Life Outcomes* **2003**, *1*, 29. [CrossRef]
23. Tan, S.M.; Benedicto, J.; Santiaguel, J.M. Prevalence of Anxiety and Depression among Filipino Patients with Chronic Obstructive Pulmonary Disease: A Multi-Center Study. *Philipp. J. Intern. Med.* **2015**, *53*, 34–48.
24. De Guzman, M.L.R.E. A Validation of the Hospital Anxiety and Depression Scale (HADS) in the Medically-Ill. *Acta. Med. Philipp.* **2013**, *47*, 53–62. [CrossRef]
25. Hedman, E.; Ljótsson, B.; Blom, K.; El Alaoui, S.; Kraepelien, M.; Rück, C.; Andersson, G.; Svanborg, C.; Lindefors, N.; Kaldo, V. Telephone versus Internet Administration of Self-Report Measures of Social Anxiety, Depressive Symptoms, and Insomnia: Psychometric Evaluation of a Method to Reduce the Impact of Missing Data. *J. Med. Internet Res.* **2013**, *15*, e229. [CrossRef]
26. Panganiban-Corales, A.T.; Medina, M.F.J. Family Resources Study: Part 1: Family Resources, Family Function and Caregiver Strain in Childhood Cancer. *Asia Pac. Fam. Med.* **2011**, *10*, 14. [CrossRef] [PubMed]
27. Trougakos, J.P.; Chawla, N.; McCarthy, J.M. Working in a Pandemic: Exploring the Impact of COVID-19 Health Anxiety on Work, Family, and Health Outcomes. *J. Appl. Psychol.* **2020**, *105*, 1234–1245. [CrossRef] [PubMed]
28. Fong, V.C.; Iarocci, G. Child and Family Outcomes Following Pandemics: A Systematic Review and Recommendations on COVID-19 Policies. *J. Pediatr. Psychol.* **2020**, *45*, 1124–1143. [CrossRef]

29. Chen, C.; Wittenberg, E.; Sullivan, S.S.; Lorenz, R.A.; Chang, Y.-P. The Experiences of Family Members of Ventilated COVID-19 Patients in the Intensive Care Unit: A Qualitative Study. *Am. J. Hosp. Palliat. Care* **2021**, *38*, 869–876. [CrossRef]
30. Drake, R.E.; Sederer, L.I.; Becker, D.R.; Bond, G.R. COVID-19, Unemployment, and Behavioral Health Conditions: The Need for Supported Employment. *Adm. Policy Ment. Health* **2021**, *48*, 388–392. [CrossRef]
31. Liu, S.; Heinzel, S.; Haucke, M.N.; Heinz, A. Increased Psychological Distress, Loneliness, and Unemployment in the Spread of COVID-19 over 6 Months in Germany. *Medicina* **2021**, *57*, 53. [CrossRef]
32. Posel, D.; Oyenubi, A.; Kollamparambil, U. Job Loss and Mental Health during the COVID-19 Lockdown: Evidence from South Africa. *PLoS ONE* **2021**, *16*, e0249352.
33. Arnout, B.A.; Al-Dabbagh, Z.S.; Al Eid, N.A.; Al Eid, M.A.; Al-Musaibeh, S.S.; Al-Miqtiq, M.N.; Alamri, A.S.; Al-Zeyad, G.M. The Effects of Corona Virus (COVID-19) Outbreak on the Individuals' Mental Health and on the Decision Makers: A Comparative Epidemiological Study. *Int. J. Med. Res. Health Sci.* **2020**, *9*, 26–47.
34. Losada-Baltar, A.; Jiménez-Gonzalo, L.; Gallego-Alberto, L.; Pedroso-Chaparro, M.D.S.; Fernandes-Pires, J.; Márquez-González, M. "We Are Staying at Home." Association of Self-Perceptions of Aging, Personal and Family Resources, and Loneliness With Psychological Distress during the Lock-Down Period of COVID-19. *J. Gerontol. B. Psychol. Sci. Soc. Sci.* **2021**, *76*, e10–e16. [CrossRef] [PubMed]
35. López, J.; Pérez-Rojo, G.; Noriega, C.; Velasco, C.; Carretero, I.; López-Frutos, P.; Galarraga, L. COVID-19 Pandemic Lockdown Responses from an Emotional Perspective: Family Function as a Differential Pattern among Older Adults. *Behav. Psychol. Psicol. Conduct.* **2021**, *29*, 331–344. [CrossRef]
36. Vanderhout, S.M.; Birken, C.S.; Wong, P.; Kelleher, S.; Weir, S.; Maguire, J.L. Family Perspectives of COVID-19 Research. *Res. Involv. Engagem.* **2020**, *6*, 69. [CrossRef]
37. Gayatri, M.; Irawaty, D.K. Family Resilience during COVID-19 Pandemic: A Literature Review. *Fam. J.* **2021**, *30*, 132–138. [CrossRef]
38. Rawal, G.; Yadav, S.; Kumar, R. Post-Intensive Care Syndrome: An Overview. *J. Transl. Intern. Med.* **2017**, *5*, 90–92. [CrossRef]
39. Ghaffari Darab, M.; Keshavarz, K.; Sadeghi, E.; Shahmohamadi, J.; Kavosi, Z. The Economic Burden of Coronavirus Disease 2019 (COVID-19): Evidence from Iran. *BMC Health Serv. Res.* **2021**, *21*, 132. [CrossRef]
40. Richards, F.; Kodjamanova, P.; Chen, X.; Li, N.; Atanasov, P.; Bennetts, L.; Patterson, B.J.; Yektashenas, B.; Mesa-Frias, M.; Tronczynski, K.; et al. Economic Burden of COVID-19: A Systematic Review. *Clin. Outcomes Res.* **2022**, *14*, 293–307. [CrossRef]
41. Tabuñar, S.M.S.; Dominado, T.M.P. Hospitalization Expenditure of COVID-19 Patients at the University of the Philippines-Philippine General Hospital (UP-PGH) with PhilHealth Coverage. *Acta. Med. Philipp.* **2021**, *55*, 216–223. [CrossRef]
42. Department of Labor and Employment National Capital Region I National Wages Productivity Commission. Available online: https://nwpc.dole.gov.ph/regionandwages/national-capital-region/ (accessed on 15 August 2022).
43. Núñez, A.; Sreeganga, S.D.; Ramaprasad, A. Access to Healthcare during COVID-19. *Int. J. Environ. Res. Public Health* **2021**, *18*, 2980. [CrossRef] [PubMed]
44. Okereke, M.; Ukor, N.A.; Adebisi, Y.A.; Ogunkola, I.O.; Favour Iyagbaye, E.; Adiela Owhor, G.; Lucero-Prisno, D.E. 3rd Impact of COVID-19 on Access to Healthcare in Low- and Middle-Income Countries: Current Evidence and Future Recommendations. *Int. J. Health Plann. Manag.* **2021**, *36*, 13–17. [CrossRef] [PubMed]
45. Singu, S.; Acharya, A.; Challagundla, K.; Byrareddy, S.N. Impact of Social Determinants of Health on the Emerging COVID-19 Pandemic in the United States. *Front. Public Health* **2020**, *8*, 406. [CrossRef] [PubMed]
46. Shadmi, E.; Chen, Y.; Dourado, I.; Faran-Perach, I.; Furler, J.; Hangoma, P.; Hanvoravongchai, P.; Obando, C.; Petrosyan, V.; Rao, K.D.; et al. Health Equity and COVID-19: Global Perspectives. *Int. J. Equity Health* **2020**, *19*, 104. [CrossRef]
47. Bjelland, I.; Krokstad, S.; Mykletun, A.; Dahl, A.A.; Tell, G.S.; Tambs, K. Does a Higher Educational Level Protect against Anxiety and Depression? The HUNT Study. *Soc. Sci. Med.* **2008**, *66*, 1334–1345. [CrossRef]
48. Erickson, J.; El-Gabalawy, R.; Palitsky, D.; Patten, S.; Mackenzie, C.S.; Stein, M.B.; Sareen, J. Educational attainment as a protective factor for psychiatric disorders: Findings from a nationally representative longitudinal study. *Depress. Anxiety* **2016**, *33*, 1013–1022. [CrossRef]
49. Carlson, R.H.; McChesney, C.S. Income Sustainability through Educational Attainment. *J. Educ. Train. Stud.* **2014**, *3*, 108–115. [CrossRef]
50. Wang, G.-Y.; Tang, S.-F. Perceived Psychosocial Health and Its Sociodemographic Correlates in Times of the COVID-19 Pandemic: A Community-Based Online Study in China. *Infect. Dis. Poverty* **2020**, *9*, 148. [CrossRef]

Journal of
Clinical Medicine

MDPI

Review

Prevalence of Depression among Healthcare Workers during the COVID-19 Outbreak: A Systematic Review and Meta-Analysis

Beatriz Olaya [1,2], María Pérez-Moreno [3], Juan Bueno-Notivol [4,*], Patricia Gracia-García [4], Isabel Lasheras [5] and Javier Santabárbara [2,5,6]

1 Research, Innovation and Teaching Unit, Parc Sanitari Sant Joan de Déu, Universitat de Barcelona, 08830 Sant Boi de Llobregat, Spain; beatriz.olaya@sjd.es
2 Centro de Investigación Biomédica en Red de Salud Mental (CIBERSAM), Ministry of Science and Innovation, 28029 Madrid, Spain; jsantabarbara@unizar.es
3 Hospitalary Pharmacy Service, Hospital Universitario Miguel Servet, Paseo Isabel la Católica, 1-3, 50009 Zaragoza, Spain; marpermor159@gmail.com
4 Psychiatry Service, Hospital Universitario Miguel Servet, Paseo Isabel la Católica, 1-3, 50009 Zaragoza, Spain; pgraciag@salud.aragon.es
5 Department of Microbiology, Pediatrics, Radiology and Public Health, Faculty of Medicine, University of Zaragoza, Building A, 50009 Zaragoza, Spain; isabel.lasheras@hotmail.es
6 Instituto de Investigación Sanitaria de Aragón (IIS Aragón), Avenue San Juan Bosco, 13, 50009 Zaragoza, Spain
* Correspondence: jbuenon@salud.aragon.es; Tel.: +34-659-743-354

Abstract: Background: There is evidence of a high psychological toll from the COVID-19 pandemic in healthcare workers. This paper was aimed at conducting a systematic review and meta-analysis of studies reporting levels of depression among healthcare workers during the COVID-19 and estimating the pooled prevalence of depression. Methods: We searched for cross-sectional studies listed on PubMed from 1 December 2019 to 15 September 2020 that reported prevalence of depression in healthcare workers, nurses, medical doctors, and COVID-19 frontline professionals. The pooled proportions of depression were calculated with random effects models. Results: We identified 57 studies from seventeen countries. The pooled prevalence of depression in healthcare workers was 24% (95% CI: 20–28%), 25% for nurses (95% CI: 18–33%), 24% for medical doctors (95% CI: 16–31%), and 43% for frontline professionals (95% CI: 28–59%). Conclusions: The proportion of depression in nurses and medical doctors during the COVID-19 pandemic was similar to that found in the general population as previously reported in other meta-analyses conducted with smaller numbers of studies. Importantly, almost half of the frontline healthcare workers showed increased levels of depression. There is need for a comprehensive, international response to prevent and treat common mental health problems in healthcare workers.

Keywords: depressive symptoms; COVID-19; nurses; medical doctors; frontline; pooled prevalence

Citation: Olaya, B.; Pérez-Moreno, M.; Bueno-Notivol, J.; Gracia-García, P.; Lasheras, I.; Santabárbara, J. Prevalence of Depression among Healthcare Workers during the COVID-19 Outbreak: A Systematic Review and Meta-Analysis. *J. Clin. Med.* **2021**, *10*, 3406. https://doi.org/10.3390/jcm10153406

Academic Editor: Emmanuel Andrès

Received: 2 July 2021
Accepted: 26 July 2021
Published: 30 July 2021

1. Introduction

The new coronavirus (SARS-CoV-2) was first identified in a wet market in Wuhan, Hubei province, China, in December 2019 [1]. This virus causes a highly infectious acute respiratory syndrome (COVID-19) that can be associated with serious pneumonia and eventually lead to death. Due to its rapid spread around the world, the World Health Organization [2] declared the COVID-19 as a pandemic in March 2020, and from its identification to this date (12th November 2020), more than 51.9 million people have been confirmed as cases worldwide, with 1.2 million deaths [3]. The enormous impact on people's physical and mental health, and on economic systems worldwide, is one of the main challenges for society in this century [4].

Healthcare workers (HCW) are a fundamental part of the global response to COVID-19. Because of their close personal exposure to patients with COVID-19, their risk of infection is very high. A recent study reports HCW to be at an 11.6 times higher risk of infection than the general population, although this risk decreases to 3.4 after accounting for the differences in testing frequency between HCW and the general community [5]. Besides this higher risk of infection, several observational studies conducted during the COVID-19 pandemic have shown that health professionals are at a higher risk of developing psychological problems [6]. Growing patient load and working under pressure in resource-deprived settings might increase psychological stress among HCW [7,8]. They are also more exposed to prolonged work shifts, lack of adequate equipment (i.e., protective equipment (PPE)), and fear of infecting themselves or relatives [9,10]. This fear, in turn, may be associated with anxiety, depression, and insomnia [11–13].

HCW thus constitute one of the groups most vulnerable to psychological distress, requiring immediate interventions to improve their wellbeing and the healthcare system capacity. Two very recent systematic reviews and meta-analyses on the prevalence of anxiety and depression have been published, reporting the pooled prevalence among HCW. The first one, conducted by Pappa et al. [14] in April 2020, included a total of thirteen cross-sectional studies (all of them conducted in China except one, from Singapore) reporting a pooled prevalence of anxiety of 23.2% and 22.8% for depression. The second [15] was based on seven studies conducted in China and found an increased risk of anxiety and depression in HCW, compared with other professionals (OR = 1.61; 95%CI 1.33 to 1.96 and OR = 1.32; 95%CI 1.09 to 1.60, respectively).

Due to the rapid, evolving nature of this health emergency, an increasing number of other studies from different countries addressing mental health problems among HCW have been published in recent months. Thus, the present study is aimed at updating and extending the previous work of Pappa et al. [14] and da Silva and Neto [15] by conducting a systematic review and meta-analysis of studies published afterwards reporting a global prevalence of anxiety and depression among HCW during the COVID-19 outbreak.

2. Materials and Methods

The present study followed the PRISMA guidelines for reporting systematic reviews and meta-analysis [16] (Supplementary Table S1).

2.1. Search Strategy

The search strategy (Supplementary Table S2) included all cross-sectional studies informing about the prevalence of depression that were published from 1 December 2019 to 15 September 2020. The search was conducted by two researchers (MPM and JBN) using MEDLINE via PubMed. Briefly, they focused on depression, although an anxiety term was additionally included to examine whether these articles also included relevant information about depression. Depression could be measured either using diagnostic tools (e.g., structured interviews) or standardized scales to assess depressive symptomatology. As our main objective was to calculate the overall prevalence of depression, in case we found a study using scales, we considered the presence of depression reported according to a certain cut-off point for that given scale. Thus, henceforth we use the term "depression" to refer to either a full-blown diagnosis or presence of depression according to a cut-off point.

Search terms also included samples of HCW, nurses, medical doctors, and/or frontline HCW. There was no language restriction. We inspected references from selected articles to detect additional studies. In case of disagreement, a third and fourth reviewer (JS and IL) were consulted to reach a consensus.

2.2. Selection Criteria

The following inclusion criteria for studies were used: (1) studies providing cross-sectional data on the proportion of depression during the COVID-19 outbreak; (2) studies conducted with samples of health care workers; (3) studies in which the assessment methods for depression were described; and (4) studies for which the full-text was available.

Studies that used other specific samples (e.g., adolescents and patients) and review articles were excluded from the present study.

We extracted the following data using a pre-designed form: country, sample size, prevalence rates of depression, proportion of women, average age, instruments used to assess depression, response rate, and sampling methods.

2.3. Assessment of Methodological Quality

Two independent reviewers (JS and JBN) rated the methodological validity of selected articles before their inclusion in the review using the Joanna Briggs Institute (JBI) standardized critical appraisal instrument for prevalence studies [17]. This tool uses nine criteria to evaluate quality with a score ranging from zero ('No') to one ('Yes').

In case of disagreement between the two reviewers, there was a discussion to resolve it between them or with a third reviewer (PGG).

2.4. Statistical Analysis

We used a generic inverse variance method with a random effect model [18]. To check heterogeneity across studies, we calculated the Hedges Q statistic (a p value < 0.10 indicates statistical significance) and the I^2 statistic and 95% confidence interval [19]. I^2 values between 25% and 50% are considered low, 50%–75% moderate, and 75% or greater high [20]. Different study designs or demographic characteristics may explain the heterogeneity. Thus, we calculated meta-regression and carried out subgroup analyses [21] to find potential sources of heterogeneity [22]. A sensitivity analysis was also made by omitting studies one by one. This allowed us to learn how each individual study influenced the overall result. Publication bias was determined by visually inspecting a funnel plot. Since funnel plots might inaccurately assess publication bias in meta-analyses of proportion studies [23], we additionally calculated Egger's [24] and Begg's tests [25], with p values < 0.05 indicating publication bias.

Despite the fact that one inclusion criterion for a given study was the use of HCW samples, we were interested in separately calculating the pooled prevalence for the following groups: HCW in general (with no distinction of the type of worker or working in the frontline), nurses, medical doctors, and frontline HCW. Frontline HCW were those who provided direct care to patients with a diagnosis of infection by COVID-19 or who worked in units where care was provided. Additionally, for practical purposes, the pediatric HCW, physical therapists, and laboratory HCW were considered as HCW. Statistical analyses were conducted with STATA statistical software (version 10.0; College Station, TX, USA) and R [26].

3. Results

Flowchart of the search strategy and study selection process is shown in Figure 1. We initially identified 354 studies. After removing duplicates and studies after the first screening, 186 articles were read in full. Finally, a total of 57 studies were included in the present meta-analysis [6,12,13,27–80].

The results are organized as follows: Table 1 shows the characteristics of those studies (46) that reported prevalence rates of depression in HCW (without distinction in the type of workers); Table 2 displays characteristics of studies reporting data from nurses (14); Table 3 characteristics for medical doctors (10); and Table 4 for frontline HCW (12).

Approximately half of the studies were conducted in China (n = 24), but we also found studies from India (n = 4), Italy (n = 3), Turkey (n = 3), Singapore (n = 2), and one study from each of the following countries: Cameroon, Croatia, Jordan, Kosovo, Libya, Nepal, Poland, Serbia, South Korea, Spain, Switzerland, and the USA. The sample size ranged from 46 to 14,825 participants, and the mean age ranged from 29 to 47 years. All studies except one included both men and women, with women predominating in most of the studies that reported this (40 out of 43). All studies used online questionnaires and all except two used non-random methods. Twenty-three studies reported response rate, ranging from 20.4% to

94.9%. All studies measured depression using standardized scales, most commonly the Patient Health Questionnaire-9 (PHQ-9, n = 21 studies), the Depression, Anxiety, and Stress Scale (DASS-21, n = 8 studies), and the Hospital Anxiety and Depression Scale (HADS, n = 8 studies).

The risk of bias ranged from 5 to 8, with a mean score of 6.95 (Supplementary Table S3, Table 1). The most common limitations were (a) recruitment of participants not appropriate (56 studies), (b) response rate not reported or large number of non-responders (33 studies), and (c) sample size too small to ensure good precision of the final estimate (19 studies).

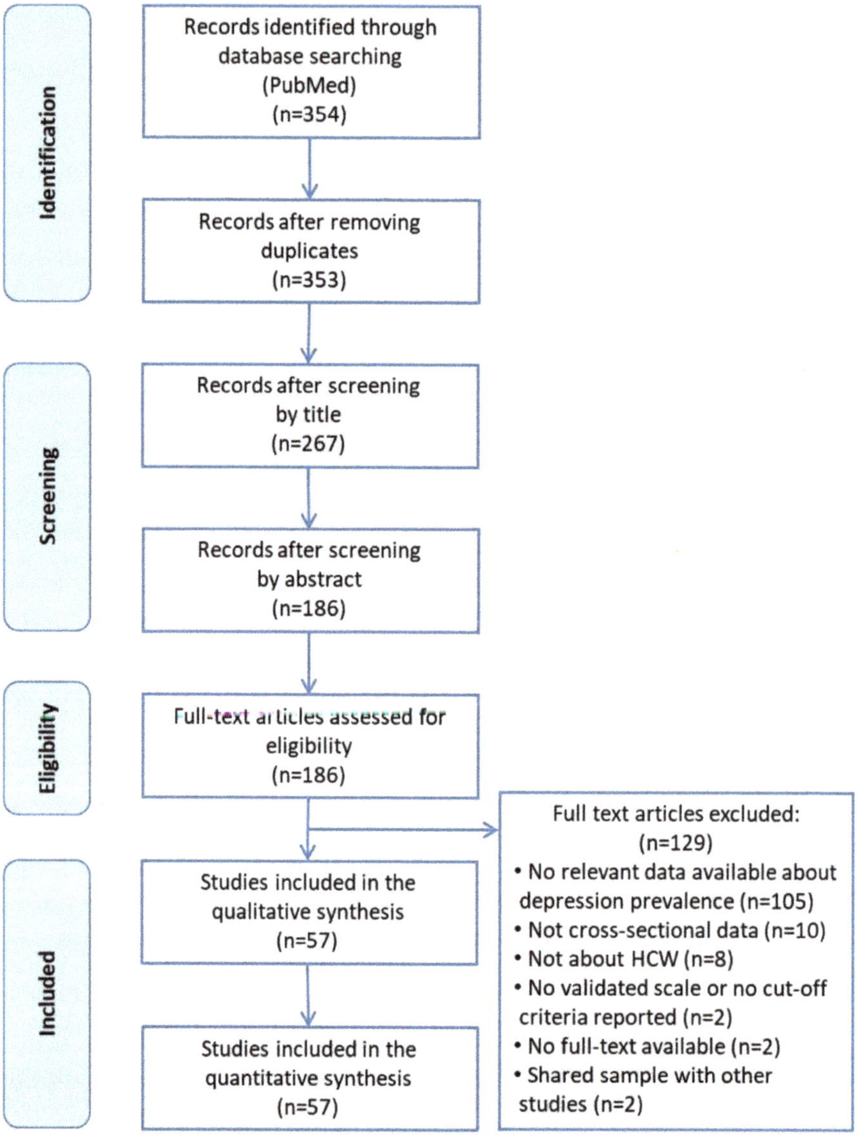

Figure 1. Flowchart of the study selection.

Table 1. Characteristics of the studies included in the meta-analysis based on samples of healthcare workers.

Author (Publication Year)	Population	Country	Mean Age (SD)	% Females (*n*)	Sample Size (*n*)	Response Rate (%)	Sampling Method	Depression Assessment	Time Frame Assessment	Diagnostic Criteria	Prevalence %	Prevalence *n*	Quality Assessment *
Chen J. et al. (2020)	HCW	China	36.54 (8.57)	68.63% (619)	902	NR	Convenience sampling	PHQ-9	Last 2 weeks	≥10	18.29%	165	7
Chen Y. et al. (2020)	Pediatric HCW	China	32.6 (6.5)	90.48% (95)	105	84.68%	NR	SDS	Past several days	≥53	29.52%	31	7
Chew et al. (2020)	HCW	India, Singapore	29 (NR)	64.3% (583)	906	90.60%	NR	DASS-21	Last week	≥14	5.30%	48	8
Di Tella et al. (2020)	HCW	Italy	42.9 (11.2)	72.4% (105)	145	NR	Convenience sampling	BDI-II	Last 2 weeks	>13	31.03%	45	6
Dosil Santamaría et al. (2020)	HCW	Spain	42.8 (10.2)	80.29% (338)	421	NR	Snowball sampling	DASS-21	Last week	≥14	16.86%	71	7
Elbay et al.(2020)	HCW	Turkey	36.05 (8.69)	56.8% (251)	442	NR	Convenience sampling	DASS-21	Last week	≥14	47.06%	208	7
Elhadi et al. (2020)	HCW	Libya	33.3 (7.4)	51.94% (387)	745	93.13%	Convenience sampling	HADS	Last week	>10	56.38%	420	8
Gallopeni et al. (2020)	HCW	Kosovo	39 (10.37)	61.32% (363)	592	NR	NR	HADS	Last week	>10	38.68%	229	7
Gupta A.K. et al. (2020)	HCW	Nepal	29.5 (6.1)	52.67% (79)	150	NR	Snowball sampling	PHQ-9	Last 2 weeks	≥10	8.00%	12	6
Gupta S. et al. (2020)	HCW	India	NR	36.12% (406)	1124	79.45%	Quota sampling	HADS	Last week	>7	31.49%	354	8
Huang & Zhao (2020)	HCW	China	NR	NR	2250	85.30%	Convenience sampling	CES-D	Last 2 weeks	>28	19.82%	446	7
Kannampallil et al. (2020)	HCW	USA	NR	54.96% (216)	393	28.58%	NR	DASS-21	Last week	≥10	27.23%	107	6
Keubo et al. (2020)	HCW	Cameroon	NR	54.45% (159)	292	NR	Snowball sampling	HADS	Last week	>10	43.49%	127	6
Khanna et al. (2020)	HCW	India	42.5 (12.05)	43.44% (1023)	2355	NR	NR	PHQ-9	Last 2 weeks	≥10	11.21%	264	7
Koksal et al. (2020)	HCW	Turkey	35.6 (8.5)	70.1% (492)	702	NR	NR	HADS	Last week	>7	36.89%	259	7
Krammer et al. (2020)	HCW	Switzerland	42.6 (13.5)	74.00% (74)	85	76.92%	Convenience sampling	PHQ-9	Last 2 weeks	≥10	15.29%	13	7
Lai et al. (2020)	HCW	China	NR	76.69% (964)	1257	68.69%	Convenience sampling	PHQ-9	Last 2 weeks	≥10	14.80%	186	8
Lam et al. (2020)	HCW	China	NR	75.21% (701)	932	59.51%	Convenience sampling	PHQ-9	Last 2 weeks	≥9	24.36%	227	7
Li et al. (2020)	HCW	China	NR	100% (4369)	4369	82.17%	Convenience sampling	PHQ-9	Last 2 weeks	≥10	14.21%	621	8
Liang et al. (2020)	HCW	China	NR	81.31% (731)	899	NR	Convenience sampling	PHQ-9	Last 2 weeks	≥10	24.25%	218	7
Lin et al. (2020)	HCW	China	NR	NR	2316	NR	Convenience sampling	PHQ-9	Last 2 weeks	>5	46.89%	1086	6
Liu et al. (2020)	Pediatric HCW	China	NR	85.52% (1737)	2031	NR	Convenience sampling	DASS-21	Last week	≥14	7.09%	144	7
Lu et al. (2020)	HCW	China	NR	77.64% (1785)	2299	94.88%	NR	HAMD	Last week	≥7	11.66%	268	8
Magnavita et al. (2020)	HCW	Italy	NR	70.10% (417)	595	73.46%	Convenience sampling	GADS	Last 2 weeks	≥2	20.34%	121	8
Naser et al. (2020)	HCW	Jordan	NR	56,1% (653)	1163	NR	Convenience sampling	PHQ-9	Last 2 weeks	≥10	44.71%	520	7
Ning et al. (2020)	HCW	China	NR	72.88% (446)	612	NR	Snowball sampling	SDS	Past several days	≥53	25.00%	153	7
Que et al. (2020)	HCW	China	31.06 (6.99)	69.06% (1578)	2285	NR	Convenience sampling	PHQ-9	Last 2 weeks	≥10	12.82%	293	7

Table 1. *Cont.*

Author (Publication Year)	Population	Country	Mean Age (SD)	% Females (*n*)	Sample Size (*n*)	Response Rate (%)	Sampling Method	Depression Assessment	Time Frame Assessment	Diagnostic Criteria	Prevalence		Quality Assessment *
											%	*n*	
Sahin et al. (2020)	HCW	Turkey	NR	66.03% (620)	939	NR	Convenience sampling	PHQ-9	Last 2 weeks	≥10	37.59%	353	7
Salopek-Žiha et al. (2020)	HCW	Croatia	NR	NR	124	NR	Convenience sampling	DASS-21	Last week	≥14	11.29%	14	5
Si et al. (2020)	HCW	China	NR	70.68% (610)	863	76.00%	Convenience sampling	DASS-21	Last week	≥14	6.03%	52	8
Song et al. (2020)	HCW	China	34 (8.2)	64.3% (NR)		NR	Convenience sampling	CES-D	Last 2 weeks	≥16	25.18%	3733	7
Stojanov et al. (2020)	HCW	Serbia	40.5 (8.37)	66.17% (133)	201	NR	NR	SDS	Past several days	≥60	15.92%	32	6
Suryavanshi et al. (2020)	HCW	India	NR	51.27% (101)	197	20.40%	Snowball sampling	PHQ-9	Last 2 weeks	≥10	22.34%	44	6
Teng et al. (2020)	HCW	China	NR	NR	338	NR	Snowball sampling	PHQ-9	Last 2 weeks	≥5	34.62%	117	6
Teo et al. (2020)	Laboratory HCW	Singapore	34 (NR)	73.77% (90/122)	103	84.43%	NR	SDS	Past several days	≥60	37.86%	39	7
Vanni et al. (2020)	HCW	Italy	47 (10.37)	65.22% (30)	46	90.20%	Convenience sampling	DASS-21	Last week	≥14	26.09%	12	7
Wang H. et al. (2020)	HCW	China	NR	85.84% (897)	1045	73.18%	Convenience sampling	HADS	Last week	>10	13.59%	142	7
Wang L.Q. et al. (2020)	HCW	China	37 (NR)	77.37% (212)	274	NR	Convenience sampling	PHQ-9	Last 2 weeks	≥10	16.06%	44	6
Wang S. et al. (2020)	Pediatric HCW	China	33.75 (8.41)	90.24% (111)	123	52.44%	Convenience sampling	SDS	Past several days	≥50	25.20%	31	7
Wang W. et al. (2020)	HCW	China	33.5 (8.89)	64.52% (1291)	2001	72.06%	Convenience sampling	HADS	Last week	>7	35.03%	701	8
Wankowicz et al. (2020)	HCW	Poland	40.25 (5.25)	52.15% (230)	441	NR	NR	PHQ-9	Last 2 weeks	>5	70.75%	312	7
Xiao et al. (2020)	HCW	China	NR	67.22% (644)	958	NR	Convenience sampling	HADS	Last week	>7	57.31%	549	6
Xiaoming et al. (2020)	HCW	China	33.25 (8.26)	77.93% (6874)	8817	90.62%	Convenience sampling	PHQ-9	Last 2 weeks	≥10	9.41%	830	8
Yang et al. (2020)	Physical therapists	South Korea	NR	47.69% (31)	65	89.04%	Convenience sampling	PHQ-9	Last 2 weeks	≥10	18.46%	12	7
Zhang et al. (2020)	HCW	China	NR	82.73% (1293)	1563	80.32%	Convenience sampling	PHQ-9	Last 2 weeks	≥10	17.21%	269	8
Zhu et al. (2020)	HCW	China	NR	85.03% (4304)	5062	77.07%	Convenience sampling	PHQ-9	Last 2 weeks	≥10	13.45%	681	8

Note. * Quality score based on the Joanna Briggs Institute (JBI) standardized critical appraisal instrument for prevalence studies [17] (see Supplementary Table S3). NR = not reported; BDI-II = Beck depression inventory-second edition; CES-D = Center for Epidemiologic Studies-Depression scale; DASS-21 = Depression, Anxiety and Stress scales; GADS = Goldberg Anxiety and Depression Scale; HADS = Hospital Anxiety and Depression Scale; HAMD = Hamilton Depression Rating Scale; PHQ-9 = Patient Health Questionnaire; SDS = Zung's Self-Rating Depression Scale.

Table 2. Characteristics of the studies included in the meta-analysis based on samples of nurses.

Author (Publication Year)	Population	Country	Mean Age (SD)	% Females (*n*)	Sample Size (*n*)	Response Rate (%)	Sampling Method	Depression Assessment	Time Frame Assessment	Diagnostic Criteria	Prevalence		Quality Assessment *
											%	*n*	
An et al. (2020)	Nurses	China	32.2 (7.61)	90.75% (1001)	1103	NR	Snowball sampling	PHQ-9	Last 2 weeks	≥10	15.96%	176	7
Dal'Bosco et al. (2020)	Nurses	Brazil	NR	79% (89.8)	88	18.49%	Convenience sampling	HADS	Last week	>7	25.00%	22	6
Gupta S. et al. (2020)	Nurses	India	NR	NR	207	79.45%	Quota sampling	HADS	Last week	>7	38.65%	80	6
Keubo et al. (2020)	Nurses	Cameroon	NR	NR	168	NR	Snowball sampling	HADS	Last week	>10	44.05%	74	5
Lai et al. (2020)	Nurses	China	NR	90.84% (694)	764	68.69%	Convenience sampling	PHQ-9	Last 2 weeks	≥10	15.45%	118	8
Liu Y. et al. (2020)	Nurses	China	NR	NR	1173	NR	Convenience sampling	DASS-21	Last week	≥14	6.31%	74	6
Ning et al. (2020)	Nurses	China	NR	97.97% (289)	295	NR	Snowball sampling	SDS	Past several days	≥53	30.17%	89	6
Pouralizadeh et al. (2020)	Nurses	Iran	36.34 (8.74)	95.2% (420)	441	NR	NR	PHQ-9	Last 2 weeks	≥10	37.41%	165	7
Que et al. (2020)	Nurses	China	35.94 (8.17)	97.75% (195)	208	NR	Convenience sampling	PHQ-9	Last 2 weeks	≥10	12.02%	25	6
Sahin et al. (2020)	Nurses	Turkey	NR	NR	254	NR	Convenience sampling	PHQ-9	Last 2 weeks	≥10	42.13%	107	5
Tu et al. (2020)	Frontline Nurses	China	34.44 (5.85)	100% (100)	100	100%	Cluster Sampling	PHQ-9	Last 2 weeks	≥5	46.00%	46	8
Wang H. et al. (2020)	Nurses	China	NR	NR	773	73.18%	Convenience sampling	HADS	Last week	>10	13.58%	105	7
Xiong et al. (2020)	Nurses	China	NR	97.31 (217)	223	61.80%	Convenience sampling	PHQ-9	Last 2 weeks	≥10	6.73%	15	7
Zhu J. et al. (2020)	Frontline Nurses	China	NR	NR	86	NR	Convenience sampling	SDS	Past several days	≥50	43.02%	37	5

Note. * Quality score based on the Joanna Briggs Institute (JBI) standardized critical appraisal instrument for prevalence studies [17] (see Supplementary Table S3). NR = not reported; DASS-21 = Depression, Anxiety and Stress scales; HADS = Hospital Anxiety and Depression Scale; PHQ-9 = Patient Health Questionnaire; SDS = Zung's Self-Rating Depression Scale.

Table 3. Characteristics of the studies included in the meta-analysis based on samples of medical doctors.

Author (Publication Year)	Population	Country	Mean Age (SD)	% Females (*n*)	Sample Size (*n*)	Response Rate (%)	Sampling Method	Depression Assessment	Time Frame Assessment	Diagnostic Criteria	Prevalence		Quality Assessment *
											%	*n*	
Almater et al. (2020)	MD	Saudi Arabia	32.9 (9.6)	43.9% (47)	107	30.60%	Convenience sampling	PHQ-9	Last 2 weeks	≥10	28.97%	31	6
Gupta S. et al. (2020)	MD	India	NR	NR	749	79.45%	Quota sampling	HADS	Last week	>7	28.17%	211	7
Keubo et al. (2020)	MD	Cameroon	NR	NR	74	NR	Snowball sampling	HADS	Last week	>10	39.19%	29	5
Lai et al. (2020)	MD	China	NR	54.77% (270)	493	68.69%	Convenience sampling	PHQ-9	Last 2 weeks	≥10	13.79%	68	8
Liu Y. et al. (2020)	MD	China	NR	NR	858	NR	Convenience sampling	DASS-21	Last week	≥14	8.16%	70	6
Ning et al. (2020)	MD	China	NR	49.53% (157)	317	NR	Snowball sampling	SDS	Past several days	≥53	20.19%	64	6
Que et al. (2020)	MD	China	33.69 (7.44)	63.49% (546)	860	NR	Convenience sampling	PHQ-9	Last 2 weeks	≥10	12.91%	111	7
Sahin et al. (2020)	MD	Turkey	NR	NR	580	NR	Convenience sampling	PHQ-9	Last 2 weeks	≥10	35.69%	207	6
Wang H. et al. (2020)	MD	China	NR	NR	149	73.18%	Convenience sampling	HADS	Last week	>10	17.45%	26	6
Zhu J. et al. (2020)	Frontline MD	China	NR	64.56% (51)	79	NR	Convenience sampling	SDS	Past several days	≥50	45.57%	36	6

Note. * Quality score based on the Joanna Briggs Institute (JBI) standardized critical appraisal instrument for prevalence studies [17] (see Supplementary Table S3). NR = not reported; DASS-21 = Depression, Anxiety and Stress scales; HADS = Hospital Anxiety and Depression Scale; PHQ-9 = Patient Health Questionnaire; SDS = Zung's Self-Rating Depression Scale.

Table 4. Characteristics of the studies included in the meta-analysis based on samples of frontline healthcare workers.

Author (Publication Year)	Population	Country	Mean Age (SD)	% Females (*n*)	Sample Size (*n*)	Response Rate (%)	Sampling Method	Depression Assessment	Time Frame Assessment	Diagnostic Criteria	Prevalence		Quality Assessment *
											%	*n*	
Cai et al. (2020)	Frontline HCW	China	30.6 (8.8)	69.82% (819)	1173	NR	Non-probabilistic sampling	PHQ-9	Last 2 weeks	≥10	14.32%	168	7
Kannampallil et al. (2020)	Frontline HCW	USA	NR	51.38% (112)	218	15.85%	NR	DASS-21	Last week	≥10	27.98%	61	5
Lai et al. (2020)	Frontline HCW	China	NR	NR	522	68.69%	Convenience sampling	PHQ-9	Last 2 weeks	≥10	18.01%	94	7
Luceño-Moreno et al. (2020)	Frontline HCW	Spain	43.88 (10.82)	86.40% (1228)	1422	92.40%	Non probabilistic sampling	HADS	Last week	≥7	51.34%	730	8
Sandesh et al. (2020)	Frontline HCW	Pakistan	NR	42.86% (48)	112	NR	Convenience sampling	DASS-21	Last week	≥14	72.32%	81	5
Stojanov et al. (2020)	Frontline HCW	Serbia	39.1 (7.3)	65.25% (77)	118	NR	NR	SDS	Past several days	≥60	17.80%	21	6
Tu et al. (2020)	Frontline Nurses	China	34.44 (5.85)	100% (100)	100	100%	Cluster Sampling	PHQ-9	Last 2 weeks	≥5	46.00%	46	8
Wang H. et al. (2020)	Frontline HCW	China	NR	NR	401	73.18%	Convenience sampling	HADS	Last week	>10	16.46%	66	7
Wang W. et al. (2020)	Frontline HCW	China	NR	59.46% (393)	661	72.06%	Convenience sampling	HADS	Last week	>7	45.99%	304	8
Wankowicz et al. (2020)	Frontline HCW	Poland	40.47 (4.93)	56.31% (116)	206	NR	NR	PHQ-9	Last 2 weeks	>5	99.51%	205	6
Zhou et al. (2020)	Frontline HCW	China	35.77 (8.13)	81.19% (492)	606	NR	NR	PHQ-9	Last 2 weeks	>5	57.59%	349	7
Zhu J. et al. (2020)	Frontline HCW	China	34.16 (8.06)	83.03% (137)	165	NR	Convenience sampling	SDS	Past several days	≥50	44.24%	73	6

Note. * Quality score based on the Joanna Briggs Institute (JBI) standardized critical appraisal instrument for prevalence studies [17] (see Supplementary Table S3). NR = not reported; DASS-21 = Depression, Anxiety and Stress scales; HADS = Hospital Anxiety and Depression Scale; PHQ-9 = Patient Health Questionnaire; SDS = Zung's Self-Rating Depression Scale.

Figure 2 shows the estimated overall prevalence of depression in HCW (24%; 95% CI: 20%–28%), 25% in nurses (95% CI: 18%–33%) (Figure 3), 24% in medical doctors (95% CI: 16%–31%) (Figure 4), and 43% in frontline HCW (95% CI: 28%–59%) (Figure 5), with significant heterogeneity between studies (Q test: $p < 0.001$) across these four categories. Additionally, the prevalence of depression in frontline HCW was significantly higher than in HCW overall ($p < 0.05$).

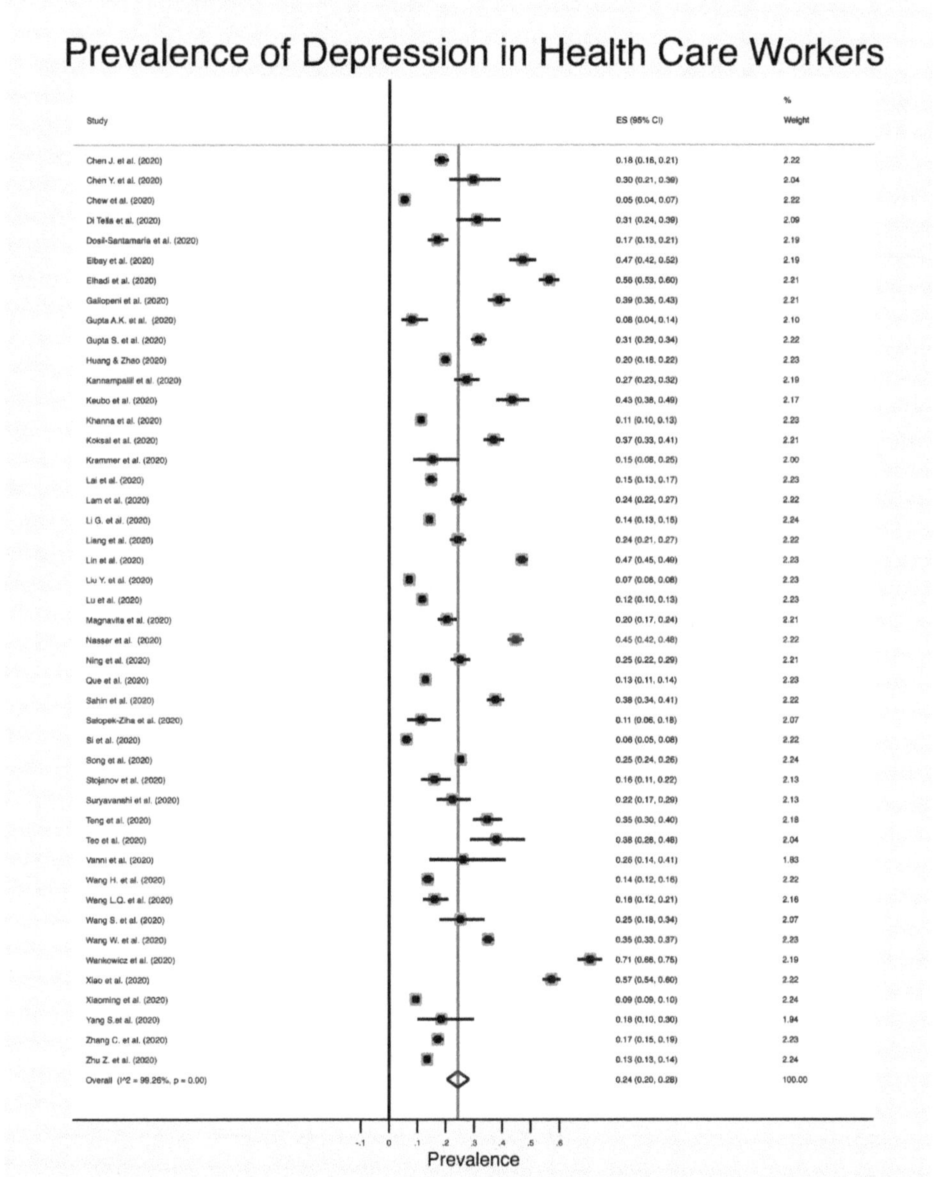

Figure 2. Forest plot for the prevalence of depression among healthcare workers.

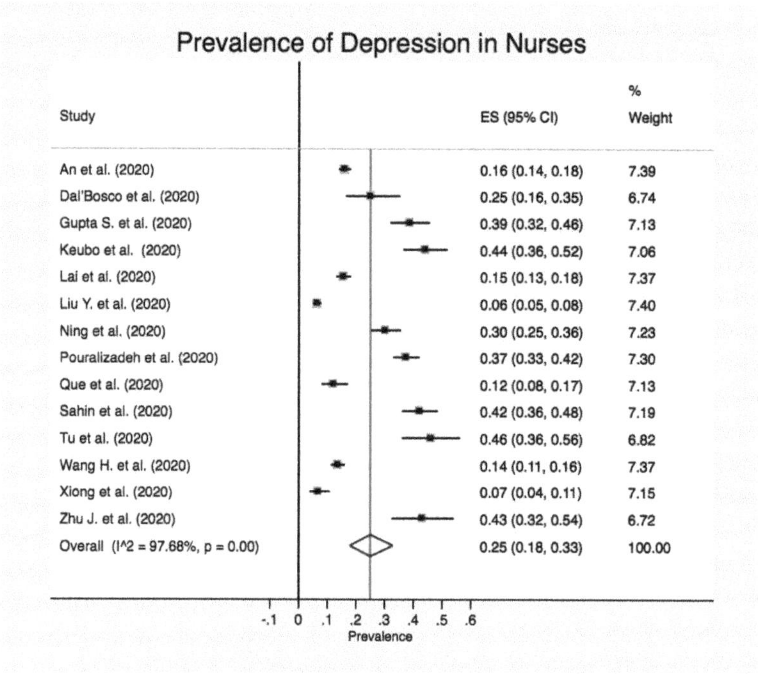

Figure 3. Forest plot for the prevalence of depression among nurses.

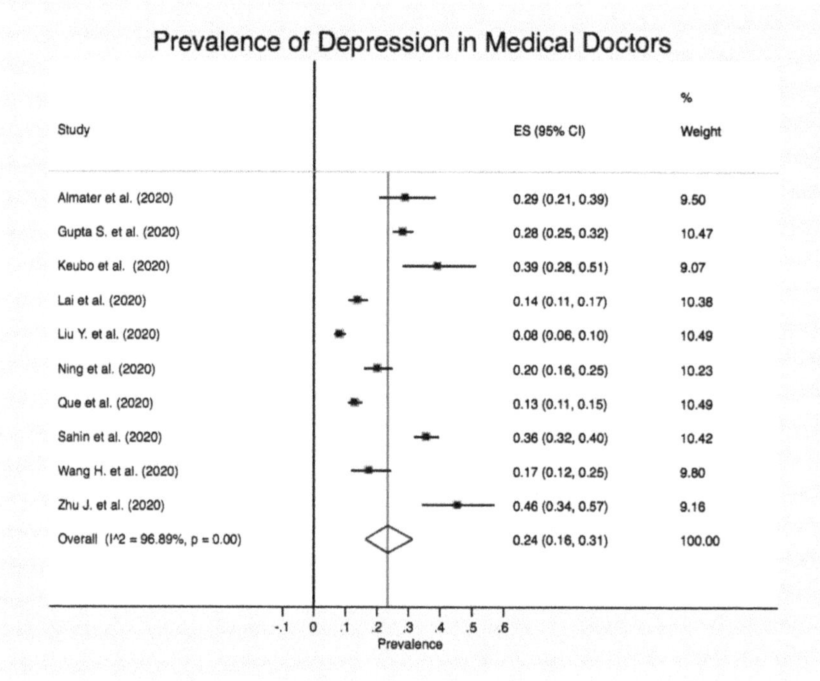

Figure 4. Forest plot for the prevalence of depression among medical doctors.

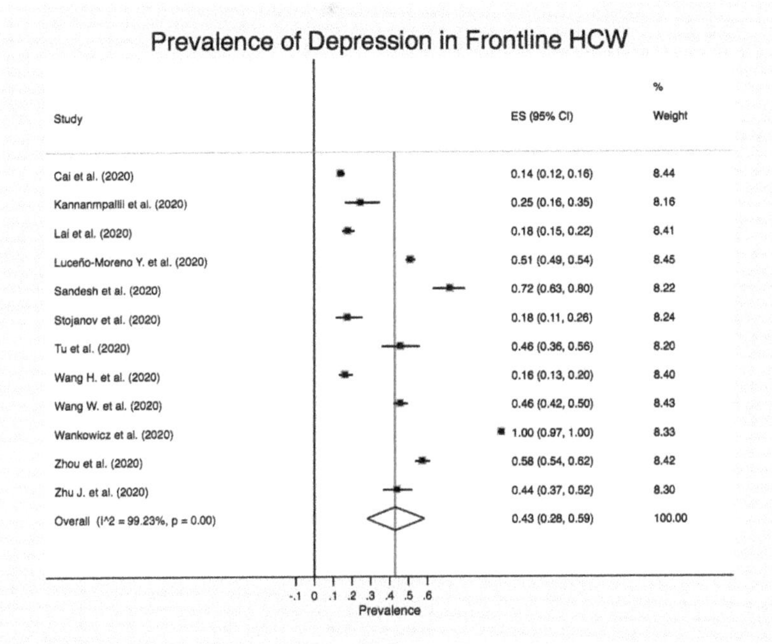

Figure 5. Forest plot for the prevalence of depression among frontline healthcare workers.

Potential sources of heterogeneity were investigated across the studies. Our subgroup analysis showed that prevalence of depression was lower in studies using the DASS-21, those carried out in China, studies using convenience sampling methods and those of high methodological quality (Table 5).

Table 5. Overall prevalence rates of depression according to study characteristics.

	Healthcare Workers			Nurses			Medical Doctors			Frontline Healthcare Workers		
	No. Studies	Prevalence (%) (95% CI)	p *	No. Studies	Prevalence (%) (95% CI)	p *	No. Studies	Prevalence (%) (95% CI)	p *	No. Studies	Prevalence (%) (95% CI)	p *
Depression assessment			0.531			0.636			0.964			0.600
PHQ-9	20	23 (17–29)		7	23 (14–34)		4	22 (11–35)		5	50 (18–81)	
HADS	43	43 (35–51)		4	29 (14–48)		3	27 (18–38)		2	51 (44–58)	
DASS-21	9	16 (9–24)		1	6 (5–8)		1	8 (6–10)		3	37 (19–57)	
SDS	5	26 (20–32)		2	33 (28–38)		2	25 (21–29)		2	32 (27–38)	
CES-D	2	24 (24–25)		-	-		-	-		-	-	
Other (BDI-II/HAMD/GADS)	3	20 (11–31)		-	-		-	-		-	-	
Country			0.087			**0.031**			0.067			0.235
China	23	21 (16–25)		8	21 (15–27)		6	18 (12–24)		7	33 (19–49)	
Other	23	28 (21–36)		6	38 (33–43)		4	32 (27–38)		5	57 (25–86)	
Sampling method			0.803			0.058			0.508			0.900
Convenience	29	23 (19–28)		8	19 (11–27)		7	22 (13–32)		5	38 (21–57)	
Other	7	25 (18–33)		5	34 (21–48)		3	28 (20–36)		3	36 (10–63)	
Quality rating			0.440			0.356			0.314			0.307
Medium (< 7)	11	28 (19–37)		8	29 (15–44)		7	27 (15–40)		5	55 (18–90)	
High (≥ 7)	35	23 (19–27)		6	21 (13–30)		3	18 (12–24)		7	34 (20–50)	

* p value obtained from univariate meta-regression. In bold, significant associations.

The exclusion of studies one-by-one from the analysis did not substantially change the overall prevalence rate of depression. Thus, no single study had a disproportional impact on the overall prevalence (data not shown).

Visual inspection of the funnel plot (Figure 6) suggested a small publication bias for the prevalence estimate in HWC, nurses, and medical doctors, confirmed by significant results in the Egger's test ($p < 0.05$). However, no publication bias was detected for frontline HCW (Egger's test: $p = 0.928$).

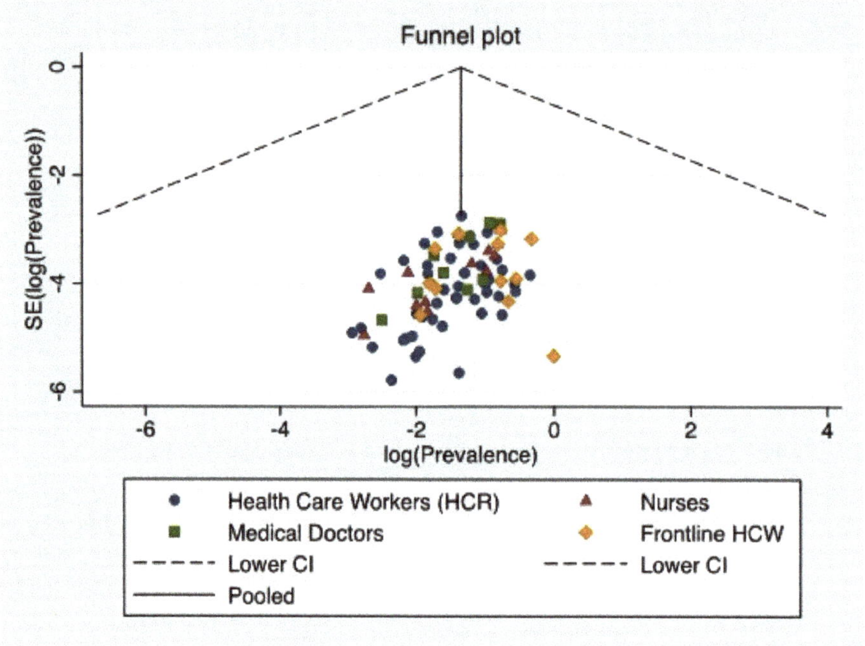

Figure 6. Funnel plot for the prevalence of depression.

4. Discussion

The present systematic review and meta-analysis identified a total of 57 cross-sectional studies reporting rates of depression among HCW. The pooled prevalence rate of depression in HCW was 24%, and when analyzing professional groups, we found that the rates were similar in nurses (25%) and medical doctors (24%), whereas up to 43% of frontline HCW report depression. The overall prevalence of depression found in HCW, nurses and medical doctors is similar to that found in a recent meta-analysis conducted from January 2020 to May 2020. This meta-analysis was based on 12 population-based studies conducted during the COVID-19 outbreak, finding that the overall prevalence was 25% in the general population [81].

Since the outbreak of COVID-19 pandemic in January 2020, the attention paid to the impact on mental health among HCW has grown exponentially, as indicated by the large number of studies found. A recent systematic review and meta-analysis of the prevalence of depression, anxiety, and insomnia among HCW during the pandemic included thirteen studies published up to 17 April 2020. In that study, the pooled prevalence of depression was 22.8%, based on ten studies [14]. A subgroup analysis for different occupational categories found that the pooled prevalence for nurses was 30.3% and for medical doctors 25.9%. These figures are slightly higher than those reported in our meta-analysis. These discrepancies might be explained by the different number of studies included. In the Pappa et al. meta-analysis, only five studies were considered in calculating separate pooled prevalence of depression for nurses and doctors, whereas our study was based on 14 and 10 studies to calculate prevalence depression in nurses and doctors, respectively. Another remarkable difference between the two meta-analyses is the origin of the samples, with the Pappa et al. study mainly focused on a Chinese population. However, our meta-analysis includes a broad range of countries from very different regions worldwide. This regional heterogeneity, along with a greater sample size, allows us to provide an updated estimation of the pooled prevalence of depression among HCW.

Our pooled prevalence of depression found in HCW (25%) is also higher compared with another systematic review and meta-analysis based on samples of HCW that reported a prevalence of 12.2% [15]. The study was conducted April–May 2020 and was based on seven cross-sectional studies, all of them conducted in China. Again, the diversity of the origin of the samples and/or the number of studies included might explain these discrepancies.

Note that all the studies included in our meta-analysis used self-reported standardized questionnaires to assess depressive symptomatology. Additionally, the use of a great variety of scales might have led to differences in the estimation of the presence of depression. In fact, our results show that those studies using the DASS-21 questionnaire reported lower prevalence rates of depression. Despite the convenience of using the same instruments and the inclusion of a diagnosis based on clinical interviews, this is not always possible in epidemiological studies.

Similarly, Muller et al. [82] conducted a rapid systematic review in May 2020 focusing on several outcomes such as mental health problems and risk or resilience factors from quantitative and qualitative data. They found a total of 19 studies, with a percentage of depression ranging from 5% to 51%, and a median of 21%. According to their systematic review, the most common risk factors for mental health problems in HCW were being a woman, being exposed to infected patients, and the worry of being infected.

An important contribution of the present meta-analysis is the calculation of the pooled prevalence of depression in frontline HCW. The prevalence is significantly higher (43%) compared with other types of HCW. The mental toll of working at the frontline during previous pandemic outbreaks, such as that of severe acute respiratory syndrome (SARS) and Middle East respiratory syndrome (MERS), has previously been reported to be high [83,84]. The fear of being infected, stigmatization and uncertainty put these workers under extraordinary stress. A qualitative study conducted among frontline HCW in Wuhan (China) pointed up the intensive work (i.e., long working hours and use of personal protective equipment), fear of infecting others or being infected, managing relationships under stressful situations, and feeling powerless to handle patients' conditions as common experiences during the COVID-19 outbreak [85].

However, factors contributing to increased vulnerability to depression among HCW as well as resilience characteristics (such as coping strategies) might be culturally different. Additionally, inequalities related to health systems and resources across high- and low-income countries might also contribute to the differing impact of COVID-19 on mental health among HCW from diverse settings. Furthermore, note that the first wave of COVID-19 was characterized by a high degree of uncertainty about the illness, its treatment, and its prognosis. Since the outbreak, there has been an intensive international response to fight the virus along with a research agenda aimed at finding effective treatments for infected patients and preventing the spread of the virus (e.g., vaccines). This means that COVID-19 is a rapid, evolving health challenge that requires up-to-date data to ensure appropriate surveillance of mental health, and specifically for vulnerable subpopulations such as HCW.

There are limitations to be considered when interpreting our results. First, the majority of studies included in the present meta-analysis used convenience samples, so representativeness of HCW might be jeopardized. Second, depression was mainly assessed by means of self-reported data drawn from questionnaires, which might have introduced biases such as social desirability [86], as well as being less accurate than clinical interviews. Third, the inclusion of cross-sectional studies makes it difficult to determine causal associations between the pandemic and depression. Fourth, some of the studies included in the calculation of the pooled prevalence for the three groups of HCW (i.e., nurses, medical doctors, and frontline HCW) might have also been included in the calculation of the pooled prevalence for HCW. Thus, caution should be taken when interpreting our results. Fifth, our systematic review was only conducted in a medical database (MEDLINE); thus, some articles, especially those related to psychology, might not be included. Finally, we found some sources of heterogeneity. For example, using convenience sampling methods, conducting studies in China, and using the DASS-21 questionnaire were associated with lower prevalence rates of depression. Related to this, half of the studies were carried out with Chinese samples, so the results of the present meta-analysis should be approached with caution. Future studies should endeavor to investigate the prevalence of depression among HCW in other countries, and use randomized sampling designs whenever possible, as well as longitudinal designs to determine the evolution of mental health problems in this population.

In summary, our meta-analysis shows that depression during the COVID-19 pandemic is a common mental condition among HCW, with the frontline HCW especially affected. A unified response to help HCW during the pandemic should be placed in the international agenda. Comprehensive psychological support, along with regular and intensive training for HCW, can help safeguard their well-being [87]. Common mental problems, such as depression, should be routinely assessed to detect those HCW at high risk of mental disorders and in need of intensive interventions to alleviate their symptomatology.

Supplementary Materials: The following are available online at https://www.mdpi.com/article/10.3390/jcm10153406/s1, Table S1: PRISMA checklist, Table S2: Search strategy in MEDLINE via Pubmed, Table S3: Quality assessment with the JBI Appraisal Checklist for Prevalence Studies.

Author Contributions: Conceptualization, B.O., J.B.-N., and J.S.; methodology, M.P.-M., J.B.-N., P.G.-G., and I.L.; software, J.S.; validation, B.O., J.B.-N., P.G.-G., and J.S.; formal analysis, J.S.; resources, J.S.; data curation, M.P.-M. and J.B.-N.; writing—original draft preparation, B.O., M.P.-M., J.B.-N., and P.G.-G.; writing—review and editing, B.O., J.B.-N., and J.S.; visualization, I.L. and J.S.; supervision, I.L. and J.S.; project administration, B.O. and J.S.; funding acquisition, B.O. All authors have read and agreed to the published version of the manuscript.

Funding: B.O. was supported by the Miguel Servet (CP20/00040) contract, funded by the Instituto de Salud Carlos III and co-funded by the European Union (ERDF/ESF, "Investing in your future").

Institutional Review Board Statement: No institutional approval was necessary for this study.

Informed Consent Statement: Not applicable to this study.

Data Availability Statement: Data sharing is not applicable to this article as no new data were created or analyzed in it.

Conflicts of Interest: We declare that P.G.-G. has received grant support from Janssen, AstraZeneca and the Ilustre Colegio de Médicos de Zaragoza; she has received honoraria from AstraZeneca and Lilly; and she has received travel support from Lilly, Almirall, Lundbeck, Rovi, Pfizer and Janssen-Cilag. None of these activities was related to the current project. The remaining authors declare no conflicts of interest.

References

1. Lu, H.; Stratton, C.W.; Tang, Y.W. Outbreak of pneumonia of unknown etiology in Wuhan, China: The mystery and the miracle. *J. Med. Virol.* **2020**, *92*, 401–402. [CrossRef]
2. World Health Organization (WHO). Director-General's Opening Remarks at the Media Briefing on COVID-19. Available online: https://www.who.int/dg/speeches/detail/who-director-general-s-opening-remarks-at-the-media-briefing-on-covid-19---11-march-2020#.XqySGbWV4O4.mailto (accessed on 12 December 2020).
3. World Health Organization (WHO). *COVID-19 Weekly Epidemiological Update*; World Health Organization (WHO): Geneva, Switzerland, 2020.
4. Campion, J.; Javed, A.; Sartorius, N.; Marmot, M. Addressing the public mental health challenge of COVID-19. *Lancet Psychiatry* **2020**, *7*, 657–659. [CrossRef]

5. Nguyen, L.H.; Drew, D.A.; Graham, M.S.; Joshi, A.D.; Guo, C.G.; Ma, W.; Mehta, R.S.; Warner, E.T.; Sikavi, D.R.; Lo, C.H.; et al. Risk of COVID-19 among front-line health-care workers and the general community: A prospective cohort study. *Lancet Public Health* **2020**, *5*, e475–e483. [CrossRef]
6. Zhang, C.; Yang, L.; Liu, S.; Ma, S.; Wang, Y.; Cai, Z.; Du, H.; Li, R.; Kang, L.; Su, M.; et al. Survey of Insomnia and Related Social Psychological Factors Among Medical Staff Involved in the 2019 Novel Coronavirus Disease Outbreak. *Front. Psychiatry* **2020**, *11*, 306. [CrossRef]
7. Rana, W.; Mukhtar, S.; Mukhtar, S. Mental health of medical workers in Pakistan during the pandemic COVID-19 outbreak. *Asian J. Psychiatry* **2020**, *51*, 102080. [CrossRef]
8. Spoorthy, M.S. Mental health problems faced by healthcare workers due to the COVID-19 pandemic—A review. *Asian J. Psychiatry* **2020**, *51*, 102119. [CrossRef]
9. Grover, S.; Sahoo, S.; Mehra, A.; Avasthi, A.; Tripathi, A.; Subramanyan, A.; Pattojoshi, A.; Rao, G.; Saha, G.; Mishra, K.; et al. Psychological impact of COVID-19 lockdown: An online survey from India. *Indian J. Psychiatry* **2020**, *62*, 354. [CrossRef]
10. Zhang, W.R.; Wang, K.; Yin, L.; Zhao, W.F.; Xue, Q.; Peng, M.; Min, B.Q.; Tian, Q.; Leng, H.X.; Du, J.L.; et al. Mental Health and Psychosocial Problems of Medical Health Workers during the COVID-19 Epidemic in China. *Psychother. Psychosomat.* **2020**, *89*, 242–250. [CrossRef]
11. Shigemura, J.; Ursano, R.J.; Morganstein, J.C.; Kurosawa, M.; Benedek, D.M. Public responses to the novel 2019 coronavirus (2019-nCoV) in Japan: Mental health consequences and target populations. *Psychiatry Clin. Neurosci.* **2020**, *74*, 281–282. [CrossRef]
12. Lu, W.; Wang, H.; Lin, Y.; Li, L. Psychological status of medical workforce during the COVID-19 pandemic: A cross-sectional study. *Psychiatry Res.* **2020**, *288*, 112936. [CrossRef]
13. Liu, Y.; Wang, L.; Chen, L.; Zhang, X.; Bao, L.; Shi, Y. Mental Health Status of Paediatric Medical Workers in China During the COVID-19 Outbreak. *Front. Psychiatry* **2020**, *11*, 702. [CrossRef]
14. Pappa, S.; Ntella, V.; Giannakas, T.; Giannakoulis, V.G.; Papoutsi, E.; Katsaounou, P. Prevalence of depression, anxiety, and insomnia among healthcare workers during the COVID-19 pandemic: A systematic review and meta-analysis. *Brain Behav. Immun.* **2020**, *88*, 901–907. [CrossRef]
15. Da Silva, F.C.T.; Neto, M.L.R. Psychological effects caused by the COVID-19 pandemic in health professionals: A systematic review with meta-analysis. *Prog. Neuro Psychopharmacol. Biol. Psychiatry* **2021**, *104*, 110062. [CrossRef]
16. Moher, D.; Liberati, A.; Tetzlaff, J.; Altman, D.G.; Altman, D.; Antes, G.; Atkins, D.; Barbour, V.; Barrowman, N.; Berlin, J.A.; et al. Preferred reporting items for systematic reviews and meta-analyses: The PRISMA statement. *PLoS Med.* **2009**, *6*, e1000097. [CrossRef] [PubMed]
17. Moola, S.; Munn, Z.; Tufanaru, C.; Aromataris, E.; Sears, K.; Sfetc, R.; Currie, M.; Lisy, K.; Qureshi, R.; Mattis, P.; et al. Chapter 7: Systematic reviews of etiology and risk. In *Joanna Briggs Institute Reviewer's Manual*; Aromataris, E., Munn, Z., Eds.; The Joanna Briggs Institute: Adelaide, Australia, 2017; pp. 219–226.
18. DerSimonian, R.; Laird, N. Meta-analysis in clinical trials. *Control. Clin. Trials* **1986**, *7*, 177–188. [CrossRef]
19. Von Hippel, P.T. The heterogeneity statistic I(2) can be biased in small meta-analyses. *BMC Med. Res. Methodol.* **2015**, *15*, 35. [CrossRef] [PubMed]
20. Higgins, J.P.T.; Thompson, S.G.; Deeks, J.J.; Altman, D.G. Measuring inconsistency in meta-analyses. *BMJ* **2003**, *327*, 557–560. [CrossRef]
21. Thompson, S.G.; Higgins, J.P.T. How should meta-regression analyses be undertaken and interpreted? *Stat. Med.* **2002**, *21*, 1559–1573. [CrossRef]
22. Egger, M.; Schneider, M.; Smith, G.D. Meta-analysis Spurious precision? Meta-analysis of observational studies. *BMJ* **1998**, *316*, 140–144. [CrossRef] [PubMed]
23. Hunter, J.P.; Saratzis, A.; Sutton, A.J.; Boucher, R.H.; Sayers, R.D.; Bown, M.J. In meta-analyses of proportion studies, funnel plots were found to be an inaccurate method of assessing publication bias. *J. Clin. Epidemiol.* **2014**, *67*, 897–903. [CrossRef]
24. Egger, M.; Smith, G.D.; Schneider, M.; Minder, C. Bias in meta-analysis detected by a simple, graphical test. *BMJ* **1997**, *315*, 629–634. [CrossRef]
25. Begg, C.B.; Mazumdar, M. Operating characteristics of a rank correlation test for publication bias. *Biometrics* **1994**, *50*, 1088–1101. [CrossRef]
26. R Development Core Team. *R: A Language and Environment for Statistical Computing*; R Foundation for Statistical Computing: Vienna, Austria, 2019.
27. Di Tella, M.; Romeo, A.; Benfante, A.; Castelli, L. Mental health of healthcare workers during the COVID-19 pandemic in Italy. *J. Eval. Clin. Pract.* **2020**, *26*, 1583–1587. [CrossRef]
28. Dosil Santamaría, M.; Ozamiz-Etxebarria, N.; Redondo Rodríguez, I.; Jaureguizar Alboniga-Mayor, J.; Picaza Gorrotxategi, M. Psychological impact of COVID-19 on a sample of Spanish health professionals. *Rev. Psiquiatr. Salud Ment.* **2020**. [CrossRef]
29. Elbay, R.Y.; Kurtulmuş, A.; Arpacıoğlu, S.; Karadere, E. Depression, anxiety, stress levels of physicians and associated factors in Covid-19 pandemics. *Psychiatry Res.* **2020**, *290*, 113130. [CrossRef]
30. Elhadi, M.; Msherghi, A.; Elgzairi, M.; Alhashimi, A.; Bouhuwaish, A.; Biala, M.; Abuelmeda, S.; Khel, S.; Khaled, A.; Alsoufi, A.; et al. Psychological status of healthcare workers during the civil war and COVID-19 pandemic: A cross-sectional study. *J. Psychosomat. Res.* **2020**, *137*, 110221. [CrossRef]

31. Gallopeni, F.; Bajraktari, I.; Selmani, E.; Tahirbegolli, I.A.; Sahiti, G.; Muastafa, A.; Bojaj, G.; Muharremi, V.B.; Tahirbegolli, B. Anxiety and depressive symptoms among healthcare professionals during the Covid-19 pandemic in Kosovo: A cross sectional study. *J. Psychosomat. Res.* **2020**, *137*, 110212. [CrossRef]
32. Gupta, A.K.; Mehra, A.; Niraula, A.; Kafle, K.; Deo, S.P.; Singh, B.; Sahoo, S.; Grover, S. Prevalence of anxiety and depression among the healthcare workers in Nepal during the COVID-19 pandemic. *Asian J. Psychiatry* **2020**, *54*, 102260. [CrossRef]
33. Gupta, S.; Prasad, A.S.; Dixit, P.K.; Padmakumari, P.; Gupta, S.; Abhisheka, K. Survey of prevalence of anxiety and depressive symptoms among 1124 healthcare workers during the coronavirus disease 2019 pandemic across India. *Med. J. Armed Forces India* **2020**, *77*, S404–S412. [CrossRef]
34. Huang, Y.; Zhao, N. Generalized anxiety disorder, depressive symptoms and sleep quality during COVID-19 outbreak in China: A web-based cross-sectional survey. *Psychiatry Res.* **2020**, *288*, 112954. [CrossRef]
35. Kannampallil, T.G.; Goss, C.W.; Evanoff, B.A.; Strickland, J.R.; McAlister, R.P.; Duncan, J. Exposure to COVID-19 patients increases physician trainee stress and burnout. *PLoS ONE* **2020**, *15*, e0237301. [CrossRef]
36. Keubo, F.R.N.; Mboua, P.C.; Tadongfack, T.D.; Tchoffo, E.F.; Tatang, C.T.; Zeuna, J.I.; Noupoue, E.M.; Tsoplifack, C.B.; Folefack, G.O. Psychological distress among health care professionals of the three COVID-19 most affected Regions in Cameroon: Prevalence and associated factors. In *Annales Medico-Psychologiques, Revue Psychiatrique*; Elsevier Masson: Hoboken, NJ, USA, 2020; Volume 179, pp. 141–146. [CrossRef]
37. Khanna, R.C.; Honavar, S.G.; Metla, A.L.; Bhattacharya, A.; Maulik, P.K. Psychological impact of COVID-19 on ophthalmologists-in-training and practising ophthalmologists in India. *Indian J. Ophthalmol.* **2020**, *68*, 994–998. [CrossRef]
38. Koksal, E.; Dost, B.; Terzi, Ö.; Ustun, Y.B.; Özdin, S.; Bilgin, S. Evaluation of Depression and Anxiety Levels and Related Factors Among Operating Theater Workers During the Novel Coronavirus (COVID-19) Pandemic. *J. Perianesth. Nurs. Off. J. Am. Soc. PeriAnesth. Nurses* **2020**, *35*, 472–477. [CrossRef]
39. Krammer, S.; Augstburger, R.; Haeck, M.; Maercker, A. Adjustment Disorder, Depression, Stress Symptoms, Corona Related Anxieties and Coping Strategies during the Corona Pandemic (COVID-19) in Swiss Medical Staff. *Psychother. Psychosomat. Med. Psychol.* **2020**, *70*, 272–282. [CrossRef]
40. Lai, J.; Ma, S.; Wang, Y.; Cai, Z.; Hu, J.; Wei, N.; Wu, J.; Du, H.; Chen, T.; Li, R.; et al. Factors Associated With Mental Health Outcomes Among Health Care Workers Exposed to Coronavirus Disease 2019. *JAMA Netw. Open* **2020**, *3*, e203976. [CrossRef] [PubMed]
41. Lam, S.C.; Arora, T.; Grey, I.; Suen, L.K.P.; Huang, E.Y.-Z.; Li, D.; Lam, K.B.H. Perceived Risk and Protection From Infection and Depressive Symptoms Among Healthcare Workers in Mainland China and Hong Kong During COVID-19. *Front. Psychiatry* **2020**, *11*, 686. [CrossRef]
42. Li, G.; Miao, J.; Wang, H.; Xu, S.; Sun, W.; Fan, Y.; Zhang, C.; Zhu, S.; Zhu, Z.; Wang, W. Psychological impact on women health workers involved in COVID-19 outbreak in Wuhan: A cross-sectional study. *J. Neurol. Neurosurg. Psychiatry* **2020**, *91*, 895–897. [CrossRef]
43. Liang, Y.; Wu, K.; Zhou, Y.; Huang, X.; Zhou, Y.; Liu, Z. Mental Health in Frontline Medical Workers during the 2019 Novel Coronavirus Disease Epidemic in China: A Comparison with the General Population. *Int. J. Environ. Res. Public Health* **2020**, *17*, 6550. [CrossRef]
44. Lin, K.; Yang, B.X.; Luo, D.; Liu, Q.; Ma, S.; Huang, R.; Lu, W.; Majeed, A.; Lee, Y.; Lui, L.M.W.; et al. The Mental Health Effects of COVID-19 on Health Care Providers in China. *Am. J. Psychiatry* **2020**, *177*, 635–636. [CrossRef]
45. Luceño-Moreno, L.; Talavera-Velasco, B.; García-Albuerne, Y.; Martín-García, J. Symptoms of Posttraumatic Stress, Anxiety, Depression, Levels of Resilience and Burnout in Spanish Health Personnel during the COVID-19 Pandemic. *Int. J. Environ. Res. Public Health* **2020**, *17*, 5514. [CrossRef] [PubMed]
46. Magnavita, N.; Tripepi, G.; Di Prinzio, R.R. Symptoms in Health Care Workers during the COVID-19 Epidemic. A Cross-Sectional Survey. *Int. J. Environ. Res. Public Health* **2020**, *17*, 5218. [CrossRef] [PubMed]
47. Almater, A.; Tobaigy, M.; Younis, A.; Alaqeel, M.; Abouammoh, M. Effect of 2019 coronavirus pandemic on ophthalmologists practicing in Saudi Arabia: A psychological health assessment. *Middle East Afr. J. Ophthalmol.* **2020**, *27*, 79–85. [CrossRef] [PubMed]
48. Naser, A.Y.; Dahmash, E.Z.; Al-Rousan, R.; Alwafi, H.; Alrawashdeh, H.M.; Ghoul, I.; Abidine, A.; Bokhary, M.A.; Al-Hadithi, H.T.; Ali, D.; et al. Mental health status of the general population, healthcare professionals, and university students during 2019 coronavirus disease outbreak in Jordan: A cross-sectional study. *Brain Behav.* **2020**, *10*, e01730. [CrossRef] [PubMed]
49. Ning, X.; Yu, F.; Huang, Q.; Li, X.; Luo, Y.; Huang, Q.; Chen, C. The mental health of neurological doctors and nurses in Hunan Province, China during the initial stages of the COVID-19 outbreak. *BMC Psychiatry* **2020**, *20*, 436. [CrossRef]
50. Pouralizadeh, M.; Bostani, Z.; Maroufizadeh, S.; Ghanbari, A.; Khoshbakht, M.; Alavi, S.A.; Ashrafi, S. Anxiety and depression and the related factors in nurses of Guilan University of Medical Sciences hospitals during COVID-19: A web-based cross-sectional study. *Int. J. Afr. Nurs. Sci.* **2020**, *13*, 100233. [CrossRef] [PubMed]
51. Que, J.; Shi, L.; Deng, J.; Liu, J.; Zhang, L.; Wu, S.; Gong, Y.; Huang, W.; Yuan, K.; Yan, W.; et al. Psychological impact of the COVID-19 pandemic on healthcare workers: A cross-sectional study in China. *Gen. Psychiatry* **2020**, *33*, e100259. [CrossRef] [PubMed]
52. Şahin, M.K.; Aker, S.; Şahin, G.; Karabekiroğlu, A. Prevalence of Depression, Anxiety, Distress and Insomnia and Related Factors in Healthcare Workers During COVID-19 Pandemic in Turkey. *J. Community Health* **2020**, *45*, 1168–1177. [CrossRef] [PubMed]

53. Salopek-Žiha, D.; Hlavati, M.; Gvozdanović, Z.; Gašić, M.; Placento, H.; Jakić, H.; Klapan, D.; Šimić, H. Differences in Distress and Coping with the COVID-19 Stressor in Nurses and Physicians. *Psychiatr. Danub* **2020**, *32*, 287–293. [CrossRef] [PubMed]
54. Sandesh, R.; Shahid, W.; Dev, K.; Mandhan, N.; Shankar, P.; Shaikh, A.; Rizwan, A. Impact of COVID-19 on the Mental Health of Healthcare Professionals in Pakistan. *Cureus* **2020**, *12*, e8974. [CrossRef] [PubMed]
55. Si, M.Y.; Su, X.Y.; Jiang, Y.; Wang, W.J.; Gu, X.F.; Ma, L.; Li, J.; Zhang, S.K.; Ren, Z.F.; Ren, R.; et al. Psychological impact of COVID-19 on medical care workers in China. *Infect. Dis. Poverty* **2020**, *9*, 113. [CrossRef] [PubMed]
56. Song, X.; Fu, W.; Liu, X.; Luo, Z.; Wang, R.; Zhou, N.; Yan, S.; Lv, C. Mental health status of medical staff in emergency departments during the Coronavirus disease 2019 epidemic in China. *Brain Behav. Immun.* **2020**, *88*, 60–65. [CrossRef] [PubMed]
57. Stojanov, J.; Malobabic, M.; Stanojevic, G.; Stevic, M.; Milosevic, V.; Stojanov, A. Quality of sleep and health-related quality of life among health care professionals treating patients with coronavirus disease-19. *Int. J. Soc. Psychiatry* **2020**, *67*, 175. [CrossRef]
58. An, Y.; Yang, Y.; Wang, A.; Li, Y.; Zhang, Q.; Cheung, T.; Ungvari, G.S.; Qin, M.-Z.; An, F.-R.; Xiang, Y.-T. Prevalence of depression and its impact on quality of life among frontline nurses in emergency departments during the COVID-19 outbreak. *J. Affect. Disord.* **2020**, *276*, 312–315. [CrossRef] [PubMed]
59. Suryavanshi, N.; Kadam, A.; Dhumal, G.; Nimkar, S.; Mave, V.; Gupta, A.; Cox, S.R.; Gupte, N. Mental health and quality of life among healthcare professionals during the COVID-19 pandemic in India. *Brain Behav.* **2020**, *10*, e01837. [CrossRef]
60. Teng, Z.; Huang, J.; Qiu, Y.; Tan, Y.; Zhong, Q.; Tang, H.; Wu, H.; Wu, Y.; Chen, J. Mental health of front-line staff in prevention of coronavirus disease 2019. *Zhong Nan Da Xue Xue Bao Yi Xue Ban J. Cent. South Univ. Med. Sci.* **2020**, *45*, 613–619. [CrossRef]
61. Teo, W.Z.Y.; Soo, Y.E.; Yip, C.; Lizhen, O.; Chun-Tsu, L. The psychological impact of COVID-19 on "hidden" frontline healthcare workers. *Int. J. Soc. Psychiatry* **2020**, 284–289. [CrossRef] [PubMed]
62. Tu, Z.H.; He, J.W.; Zhou, N. Sleep quality and mood symptoms in conscripted frontline nurse in Wuhan, China during COVID-19 outbreak: A cross-sectional study. *Medicine* **2020**, *99*, e20769. [CrossRef]
63. Vanni, G.; Materazzo, M.; Santori, F.; Pellicciaro, M.; Costesta, M.; Orsaria, P.; Cattadori, F.; Pistolese, C.A.; Perretta, T.; Chiocchi, M.; et al. The Effect of Coronavirus (COVID-19) on Breast Cancer Teamwork: A Multicentric Survey. *In Vivo* **2020**, *34*, 1685–1694. [CrossRef]
64. Wang, H.; Huang, D.; Huang, H.; Zhang, J.; Guo, L.; Liu, Y.; Ma, H.; Geng, Q. The psychological impact of COVID-19 pandemic on medical staff in Guangdong, China: A cross-sectional study. *Psychol. Med.* **2020**, 1–9. [CrossRef]
65. Wang, L.Q.; Zhang, M.; Liu, G.M.; Nan, S.Y.; Li, T.; Xu, L.; Xue, Y.; Wang, L.; Qu, Y.D.; Liu, F. Psychological impact of coronavirus disease (2019) (COVID-19) epidemic on medical staff in different posts in China: A multicenter study. *J. Psychiatr. Res.* **2020**, *129*, 198–205. [CrossRef]
66. Wang, S.; Xie, L.; Xu, Y.; Yu, S.; Yao, B.; Xiang, D. Sleep disturbances among medical workers during the outbreak of COVID-2019. *Occup. Med.* **2020**, *70*, 364–369. [CrossRef]
67. Wang, W.; Song, W.; Xia, Z.; He, Y.; Tang, L.; Hou, J.; Lei, S. Sleep Disturbance and Psychological Profiles of Medical Staff and Non-Medical Staff During the Early Outbreak of COVID-19 in Hubei Province, China. *Front. Psychiatry* **2020**, *11*, 733. [CrossRef]
68. Wańkowicz, P.; Szylińska, A.; Rotter, I. Assessment of Mental Health Factors among Health Professionals Depending on Their Contact with COVID-19 Patients. *Int. J. Environ. Res. Public Health* **2020**, *17*, 5849. [CrossRef] [PubMed]
69. Cai, Q.; Feng, H.; Huang, J.; Wang, M.; Wang, Q.; Lu, X.; Xie, Y.; Wang, X.; Liu, Z.; Hou, B.; et al. The mental health of frontline and non-frontline medical workers during the coronavirus disease 2019 (COVID-19) outbreak in China: A case-control study. *J. Affect. Disord.* **2020**, *275*, 210–215. [CrossRef]
70. Xiao, X.; Zhu, X.; Fu, S.; Hu, Y.; Li, X.; Xiao, J. Psychological impact of healthcare workers in China during COVID-19 pneumonia epidemic: A multi-center cross-sectional survey investigation. *J. Affect. Disord.* **2020**, *274*, 405–410. [CrossRef] [PubMed]
71. Xiaoming, X.; Ming, A.; Su, H.; Wo, W.; Jianmei, C.; Qi, Z.; Hua, H.; Xuemei, L.; Lixia, W.; Jun, C.; et al. The psychological status of 8817 hospital workers during COVID-19 Epidemic: A cross-sectional study in Chongqing. *J. Affect. Disord.* **2020**, *276*, 555–561. [CrossRef] [PubMed]
72. Xiong, H.; Yi, S.; Lin, Y. The Psychological Status and Self-Efficacy of Nurses During COVID-19 Outbreak: A Cross-Sectional Survey. *Inquiry* **2020**, *57*, 46958020957114. [CrossRef]
73. Yang, S.; Kwak, S.G.; Ko, E.J.; Chang, M.C. The Mental Health Burden of the COVID-19 Pandemic on Physical Therapists. *Int. J. Environ. Res. Public Health* **2020**, *17*, 3723. [CrossRef]
74. Zhou, Y.; Wang, W.; Sun, Y.; Qian, W.; Liu, Z.; Wang, R.; Qi, L.; Yang, J.; Song, X.; Zhou, X.; et al. The prevalence and risk factors of psychological disturbances of frontline medical staff in china under the COVID-19 epidemic: Workload should be concerned. *J. Affect. Disord.* **2020**, *277*, 510–514. [CrossRef]
75. Zhu, J.; Sun, L.; Zhang, L.; Wang, H.; Fan, A.; Yang, B.; Li, W.; Xiao, S. Prevalence and Influencing Factors of Anxiety and Depression Symptoms in the First-Line Medical Staff Fighting Against COVID-19 in Gansu. *Front. Psychiatry* **2020**, *11*, 386. [CrossRef]
76. Zhu, Z.; Xu, S.; Wang, H.; Liu, Z.; Wu, J.; Li, G.; Miao, J.; Zhang, C.; Yang, Y.; Sun, W.; et al. COVID-19 in Wuhan: Sociodemographic characteristics and hospital support measures associated with the immediate psychological impact on healthcare workers. *EClinicalMedicine* **2020**, *24*, 100443. [CrossRef]
77. Chen, J.; Liu, X.; Wang, D.; Jin, Y.; He, M.; Ma, Y.; Zhao, X.; Song, S.; Zhang, L.; Xiang, X.; et al. Risk factors for depression and anxiety in healthcare workers deployed during the COVID-19 outbreak in China. *Soc. Psychiatry Psychiatr. Epidemiol.* **2020**, *56*, 47–55. [CrossRef] [PubMed]

78. Chen, Y.; Zhou, H.; Zhou, Y.; Zhou, F. Prevalence of self-reported depression and anxiety among pediatric medical staff members during the COVID-19 outbreak in Guiyang, China. *Psychiatry Res.* **2020**, *288*, 113005. [CrossRef]
79. Chew, N.W.S.; Lee, G.K.H.; Tan, B.Y.Q.; Jing, M.; Goh, Y.; Ngiam, N.J.H.; Yeo, L.L.L.; Ahmad, A.; Ahmed Khan, F.; Napolean Shanmugam, G.; et al. A multinational, multicentre study on the psychological outcomes and associated physical symptoms amongst healthcare workers during COVID-19 outbreak. *Brain. Behav. Immun.* **2020**, *88*, 559–565. [CrossRef] [PubMed]
80. Dal'Bosco, E.B.; Messias Floriano, L.S.; Skupien, S.V.; Arcaro, G.; Martins, A.R.; Correa Anselmo, A.C. Mental health of nursing in coping with COVID-19 at a regional university hospital. *Rev. Bras. Enferm.* **2020**, *73*. [CrossRef]
81. Bueno-Notivol, J.; Gracia-García, P.; Olaya, B.; Lasheras, I.; López-Antón, R.; Santabárbara, J. Prevalence of depression during the COVID-19 outbreak: A meta-analysis of community-based studies. *Int. J. Clin. Health Psychol.* **2020**, 21–100196. [CrossRef]
82. Muller, A.E.; Hafstad, E.V.; Himmels, J.P.W.; Smedslund, G.; Flottorp, S.; Stensland, S.; Stroobants, S.; Van de Velde, S.; Vist, G.E. The mental health impact of the covid-19 pandemic on healthcare workers, and interventions to help them: A rapid systematic review. *medRxiv* **2020**. [CrossRef]
83. Wu, P.; Fang, Y.; Guan, Z.; Fan, B.; Kong, J.; Yao, Z.; Liu, X.; Fuller, C.J.; Susser, E.; Lu, J.; et al. The psychological impact of the SARS epidemic on hospital employees in China: Exposure, risk perception, and altruistic acceptance of risk. *Can. J. Psychiatry* **2009**, *54*, 302–311. [CrossRef] [PubMed]
84. Lee, S.M.; Kang, W.S.; Cho, A.R.; Kim, T.; Park, J.K. Psychological impact of the 2015 MERS outbreak on hospital workers and quarantined hemodialysis patients. *Compr. Psychiatry* **2018**, *87*, 123–127. [CrossRef]
85. Liu, Q.; Luo, D.; Haase, J.E.; Guo, Q.; Wang, X.Q.; Liu, S.; Xia, L.; Liu, Z.; Yang, J.; Yang, B.X. The experiences of health-care providers during the COVID-19 crisis in China: A qualitative study. *Lancet Glob. Health* **2020**, *8*, e790–e798. [CrossRef]
86. Ahmed, M.Z.; Ahmed, O.; Aibao, Z.; Hanbin, S.; Siyu, L.; Ahmad, A. Epidemic of COVID-19 in China and associated Psychological Problems. *Asian J. Psychiatry* **2020**, *51*, 102092. [CrossRef] [PubMed]
87. Tomlin, J.; Dalgleish-Warburton, B.; Lamph, G. Psychosocial Support for Healthcare Workers During the COVID-19 Pandemic. *Front. Psychol.* **2020**, *11*, 1960. [CrossRef] [PubMed]

Journal of
Clinical Medicine

MDPI

Article

Influence of the Cumulative Incidence of COVID-19 Cases on the Mental Health of the Spanish Out-of-Hospital Professionals

Raúl Soto-Cámara [1,2,3], Susana Navalpotro-Pascual [3,4,5,*], José Julio Jiménez-Alegre [3,4,6], Noemí García-Santa-Basilia [2,3], Henar Onrubia-Baticón [2,3], José M. Navalpotro-Pascual [3,4], Israel John Thuissard [3,7], Juan José Fernández-Domínguez [3,4,7,8], María Paz Matellán-Hernández [2,3], Elena Pastor-Benito [3,4], Carlos Eduardo Polo-Portes [3,4,7], Rosa M. Cárdaba-García [2,3,9,*] and on behalf of the IMPSYCOVID-19 Study Group †

1 Department of Health Sciences, University of Burgos, 09001 Burgos, Spain; rscamara@ubu.es (R.S.-C.); ngarcia@saludcastillayleon.es (N.G.-S.-B.); monrubia@saludcastillayleon.es (H.O.-B.); mmatellanh@saludcastillayleon.es (M.P.M.-H.)
2 Emergency Medical Service of Castilla y León—Sacyl, 47007 Valladolid, Spain
3 Red de Investigación de Emergencias Prehospitalarias (RINVEMER), Sociedad Española de Urgencias y Emergencias (SEMES), 28020 Madrid, Spain; juljimal@gmail.com (J.J.J.-A.); chemanp@gmail.com (J.M.N.-P.); israeljohn.thuissard@universidadeuropea.es (I.J.T.); jjfernandezd@gmail.com (J.J.F.-D.); elenapastorbenito@gmail.com (E.P.-B.); carlospolo1763@hotmail.com (C.E.P.-P.)
4 Emergency Medical Service of Madrid—SUMMA 112, 28045 Madrid, Spain
5 Nursing Department, Faculty of Medicine, Autonomous University of Madrid, 28029 Madrid, Spain
6 Faculty of Medicine, Alfonso X El Sabio University, 28691 Madrid, Spain
7 Department of Medicine, Faculty of Biomedical and Health Sciences, European University of Madrid, 28670 Madrid, Spain
8 Emergency Service, HLA Moncloa University Hospital, 28008 Madrid, Spain
9 Nursing Department, Faculty of Nursing, University of Valladolid, 47005 Valladolid, Spain
* Correspondence: snavalpotro@gmail.com (S.N.-P.); rosamaria.cardaba@uva.es (R.M.C.-G.)
† Membership of the IMPSYCOVID-19 Study Group: Juan Francisco Bejarano-Ramírez, María Elena Castejón-de-la-Encina, Fernando de-Miguel-Saldaña, Patricia Fernán-Pérez, Rafael Martín-Sánchez, Carmen María Martínez-Caballero, Beatriz Merino-Reguera, María Molina-Oliva, Almudena Morales-Sánchez, Marta Moya-Rodríguez-Carretero, Ana María Requés-Marugán, Leticia Sánchez-del-Río.

Citation: Soto-Cámara, R.; Navalpotro-Pascual, S.; Jiménez-Alegre, J.J.; García-Santa-Basilia, N.; Onrubia-Baticón, H.; Navalpotro-Pascual, J.M.; Thuissard, I.J.; Fernández-Domínguez, J.J.; Matellán-Hernández, M.P.; Pastor-Benito, E.; et al. Influence of the Cumulative Incidence of COVID-19 Cases on the Mental Health of the Spanish Out-of-Hospital Professionals. *J. Clin. Med.* **2022**, *11*, 2227. https://doi.org/10.3390/jcm11082227

Academic Editor: Mauro Giovanni Carta

Received: 29 March 2022
Accepted: 13 April 2022
Published: 15 April 2022

Abstract: This study aimed to analyze the psychological affectation of health professionals (HPs) of Spanish Emergency Medical Services (EMSs) according to the cumulative incidence (CI) of COVID-19 cases in the regions in which they worked. A cross-sectional descriptive study was designed, including all HPs working in any EMS of the Spanish geography between 1 February 2021 and 30 April 2021. Their level of stress, anxiety and depression (DASS-21) and the perception of self-efficacy (G-SES) were the study's main results. A 2-factor analysis of covariance was used to determine if the CI regions of COVID-19 cases determined the psychological impact on each of the studied variables. A total of 1710 HPs were included. A third presented psychological impairment classified as severe. The interaction of CI regions with the studied variables did not influence their levels of stress, anxiety, depression or self-efficacy. Women, younger HPs or those with less EMS work experience, emergency medical technicians (EMT), workers who had to modify their working conditions or those who lived with minors or dependents suffered a greater impact from the COVID-19 pandemic in certain regions. These HPs have shown high levels of stress, anxiety, depression and medium levels of self-efficacy, with similar data in the different geographical areas. Psychological support is essential to mitigate their suffering and teach them to react to adverse events.

Keywords: coronavirus infections; health personnel; emergency medical services; psychological stress; anxiety; depression; self-efficacy; incidence

1. Introduction

The declaration of the disease caused by the virus SARS-CoV-2, named COVID-19, as "The Sixth International Public Health Emergency" and the proclamation of the resulting situation as a pandemic by the World Health Organization (WHO) has produced important changes at the economic, social and health levels in all countries [1,2]. As in other areas, in Spain, this affectation has not remained uniform over time but has fluctuated depending on the cumulative incidence (CI) of cases in the different waves and geographical regions. For this, the Center for the Coordination of Health Alerts and Emergencies of the Ministry of Health and the National Epidemiological Surveillance Network of the National Center for Epidemiology of the Carlos III Health Institute have been designated as the organizations in charge of collecting CI information in the different Spanish regions and monitoring possible change from the start of the COVID-19 pandemic to the present [3,4].

During this period, numerous studies have analyzed the impact of the COVID-19 pandemic on the mental health of the general population and certain sectors [5,6]. Health professionals (HPs) have been among the most affected groups, focusing most of this research on primary care or hospital workers and specific national care models [7–11]. HPs have faced very intense and stressful work situations, such as work overload, prolonged work shifts, fewer hours of rest, no clear and defined protocols for action, strict safety instructions and measures, the constant need for concentration and vigilance, the lack of personal protective equipment and reduced social contact, as well as having to perform tasks for which many professionals have not been prepared [12,13]. This situation of stress has put both the physical and mental health of the HPs at risk. Their general well-being has been altered, and they have started to show high levels of anxiety and depression, other emotional disorders, sleep problems, difficulty in interpersonal relations, dysfunctional cognitive reactions, substances use behaviors, post-traumatic stress, and even vicarious traumatization stemming from compassion towards the patients that they were treating [14–17].

Generally, emergency medical service (EMS) is the department in charge of out-of-hospital care for critically ill patients in most countries. During the COVID-19 pandemic, this service had had to develop new policies, procedures, and protocols to address the consequences of this epidemiological situation, characterized by an increase in the volume of calls and the care of patients with suspected signs or confirmed cases [18]. However, the specific scientific research referring to out-of-hospital EMSs has been very limited [18,19], even though they continue to be one of the frontline healthcare providers. Like HPs in other settings, the findings of these studies have shown a negative impact of the COVID-19 pandemic on the mental health of out-of-hospital workers, with an increase in the prevalence of disorders due to stress, anxiety, depression, insomnia or burnout [18,19].

For all these reasons, the objective of the present study was to analyze the level of psychological affectation of the HPs of the Spanish EMSs, according to the CI of COVID-19 cases of the geographical regions in which they worked.

2. Materials and Methods

2.1. Study Design-Participants

A cross-sectional descriptive study was designed. The study population was all HPs working in any EMS in the Spanish geography between 1 February and 30 April 2021. Not accepting voluntary participation in the study or not completing the entire questionnaire were considered exclusion criteria.

For the estimation of the sample size, it was considered that 23,467 HPs worked in EMS in Spain in 2020, according to data from the Statistical Portal of the Primary Care Information System of the Ministry of Health [20]. It was necessary to recruit at least 1066 subjects to achieve a confidence level of 95% and an accuracy of 3%, considering a 15% possible loss.

2.2. Procedure—Data Collection

Participants were selected using non-probabilistic snowball sampling. An online questionnaire was used for data collection. The link to the questionnaire was distributed through the Prehospital Emergency Research Network (RINVEMER) of the Spanish Society of Emergency Medicine (SEMES) and the managers of the different EMSs. In the first part of the questionnaire, the participants were informed of the characteristics and objectives of the study and its anonymous and voluntary nature. Its completed return implied the person's informed consent to participate in the research. To guarantee the anonymity of the HPs, no personal data was collected that could allow their identification, even in those cases in which they specifically requested feedback on the results obtained, for which a personal alphanumeric code was created. Participants could withdraw from the study at any time without giving any reason. The time required to answer the questionnaire was approximately 15–20 min. All doubts were resolved by email.

The research protocol was approved by the Medicine Ethics and Research Committee of the East Valladolid Health Area (PI-20-2052), respecting the principles of the Declaration of Helsinki and its successive revisions [21].

2.3. Main Outcomes—Instruments

The study's main results were the level of stress, anxiety and depression of the HPs and their perception of self-efficacy.

The reduced version of the Depression Anxiety Stress Scale (DASS-21) was used as a self-reported instrument to assess the intensity of 21 different symptoms associated with a negative emotional state [22]. It consists of 3 subscales, with 7 items each one: (i) stress, which evaluates tension, irritability, nervousness, impatience, agitation, and negative affect; (ii) anxiety, which assesses physiological activation, musculoskeletal symptoms and subjective sensation of anxiety; and (iii) depression, which evaluates hopelessness, dysphoria, sadness, anhedonia, low self-esteem, and low positive affect. The HPs must indicate the frequency with which they have experienced these symptoms in the previous 2 weeks using a 4-point Likert scale (0: Never; 3: Always). In each subscale, the total score is obtained by adding the points of each item and multiplying it by 2. The score of the subscales ranges between 0 and 42, so the higher the value, the greater the degree of symptomatology. Similarly, this score can be categorized as normal, mild, moderate, severe or extremely severe. Its adaptation and validation to the Spanish population were carried out by Bados et al., with acceptable psychometric properties [23]. It has been widely used to assess the psychological impact of the COVID-19 pandemic on the general population [6] and HPs [18] as it has good discriminant validity in screening for mental disorders [24].

To evaluate the person's perception of their ability to adequately handle different stressful situations, the Spanish adaptation of the General Self-Efficacy Scale (G-SES) was used [25,26]. It is made up of 10 items, with 10 response options (1: Never; 10: Always). The score ranges between 10 and 100, associating higher values with greater perceived self-efficacy. It presents good psychometric properties, with predictive capacity on coping styles, and internal consistency of 0.87 [26].

Other variables were also collected through an ad hoc questionnaire: sex, age, living with minors or dependent persons, professional category, previous work experience in EMS, change in working conditions, previous diagnosis of COVID-19 or CI of COVID-19 cases. For analytical purposes and based on the CI per 100,000 inhabitants defined by the Health Authorities on 1 February 2021, the Spanish geography was divided into 3 areas: region with low CI if $\leq$4999 cases, region with medium CI if 5000–6999 cases, and region with high CI if $\geq$7000 cases [27] (Figure 1).

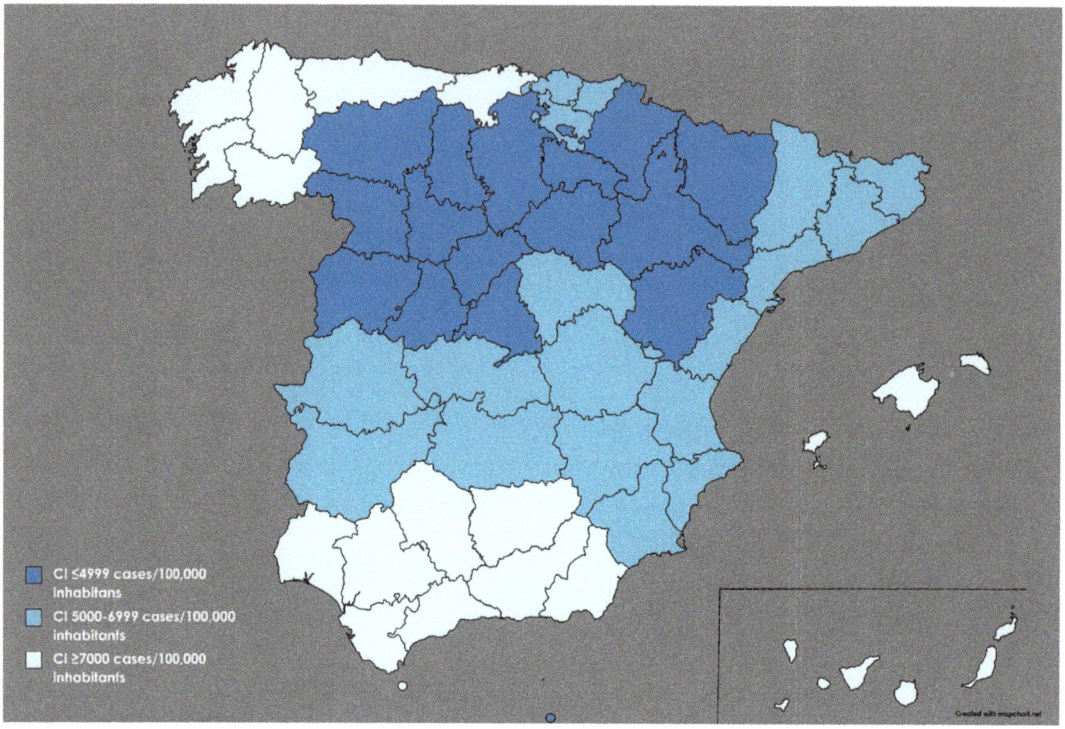

Figure 1. Distribution of the CI regions of COVID-19 cases per 100,000 inhabitants.

2.4. Statistical Analysis

Categorical variables were summarized as absolute frequencies and percentages, while quantitative ones were in terms of mean and standard deviation (SD). The compliance of the normality criteria of the quantitative variables was evaluated using the Kolmogorov–Smirnov test; in those cases in which they did not follow a normal distribution, the criteria proposed by Blanca et al. were considered [28]. To contrast the levels of stress, anxiety, depression and self-efficacy in regions with the same CI of COVID-19 cases or between the 3 regions considered, the χ^2 test, the Student's *t*-test for independent samples, the one-way analysis of variance or the Pearson's correlation were calculated, depending on the nature of the variables. For multiple comparisons, post hoc tests were corrected by Bonferroni adjustment. In addition, to find out if the different regions were a determining factor in the psychological impact of each of the variables, a 2-factor analysis of covariance (study variables × region) was performed. Statistical significance was considered if $p < 0.05$. Statistical analysis was carried out with SPSS version 25.0 software (IBM-Inc, Chicago, IL, USA).

3. Results

The sample consisted of 1710 participants; 50.58% were women, with a mean age of 43.54 years (SD ± 9.94). The most represented professional category was emergency medical technicians (EMT) (n = 765), followed by doctors (n = 474) and nurses (n = 453), with a mean work experience in EMS of 15.22 years (SD ±9.15). In relation to the mental health of these HPs, 37.39% (n = 639), 39.36% (n = 673) and 30.46% (n = 521) presented levels of stress, anxiety and depression categorized as severe or extremely severe. The mean scores obtained in stress, anxiety, depression and self-efficacy were 20.61 (SD ± 11.08), 13.08

(SD ± 11.17), 15.74 (SD ± 11.11) and 70.78 (SD ± 15.75), respectively. The distribution of their descriptive characteristics in the different CI regions is summarized in Table 1.

Table 1. Descriptive characteristics of the sample based on the CI of COVID-19 cases from the different regions.

	Regions		
	Low CI	**Medium CI**	**High CI**
Sex			
Male	250 (14.62)	330 (19.30)	265 (15.50)
Female	261 (15.26)	315 (18.42)	289 (16.90)
Age (years)	43.57 ± 9.71	42.76 ± 10.42	44.42 ± 9.50
Professional category			
Physician	151 (8.83)	183 (10.70)	140 (8.19)
Nurse	152 (8.89)	157 (9.18)	144 (8.42)
EMT	204 (11.93)	303 (17.72)	258 (15.09)
Others	3 (0.18)	4 (0.23)	11 (0.64)
EMS work experience (years)	15.00 ± 9.09	14.89 ± 9.45	15.80 ± 8.83
Change of working conditions			
Yes	286 (16.72)	344 (20.12)	290 (16.96)
No	224 (13.10)	302 (17.66)	264 (15.44)
Previous diagnosis of COVID-19			
Yes	442 (25.85)	468 (27.37)	407 (23.80)
No	85 (4.97)	147 (8.60)	161 (9.41)
Living with minors/dependents			
Yes	270 (15.79)	363 (21.23)	283 (16.55)
No	234 (13.68)	274 (16.02)	286 (16.73)
Stress	21.10 ±10.94	20.86 ± 10.76	19.88 ± 11.56
Anxiety	13.34 ± 11.08	13.16 ± 11.00	12.74 ± 11.46
Depression	16.19 ± 10.50	15.77 ± 11.17	15.31 ± 11.58
Self-efficacy	71.24 ± 15.31	70.42 ± 15.34	70.81 ± 16.62

Values are expressed as mean ± standard deviation or frequencies (percentages). Abbreviations: CI—Cumulative Incidence; EMT—Emergency Medical Technicians; EMS—Emergency Medical Service; COVID-19—Coronavirus Disease-19.

In areas with medium or high CI, women presented greater stress, anxiety, and depression; men who worked in areas with low CI reported less stress than those employed in areas with a higher number of COVID-19 cases. Regarding self-efficacy, men perceived higher values in areas with low CI. The interaction of gender and region did not affect the psychological variables analyzed (Table 2).

Table 2. Level of stress, anxiety, depression and self-efficacy according to sex and the CI regions of COVID-19 cases.

Regions	**Sex**		***p*-Value (Sex × Region)**
	Male	**Female**	
	Stress		
Low CI	20.23 ± 11.17 [&,a]	20.01 ± 10.61	
Medium CI	18.92 ± 10.49 [***,&]	22.87 ± 10.70 [***]	0.135
High CI	17.71 ± 11.67 [**,&,a]	21.94 ± 11.05 [**]	
	Anxiety		
Low CI	12.36 ± 11.22 [*]	14.33 ± 10.87 [*]	
Medium CI	11.76 ± 10.45 [**]	14.57 ± 11.35 [**]	0.442
High CI	10.83 ± 11.13 [**]	14.54 ± 11.49 [**]	
	Depression		
Low CI	15.66 ± 10.68	16.75 ± 10.28	
Medium CI	14.69 ± 10.62 [**]	16.85 ± 11.62 [**]	0.155
High CI	13.41 ± 11.11 [***]	17.10 ± 11.72 [***]	
	Self-efficacy		
Low CI	73.34 ± 14.60 [**]	69.46 ± 15.32 [**]	
Medium CI	71.32 ± 15.28	69.54 ± 15.37	0.282
High CI	71.23 ± 16.66	70.33 ± 16.55	

Values are expressed as mean ± standard deviation. Abbreviation: CI—Cumulative Incidence. * $p < 0.05$ between sexes in the same CI region. ** $p < 0.01$ between sexes in the same CI region. *** $p < 0.001$ between sexes in the same CI region. & $p < 0.05$ between CI regions in the same sex. [a] $p < 0.05$ in the post-hoc analysis (Bonferroni test).

EMTs who worked in regions with low or high CI reported negative emotional states compatible with stress or depression more frequently than other professional categories. Their anxiety levels were also significantly higher in the three areas, regardless of the number of COVID-19 cases. The professional category and region combination did not influence the mean scores obtained on the DASS-21 and the G-SES (Table 3).

Table 3. Level of stress, anxiety, depression and self-efficacy according to professional categories and the CI regions of COVID-19 cases.

Regions	Professional Categories				p-Value (Category × Region)
	Physician	Nurse	EMT	Other	
			Stress		
Low CI	18.36 ± 10.70 ^{**,a}	20.12 ± 10.70 **	23.08 ± 11.30 ^{**,a}	16.67 ± 8.33 **	
Medium CI	19.82 ± 10.80	21.08 ± 10.64	21.36 ± 10.84	21.00 ± 6.00	0.413
High CI	18.77 ± 11.41 **	18.11 ± 11.76 ^{**,b}	21.64 ± 11.27 ^{**,b}	16.18 ± 12.79 **	
			Anxiety		
Low CI	11.89 ± 10.28 ^{**,a}	10.66 ± 10.25 ^{**,b}	16.35 ± 11.50 ^{**,a,b}	8.00 ± 5.29 **	
Medium CI	11.96 ± 10.7 *	11.66 ± 10.65 ^{*,b}	14.65 ± 11.20 ^{*,b}	13.50 ± 9.00 *	0.701
High CI	10.96 ± 11.18 ^{***,a}	10.49 ± 11.27 ^{***,b}	15.00 ± 11.30 ^{***,a,b}	11.64 ± 12.80 ***	
			Depression		
Low CI	14.76 ± 11.19 ^{**,a}	15.07 ± 10.50 **	18.12 ± 10.42 ^{**,a}	6.67 ± 1.15 **	
Medium CI	14.89 ± 11.89	14.57 ± 10.87	16.90 ± 11.12	17.00 ± 8.41	0.504
High CI	13.97 ± 11.07 ^{**,a}	13.64 ± 12.05 ^{**,b}	17.18 ± 11.44 ^{**,a,b}	10.18 ± 8.65 **	
			Self-efficacy		
Low CI	70.17 ± 16.19	72.48 ± 14.19	71.83 ± 15.43	78.00 ± 7.55	
Medium CI	70.31 ± 14.70	70.43 ± 15.96	70.59 ± 15.36	59.50 ± 20.29	0.192
High CI	70.80 ± 17.42	72.80 ± 16.18	69.45 ± 16.53	77.00 ± 11.17	

Values are expressed as mean ± standard deviation. Abbreviation: CI—Cumulative Incidence; EMT—Emergency Medical Technicians. * $p < 0.05$ between professional categories in the same CI region. ** $p < 0.01$ between professional categories in the same CI region. *** $p < 0.001$ between professional categories in the same CI region. [a,b] $p < 0.05$ in the post-hoc analysis (Bonferroni test).

HPs who were forced to change their work schedule, location, or dedication reported higher levels of stress, anxiety and depression in the three regions of CI. When the psychological impact of the COVID-19 pandemic was analyzed, considering the need or not for changes in working conditions, it was concluded that the different regions were not a determining factor (Table 4).

Table 4. Level of stress, anxiety, depression and self-efficacy according to change in working conditions and the CI regions of COVID-19 cases.

Regions	Change of Working Conditions		p-Value (Change × Region)
	Yes	No	
	Stress		
Low CI	22.32 ± 10.68 *	19.74 ± 11.14 *	
Medium CI	22.55 ± 10.42 ***	18.91 ± 10.85 ***	0.359
High CI	21.98 ± 11.60 ***	17.60 ± 11.09 ***	
	Anxiety		
Low CI	14.34 ± 10.94 *	12.15 ± 11.15 *	
Medium CI	14.95 ± 11.28 ***	11.14 ± 10.37 ***	0.408
High CI	14.50 ± 11.92 ***	10.78 ± 10.65 ***	
	Depression		
Low CI	17.40 ± 10.63 **	14.69 ± 10.16 **	
Medium CI	16.97 ± 11.29 **	14.41 ± 11.94 **	0.501
High CI	17.18 ± 11.85 ***	13.22 ± 10.94 ***	
	Self-efficacy		
Low CI	70.77 ± 15.65	71.80 ± 14.93	
Medium CI	69.56 ± 15.51	71.36 ± 15.16	0.876
High CI	69.89 ± 16.69	71.87 ± 16.54	

Values are expressed as mean ± standard deviation. Abbreviation: CI—Cumulative Incidence. * $p < 0.05$ between professional categories in the same CI region. ** $p < 0.01$ between professional categories in the same CI region. *** $p < 0.001$ between professional categories in the same CI region.

Having a previous diagnosis of COVID-19 or living with minors and/or dependents was not related to significant changes in the values of stress, anxiety, depression and self-efficacy, except for a higher level of anxiety among those HPs with vulnerable dependents in regions with low CI. In both cases, when the interaction of these variables with the CI region was analyzed, no influence was observed on the psychological parameters (Tables 5 and 6).

Table 5. Level of stress, anxiety, depression and self-efficacy according to the previous diagnosis of COVID-19 and the CI regions of COVID-19 cases.

Regions	Previous Diagnosis of COVID-19		p-Value (Diagnosis × Region)
	Yes	No	
		Stress	
Low CI	20.95 ± 10.77	22.72 ± 11.33	
Medium CI	20.18 ± 10.76	22.03 ± 9.74	0.695
High CI	19.39 ± 11.72	20.56 ± 11.07	
		Anxiety	
Low CI	13.10 ± 10.84	15.61 ± 11.77	
Medium CI	12.41 ± 10.86	14.07 ± 10.49	0.790
High CI	12.32 ± 11.54	13.53 ± 11.57	
		Depression	
Low CI	16.25 ± 10.51	16.69 ± 9.95	
Medium CI	15.12 ± 11.08	16.98 ± 10.91	0.740
High CI	14.87 ± 11.71	15.94 ± 11.44	
		Self-efficacy	
Low CI	70.59 ± 14.82	74.48 ± 15.37	
Medium CI	69.87 ± 15.30	70.72 ± 15.38	0.329
High CI	70.83 ± 17.15	70.80 ± 14.96	

Values are expressed as mean ± standard deviation. Abbreviation: COVID-19—Coronavirus Disease-19; CI—Cumulative Incidence.

Table 6. Level of stress, anxiety, depression and self-efficacy according to living with minors/dependents and the CI regions of COVID-19 cases.

Regions	Living with Minors/Dependents		p-Value (Minor/Dependent × Region)
	Yes	No	
		Stress	
Low CI	20.37 ± 10.60	22.52 ± 11.26	
Medium CI	20.14 ± 10.78	21.78 ± 10.56	0.674
High CI	19.45 ± 11.33	20.18 ± 11.68	
		Anxiety	
Low CI	12.43 ± 10.39 *	14.77 ± 11.64 *	
Medium CI	12.57 ± 10.97	13.94 ± 11.03	0.260
High CI	12.63 ± 10.99	11.69 ± 11.82	
		Depression	
Low CI	16.33 ± 10.31	16.21 ± 10.61	
Medium CI	15.91 ± 11.53	15.62 ± 10.91	0.959
High CI	15.51 ± 11.49	14.99 ± 11.63	
		Self-efficacy	
Low CI	71.14 ± 15.15	70.78 ± 15.84	
Medium CI	70.01 ± 15.42	70.94 ± 15.30	0.520
High CI	69.96 ± 16.95	71.86 ± 15.99	

Values are expressed as mean ± standard deviation. Abbreviation: CI—Cumulative Incidence. * $p < 0.05$ between professional categories in the same CI region.

Both HPs' age and EMS work experience were indirectly and weakly correlated with stress levels, anxiety, depression and self-efficacy, regardless of the number of COVID-19 cases in the region they worked (Table 7).

Table 7. Level of stress, anxiety, depression and self-efficacy according to age, EMS work experience and the CI regions of COVID-19 cases.

	Regions	Stress	Anxiety	Depression	Self-Efficacy
Age	Low CI	−0.109 *	−0.104 *	−0.097 *	0.001
	Medium CI	−0.140 ***	−0.176 ***	−0.183 ***	−0.045
	High CI	−0.087 *	−0.101 *	−0.109 **	−0.028
EMS work experience	Low CI	−0.099 *	−0.122 **	−0.094 *	0.085
	Medium CI	−0.144 ***	−0.150 ***	0.206 ***	0.002
	High CI	−0.087 *	−0.133 **	−0.092 *	−0.008

Values are expressed as Spearman's r. Abbreviation: IA—Cumulative Incidence; EMS: Emergency Medical Service; * $p < 0.05$. ** $p < 0.01$. *** $p < 0.001$.

4. Discussion

This study is proposed to identify the impact of the COVID-19 pandemic on the mental health of HPs in Spanish EMSs and its influence on certain socio-demographic and labor variables, according to the number of cases registered in each region. The interaction of the CI regions with the other study variables considered has not altered the levels of stress, anxiety, depression and self-efficacy of the HPs, unlike what was observed by Brillon et al. [29]. However, in certain regions, a greater impact of the COVID-19 pandemic was observed on women, younger HPs or those with less EMS work experience, EMTs, workers who had to modify their working conditions or those who lived with minors or dependents.

Around a third of the participants presented severe or extremely severe levels of stress, anxiety and depression, data higher than those reported by HPs from other care settings [9,30–32]. Working on the front line, in areas where the unpredictability of the attended cases is greater or in environments with a high probability of contagion, as is the case of the EMSs, is becoming a risk factor for the development of negative responses to challenging situations [33,34]. The high number of HPs with scores in psychopathological alarm ranges should be considered a warning sign of the future psychosocial consequences of the acute phase of the COVID-19 pandemic, such as post-traumatic stress or burnout [35,36].

In this study, the levels of stress, anxiety or depression of the HPs have not been influenced by the number of COVID-19 cases declared in the different geographical areas. However, several authors have shown the existence of an "epicentric effect," which explains a higher prevalence of these psychological conditions the closer the HPs are to the most affected regions [29,34,37–40]. Continuous exposure to stressful elements for long periods of time, lack of social support, or living the same reality as the patients have contributed to exacerbating this effect among HPs from regions with high CI [29].

A higher level of stress and emotional burden has been observed in women who worked in regions with medium or high CI and lower use of coping strategies. The less time dedicated to self-care or self-compassion and the high work pressure during the health emergency has led to the appearance and maintenance of this situation [41,42]. All this has been favored by factors such as gender discrimination, the progressive feminization of the health sector, the difficulties in reconciling work and family, the traditional assumption of the role of primary caregiver at home, the lack of sufficient support systems, the greater empathy in providing care, or the greater ability to express feelings to others and develop emotional responses to stressful events [41,43–47]. The lower psychological affectation of men, especially in regions with low CI, is related to their relative underreporting of symptoms and underuse of health services [48,49] and the widespread use of coping strategies focused on the problem. These strategies limit the ability to recognize their emotional difficulties and become aware of their own experiences [50].

Younger HPs and those with less EMS work experience were more vulnerable to developing symptoms compatible with stress, anxiety, or depression disorders, regardless of geographic area. Some authors have speculated that these workers, whatever their professional role, have less self-confidence and less resistance at a psychological level, and a greater degree of uncertainty in how to act in unforeseen and/or complex situations [37,41,51,52].

The psychological well-being of all participants has been affected during the COVID-19 pandemic. This finding suggests their great personal and emotional involvement, being more notable in the EMTs who worked in areas with low and high CI. The lesser affectation of doctors and nurses could be related to the use of coping strategies based on intellectualization and denial and greater resistance to somatization, related to personal achievements, professional experience or self-awareness [53,54].

The modification of working conditions increased the vulnerability of HPs to stress, anxiety and depression in all regions. The reorganization and restructuring of the EMSs and the adaptation of the workplace for health reasons may be the main causes of these changes. The sudden outbreak of COVID-19 has caused unpredictable changes in the work of HPs, with an increase in the demand for care, greater contact with patients suffering from serious and complex diseases, a reduction in rest times and a lack of socio-occupational support [29,55,56]. To deal with this situation, the EMSs have created units specifically dedicated to the care of patients with COVID-19 and have moved part of the HPs from one job to another [29,52]. The adaptation of these displaced HPs to this new context, in constant change, has caused them an additional mental burden [52]. On the other hand, some authors have observed a greater impact of the COVID-19 pandemic on HPs whose workplace had to be adapted. Among the possible explanations for this result are fear and lack of information about the interaction of their previous diseases with SARS-CoV-2 infection and its possible consequences in the medium and long term [57–60]. Furthermore, HPs with previous mental diseases are more likely to present this type of psychological symptoms [61].

Only HPs who lived with vulnerable people in regions with low CI had higher anxiety levels. This finding can be attributed to the fear of becoming infected and the consequent risk of transmitting the disease to their relatives [9,31,62].

The psychological discomfort of HPs must be considered beyond a merely individual level, as it directly impacts patient care. The most distressed HPs participate less in the therapeutic relationship, make more mistakes and even compromise clinical results [40]. Based on this premise, the need for health authorities to design psychological support strategies in which HPs reflect on their psycho-emotional reactions to adverse events is reinforced [63].

These results must be interpreted within the context of their limitations. It has not been possible to determine a causal relationship between variables due to the study's cross-sectional nature. Psychological distress has been assessed only through self-report measures administered online, limiting access to HPs less accustomed to the use of new technologies. The use of non-probabilistic snowball sampling may have induced a self-selection bias by favoring the participation of HPs who are particularly sensitive to the issue and those who have a greater degree of affectation. Data collection lasted 12 weeks. This fact may have affected the quality of the responses since the CI of COVID-19 cases, and the perception related to the infection have differed between the first and last day. The lack of studies on this topic in the out-of-hospital setting has hindered comparing and contrasting the results obtained. Among its strengths is the collection of data from a large sample of HPs from all EMSs of the Spanish geography and the use of validated questionnaires with excellent psychometric properties.

5. Conclusions

The HPs from the Spanish EMSs present high levels of stress, anxiety, depression and medium levels of self-efficacy. Similar data were observed in different geographical areas. A greater impact of the COVID-19 pandemic has been observed on women, younger HPs or those with less EMS work experience, EMTs, workers who had to modify their working conditions or those who lived with minors or dependents in certain regions. In these HPs, psychological support is essential to mitigate their suffering, helping them to reflect on their psycho-emotional reactions to adverse events.

Author Contributions: Conceptualization, R.S.-C. and S.N.-P.; methodology, R.S.-C., S.N.-P., J.J.J.-A., N.G.-S.-B., H.O.-B. and J.M.N.-P.; software, R.S.-C., J.M.N.-P. and I.J.T.; validation, R.S.-C., S.N.-P. and R.M.C.-G.; formal analysis, R.S.-C., S.N.-P., J.J.J.-A., N.G.-S.-B., H.O.-B., J.M.N.-P., I.J.T., J.J.F.-D., M.P.M.-H., E.P.-B., C.E.P.-P. and R.M.C.-G.; investigation, R.S.-C., S.N.-P., J.J.J.-A., N.G.-S.-B., H.O.-B., J.M.N.-P., I.J.T., J.J.F.-D., M.P.M.-H., E.P.-B., C.E.P.-P. and R.M.C.-G.; resources, J.J.F.-D. and S.N.-P.; writing—original draft preparation, R.S.-C., S.N.-P., J.J.J.-A., N.G.-S.-B., H.O.-B. and J.M.N.-P.; writing—review and editing, R.S.-C., R.M.C.-G. and S.N.-P.; visualization, R.S.-C., S.N.-P., J.J.J.-A., N.G.-S.-B., H.O.-B., J.M.N.-P., I.J.T., J.J.F.-D., M.P.M.-H., E.P.-B., C.E.P.-P. and R.M.C.-G.; supervision, R.S.-C. and S.N.-P.; project administration, S.N.-P.; funding acquisition, J.J.F.-D. and S.N.-P. All authors have read and agreed to the published version of the manuscript.

Funding: This research was funded by Fundación ASISA and Sociedad Española de Urgencias y Emergencias (SEMES).

Institutional Review Board Statement: The study was conducted in accordance with the Declaration of Helsinki and approved by the Institutional Review Board of East Valladolid Health Area (PI-20-2052).

Informed Consent Statement: Informed consent was obtained from all subjects involved in the study.

Data Availability Statement: Data for this study are available by contacting the corresponding authors.

Acknowledgments: European University of Madrid (Spain), for the statistical analysis.

Conflicts of Interest: The authors declare no conflict of interest. The funders had no role in the design of the study; in the collection, analyses, or interpretation of data; in the writing of the manuscript, or in the decision to publish the results.

References

1. WHO Director-General's Opening Remarks at the Media Briefing on COVID-19. 11 March 2020. World Health Organization (WHO). Available online: https://www.who.int/director-general/speeches/detail/who-director-general-s-opening-remarks-at-the-media-briefing-on-covid-19---11-march-2020 (accessed on 29 September 2021).
2. García-Iglesias, J.J.; Gómez-Salgado, J.; Martín-Pereira, J.; Fagundo-Rivera, J.; Ayuso-Murillo, D.; Martínez-Riera, J.R.; Ruiz-Frutos, C. Impact of SARS-CoV-2 (COVID-19) on the Mental Health of Healthcare Professionals: A Systematic Review. *Rev. Esp. Salud Publica* **2020**, *94*, e202007088. [PubMed]
3. Centro de Coordinación de Alertas y Emergencias Sanitarias. Actualización nº 580—Enfermedad por el Coronavirus (COVID-19). Ministerio de Sanidad. Available online: https://www.sanidad.gob.es/profesionales/saludPublica/ccayes/alertasActual/nCov/documentos/Actualizacion_580_COVID-19.pdf (accessed on 9 March 2022).
4. Centro Nacional de Epidemiología. Instituto de Salud Carlos III. Available online: https://www.isciii.es/QueHacemos/Servicios/VigilanciaSaludPublicaRENAVE/Paginas/default.aspx (accessed on 9 March 2022).
5. Xiong, J.; Lipsitz, O.; Nasri, F.; Lui, L.M.W.; Gill, H.; Phan, L.; Chen-Li, D.; Iacobucci, M.; Ho, R.; Majeed, A.; et al. Impact of COVID-19 Pandemic on Mental Health in the General Population: A Systematic Review. *J. Affect. Disord.* **2020**, *277*, 55–64. [CrossRef] [PubMed]
6. Rodríguez-Fernández, P.; González-Santos, J.; Santamaría-Peláez, M.; Soto-Cámara, R.; Sánchez-González, E.; González-Bernal, J.J. Psychological Effects of Home Confinement and Social Distancing Derived from COVID-19 in the General Population—A Systematic Review. *Int. J. Environ. Res. Public Health* **2021**, *18*, 6528. [CrossRef] [PubMed]
7. Torrente, M.; Sousa, P.A.C.; Sánchez-Ramos, A.; Pimentao, J.; Royuela, A.; Franco, F.; Collazo-Lorduy, A.; Menasalvas, E.; Provencio, M. To Burn-Out or Not to Burn-Out: A Cross-Sectional Study in Healthcare Professionals in Spain during COVID-19 Pandemic. *BMJ Open* **2021**, *11*, e044945. [CrossRef]
8. Luceño Moreno, L.; Talavera Velasco, B.; García Albuerne, Y.; Martín García, J. Symptoms of Posttraumatic Stress, Anxiety, Depression, Levels of Resilience and Burnout in Spanish Health Personnel during the COVID-19 Pandemic. *Int. J. Environ. Res. Public Health* **2020**, *17*, 5514. [CrossRef]
9. Dosil Santamaría, M.; Ozamiz-Etxebarria, N.; Redondo Rodríguez, I.; Jaureguizar Alboniga-Mayor, J.; Picaza Gorrotxategi, M. Psychological Impact of COVID-19 on a Sample of Spanish Health Professionals. *Rev. Psiquiatr. Salud Ment.* **2021**, *14*, 106–112. [CrossRef]
10. González-Sanguino, C.; Ausín, B.; Castellanos, M.A.; Saiz, J.; López-Gómez, A.; Ugidos, C.; Muñoz, C. Mental Health Consequences during the Initial Stage of the 2020 Coronavirus Pandemic (COVID-19) in Spain. *Brain Behav. Immun.* **2020**, *87*, 172–176. [CrossRef]

11. Alonso, J.; Vilagut, G.; Mortier, P.; Ferrer, M.; Alayo, I.; Aragón-Peña, A.; Aragonés, E.; Campos, M.; Cura-González, I.D.; Emparanza, J.I. Mental Health Impact of the First Wave of COVID-19 Pandemic on Spanish Healthcare Workers: A Large Cross-Sectional Survey. *Rev. Psiquiatr. Salud Ment.* **2021**, *14*, 90–105. [CrossRef]
12. Vieta, E.; Pérez, V.; Arango, C. Psychiatry in the Aftermath of COVID-19. *Rev. Psiquiatr. Salud Ment.* **2020**, *13*, 105–110. [CrossRef]
13. Brooks, S.K.; Webster, R.K.; Smith, L.E.; Woodland, L.; Wessely, S.; Greenberg, N.; Rubin, G.J. The Psychological Impact of Quarantine and How to Reduce It: Rapid Review of the Evidence. *Lancet* **2020**, *395*, 912–920. [CrossRef]
14. Shreffler, J.; Petrey, J.; Huecker, M. The Impact of COVID-19 on Healthcare Worker Wellness: A Scoping Review. *West. J. Emerg. Med.* **2020**, *21*, 1059–1066. [CrossRef]
15. Vindegaard, N.; Benros, M.E. COVID-19 Pandemic and Mental Health Consequences: Systematic Review of the Current Evidence. *Brain Behav. Immun.* **2020**, *89*, 531–542. [CrossRef]
16. Pappa, S.; Ntella, V.; Giannakas, T.; Giannakoulis, V.G.; Papoutsi, E.; Katsaounou, P. Prevalence of Depression, Anxiety, and Insomnia among Healthcare Workers during the COVID-19 Pandemic: A Systematic Review and Meta-analysis. *Brain Behav. Immun.* **2020**, *88*, 901–907. [CrossRef]
17. Luan, R.; Pu, W.; Dai, L.; Yang, R.; Wang, P. Comparison of Psychological Stress Levels and Associated Factors among Healthcare Workers, Frontline Workers, and the General Public during the Novel Coronavirus Pandemic. *Front. Psychiatry* **2020**, *11*, 583971. [CrossRef]
18. Soto-Cámara, R.; García-Santa-Basilia, N.; Onrubia-Baticón, H.; Cárdaba-García, R.M.; Jiménez-Alegre, J.J.; Requés-Marugán, A.M.; Molina-Oliva, M.; Fernández-Domíguez, J.J.; Matellán-Hernandez, M.P.; Morales-Sánchez, A.; et al. Psychological Impact of the COVID-19 Pandemic on Out-of-Hospital Health Professionals: A Living Systematic Review. *J. Clin. Med.* **2021**, *10*, 5578. [CrossRef]
19. Martínez-Caballero, C.M.; Cárdaba-García, R.M.; Varas-Manovel, R.; García-Sanz, L.M.; Martínez-Piedra, J.; Fernández-Carbajo, J.J.; Pérez-Pérez, L.; Madrigal-Fernández, M.A.; Barba-Pérez, M.A.; Olea, E.; et al. Analyzing the Impact of COVID-19 Trauma on Developing Post-Traumatic Stress Disorder among Emergency Medical Workers in Spain. *Int. J. Environ. Res. Public Health* **2021**, *18*, 9132. [CrossRef]
20. Sistema de información de Atención Primaria (SIAP). Ministerio de Sanidad. Available online: https://pestadistico.inteligenciadegestion.mscbs.es/publicoSNS/C/sistema-de-informacion-de-atencion-primaria-siap/urgencias-y-emergencias-112-061/profesionales (accessed on 9 March 2022).
21. World Medical Association. World Medical Association Declaration of Helsinki Ethical Principles for Medical Research Involving Human Subjects. *J. Am. Med. Ass.* **2013**, *310*, 2191–2194. [CrossRef]
22. Lovibond, P.F.; Lovibond, S.H. The Structure of Negative Emotional States: Comparison of the Depression Anxiety Stress Scales (DASS) with the Beck Depression and Anxiety Inventories. *Behav. Res. Ther.* **1995**, *33*, 335–343. [CrossRef]
23. Bados, A.; Solanas, R.; Andrés, R. Psychometric Properties of the Spanish Version of Depression, Anxiety and Stress Scales (DASS). *Psicothema* **2005**, *17*, 679–683.
24. Mitchell, M.C.; Burns, N.R.; Dorstyn, D.S. Screening for Depression and Anxiety in Spinal Cord Injury with DASS-21. *Spinal Cord.* **2008**, *46*, 547–551. [CrossRef]
25. Baessler, J.; Schwarcer, R. Evaluación de la Autoeficacia: Adaptación Española de la Escala de Autoeficacia General. *Ansiedad Estrés* **1996**, *2*, 1–8.
26. Sanjuán Suárez, P.; Pérez García, A.M.; Bermúdez Moreno, J. Escala de Autoeficacia General: Datos Psicométricos de la Adaptación para Población Española. *Psicothema* **2000**, *12*, 509–513.
27. Centro de Coordinación de Alertas y Emergencias Sanitarias. Actualización nº 302—Enfermedad por el coronavirus (COVID-19). Ministerio de Sanidad. 2022. Available online: https://www.mscbs.gob.es/profesionales/saludPublica/ccayes/alertasActual/nCov/documentos/Actualizacion_302_COVID-19.pdf (accessed on 9 March 2022).
28. Blanca, M.J.; Alarcón, R.; Arnau, J.; Bono, R.; Bendayan, R. Non-Normal Data: Is ANOVA still a Valid Option? *Psicothema* **2017**, *29*, 552–557. [CrossRef] [PubMed]
29. Brillon, P.; Philippe, F.L.; Paradis, A.; Geoffroy, M.C.; Orri, M.; Ouellet-Morin, I. Psychological Distress of Mental Health Workers during the COVID-19 Pandemic: A Comparison with the General Population in High- and Low-Incidence Regions. *J. Clin. Psychol.* **2021**, *78*, 602–621. [CrossRef]
30. Hammond, N.E.; Crowe, L.; Abbenbroek, B.; Elliott, R.; Tian, D.H.; Donaldson, L.H.; Fitzgerald, E.; Flower, O.; Grattan, S.; Harris, R.; et al. Impact of the Coronavirus Disease 2019 Pandemic on Critical Care Healthcare Workers' Depression, Anxiety, and Stress Levels. *Aust. Crit. Care* **2021**, *34*, 146–154. [CrossRef]
31. Hammami, A.S.; Jellazi, M.; Mahjoub, L.; Fedhila, M.; Ouali, S. Psychological Impact of the COVID-19 Pandemic on Healthcare Professionals in Tunisia: Risk and Protective Factors. *Front. Psychol.* **2021**, *12*, 754047. [CrossRef]
32. Hummel, S.; Oetjen, N.; Du, J.; Posenato, E.; Resende de Almeida, R.M.; Losada, R.; Ribeiro, O.; Frisardi, V.; Hopper, L.; Rashid, A.; et al. Mental Health among Medical Professionals during the COVID-19 Pandemic in Eight European Countries: Cross-Sectional Survey Study. *J. Med. Internet Res.* **2021**, *23*, e24983. [CrossRef]
33. Kang, L.; Li, Y.; Hu, S.; Chen, M.; Yang, C.; Yang, B.X.; Wang, Y.; Hu, J.; Lai, J.; Ma, X.; et al. The Mental Health of Medical Workers in Wuhan, China Dealing With the 2019 Novel Coronavirus. *Lancet Psychiatry* **2020**, *7*, e14. [CrossRef]
34. Lai, J.; Ma, S.; Wang, Y.; Cai, Z.; Hu, J.; Wei, N.; Wu, J.; Du, H.; Chen, T.; Li, R.; et al. Factors Associated with Mental Health Outcomes among Health Care Workers Exposed to Coronavirus Disease 2019. *JAMA Netw. Open* **2020**, *3*, e203976. [CrossRef]

35. Vagni, M.; Maiorano, T.; Giostra, V.; Pajardi, D. Coping with COVID-19: Emergency Stress, Secondary Trauma and Self-efficacy in Healthcare and Emergency Workers in Italy. *Front. Psychol.* **2020**, *11*, 566912. [CrossRef]
36. Vagni, M.; Maiorano, T.; Giostra, V.; Pajardi, D. Protective Factors against Emergency Stress and Burnout in Healthcare and Emergency Workers during Second Wave of COVID-19. *Soc. Sci.* **2021**, *10*, 178. [CrossRef]
37. Romero, C.S.; Delgado, C.; Catalá, J.; Ferrer, C.; Errando, C.; Iftimi, A.; Benito, A.; de-Andrés, J.; Otero, M. COVID-19 Psychological Impact in 3109 Healthcare Workers in Spain: The PSIMCOV Group. *Psychol. Med.* **2020**, *52*, 1–7. [CrossRef]
38. Carmassi, C.; Dell'Oste, V.; Bui, E.; Foghi, C.; Bertelloni, C.A.; Atti, A.R.; Buselli, R.; di Paolo, M.; Goracci, A.; Malacarne, P.; et al. The Interplay between Acute Post-traumatic Stress, Depressive and Anxiety Symptoms on Healthcare Workers Functioning during the COVID-19 Emergency: A Multicenter Study Comparing Regions with Increasing Pandemic Incidence. *J. Affect. Disord.* **2022**, *298 Pt A*, 209–216. [CrossRef]
39. Carmassi, C.; Foghi, C.; Dell'Oste, V.; Cordone, A.; Bertelloni, C.A.; Bui, E.; Dell´Osso, L. PTSD Symptoms in Healthcare Workers Facing the Three Coronavirus Outbreaks: What Can We Expect after the COVID-19 Pandemic. *Psychiatry Res.* **2020**, *292*, 113312. [CrossRef]
40. Conti, C.; Fontanesi, L.; Lanzara, R.; Rosa, I.; Porcelli, P. Fragile Heroes. The Psychological Impact of the COVID-19 Pandemic on Health-care Workers in Italy. *PLoS ONE* **2020**, *15*, e0242538. [CrossRef]
41. Mullen, K. Barriers to Work-life Balance for Hospital Nurses. *Workplace Health Saf.* **2015**, *63*, 96–99. [CrossRef]
42. Trockel, M.T.; Hamidi, M.S.; Menon, N.K.; Rowe, S.G.; Dudley, J.C.; Stewart, M.T.; Geisler, C.Z.; Bohman, B.D.; Shanafelt, T.D. Self-valuation: Attending to the Most Important Instrument in the Practice of Medicine. *Mayo Clin. Proc.* **2019**, *94*, 2022–2031. [CrossRef]
43. Greinacher, A.; Nikendei, A.; Kottke, R.; Wiesbeck, J.; Herzog, W.; Nikendei, C. Secondary Traumatization, Psychological Stress, and Resilience in Psychosocial Emergency Care Personnel. *Int. J. Environ. Res. Public Health* **2019**, *16*, 3213. [CrossRef]
44. Mansueto, G.; Lopes, F.L.; Grassi, L.; Cosci, F. Impact of COVID-19 Outbreak on Italian Healthcare Workers versus General Population: Results from an Online Survey. *Clin. Psychol. Psychother.* **2021**, *28*, 1334–1345. [CrossRef]
45. Rossi, R.; Socci, V.; Pacitti, F.; Di Lorenzo, G.; Di Marco, A.; Siracusano, A.; Rossi, A. Mental Health Outcomes among Frontline and Second-line Health Care Workers during the Coronavirus Disease 2019 (COVID-19) Pandemic in Italy. *JAMA Netw. Open* **2020**, *3*, e2010185. [CrossRef]
46. Sanford, J.; Agrawal, A.; Miotto, K. Psychological Distress among Women Healthcare Workers: A Health System's Experience Developing Emotional Support Services during the COVID-19 Pandemic. *Front. Glob. Womens Health* **2021**, *2*, 614723. [CrossRef] [PubMed]
47. Robinson, G.E. Stresses on Women Physicians: Consequences and Coping Techniques. *Depress. Anxiety* **2003**, *17*, 180–189. [CrossRef] [PubMed]
48. Galdas, P.M.; Cheater, F.; Marshall, P. Men and Health Help-seeking Behaviour: Literature Review. *J. Adv. Nurs.* **2005**, *49*, 616–623. [CrossRef] [PubMed]
49. Seidler, Z.E.; Dawes, A.J.; Rice, S.M.; Oliffe, J.L.; Dhillon, H.M. The Role of Masculinity in Men's help-seeking for Depression: A Systematic Review. *Clin. Psychol. Rev.* **2016**, *49*, 106–118. [CrossRef]
50. Kelly, M.M.; Tyrka, A.R.; Price, L.H.; Carpenter, L.L. Sex Differences in the Use of Coping Strategies: Predictors of Anxiety and Depressive Symptoms. *Depress. Anxiety* **2008**, *25*, 839–846. [CrossRef]
51. Huang, Y.; Zhao, N. Generalized Anxiety Disorder, Depressive Symptoms and Sleep Quality during COVID-19 Outbreak in China: A Web-based Cross-sectional Survey. *Psychiatry Res.* **2020**, *288*, 112954. [CrossRef]
52. Su, Q.; Ma, X.; Liu, S.; Liu, S.; Goodman, B.A.; Yu, M.; Guo, W. Adverse Psychological Reactions and Psychological Aids for Medical Staff during the COVID-19 Outbreak in China. *Front. Psychiatry* **2021**, *12*, 580067. [CrossRef]
53. Zwack, J.; Schweitzer, J. If Every Fifth Physician is Affected by Burnout, What about the Other Four? Resilience Strategies of Experienced Physicians. *Acad. Med.* **2013**, *88*, 382–389. [CrossRef]
54. Luo, M.; Guo, L.; Yu, M.; Jiang, W.; Wang, H. The Psychological and Mental Impact of Coronavirus Disease 2019 (COVID-19) on Medical Staff and General Public—A Systematic Review and Meta-analysis. *Psychiatry Res.* **2020**, *291*, 113190. [CrossRef]
55. Liu, S.; Yang, L.; Zhang, C.; Xiang, Y.T.; Liu, Z.; Hu, S.; Zhang, B. Online Mental Health Services in China during the COVID-19 Outbreak. *Lancet Psychiatry* **2020**, *7*, e17–e18. [CrossRef]
56. Wu, W.; Zhang, Y.; Wang, P.; Zhang, L.; Wang, G.; Lei, G.; Xiao, O.; Cao, X.; Bian, Y.; Xie, S.; et al. Psychological Stress of Medical Staffs during Outbreak of COVID-19 and Adjustment Strategy. *J. Med. Virol.* **2020**, *92*, 1962–1970. [CrossRef]
57. Zhang, W.R.; Wang, K.; Yin, L.; Zhao, W.F.; Xue, Q.; Peng, M.; Min, B.Q.; Tian, Q.; Leng, H.X.; Du, J.L.; et al. Mental Health and Psychosocial Problems of Medical Health Workers during the COVID-19 Epidemic in China. *Psychother. Psychosom.* **2020**, *89*, 242–250. [CrossRef]
58. Wei, Y.Y.; Wang, R.R.; Zhang, D.W.; Tu, Y.H.; Chen, C.S.; Ji, S.; Li, C.X.; Li, X.Y.; Zhou, M.X.; Cao, W.S.; et al. Risk Factors for Severe COVID-19: Evidence from 167 Hospitalized Patients in Anhui, China. *J. Infect.* **2020**, *81*, e89–e92. [CrossRef]
59. Wolff, D.; Nee, S.; Hickey, N.S.; Marschollek, M. Risk Factors for Covid-19 Severity and Fatality: A Structured Literature Review. *Infection* **2021**, *49*, 15–28. [CrossRef]
60. Zhu, Z.; Xu, S.; Wang, H.; Liu, Z.; Wu, J.; Li, G.; Miao, J.; Zhang, C.; Yang, Y.; Sun, W.; et al. COVID-19 in Wuhan: Sociodemographic Characteristics and Hospital Support Measures Associated with the Immediate Psychological Impact on Healthcare Workers. *EClinicalMedicine* **2020**, *24*, 100443. [CrossRef]

61. Young, K.P.; Kolcz, D.L.; O'Sullivan, D.M.; Ferrand, J.; Fried, J.; Robinson, K. Health Care Workers' Mental Health and Quality of Life During COVID-19: Results from a Mid-pandemic, National Survey. *Psychiatr. Serv.* **2021**, *72*, 122–128. [CrossRef]
62. Wong, T.W.; Yau, J.K.Y.; Chan, C.L.W.; Kwong, R.S.Y.; Ho, S.M.Y.; Lau, C.C.; Lau, F.L.; Lit, C.H. The Psychological Impact of Severe Acute Respiratory Syndrome Outbreak on Healthcare Workers in Emergency Departments and How They Cope. *Eur. J. Emerg. Med.* **2005**, *12*, 13–18. [CrossRef]
63. Kisely, S.; Warren, N.; McMahon, L.; Dalais, C.; Henry, I.; Siskind, D. Occurrence, Prevention, and Management of the Psychological Effects of Emerging Virus Outbreaks on Healthcare Workers: Rapid Review and Meta-analysis. *BMJ* **2020**, *369*, m1642. [CrossRef]

Journal of
Clinical Medicine

MDPI

Article

The "Healthcare Workers' Wellbeing [Benessere Operatori]" Project: A Longitudinal Evaluation of Psychological Responses of Italian Healthcare Workers during the COVID-19 Pandemic

Gaia Perego [1,*], Federica Cugnata [2,3], Chiara Brombin [2,3], Francesca Milano [4], Emanuele Preti [1], Rossella Di Pierro [1], Chiara De Panfilis [5], Fabio Madeddu [1] and Valentina Elisabetta Di Mattei [2,4]

1 Department of Psychology, University of Milano-Bicocca, 20126 Milan, Italy; emanuele.preti@unimib.it (E.P.); rossella.dipierro@unimib.it (R.D.P.); fabio.madeddu@unimib.it (F.M.)
2 School of Psychology, Vita-Salute San Raffaele University, 20132 Milan, Italy; cugnata.federica@hsr.it (F.C.); brombin.chiara@hsr.it (C.B.); dimattei.valentina@hsr.it (V.E.D.M.)
3 University Centre for Statistics in the Biomedical Sciences (CUSSB), Vita-Salute San Raffaele University, 20132 Milan, Italy
4 Clinical and Health Psychology Unit, IRCCS San Raffaele Scientific Institute, 20132 Milan, Italy; milano.francesca96@gmail.com
5 Department of Medicine and Surgery, University of Parma, 43121 Parma, Italy; chiara.depanfilis@unipr.it
* Correspondence: g.perego23@campus.unimib.it

Abstract: Background: COVID-19 forced healthcare workers to work in unprecedented and critical circumstances, exacerbating already-problematic and stressful working conditions. The "Healthcare workers' wellbeing (Benessere Operatori)" project aimed at identifying psychological and personal factors, influencing individuals' responses to the COVID-19 pandemic. Methods: 291 healthcare workers took part in the project by answering an online questionnaire twice (after the first wave of COVID-19 and during the second wave) and completing questions on socio-demographic and work-related information, the Depression Anxiety Stress Scale-21, the Insomnia Severity Index, the Impact of Event Scale-Revised, the State-Trait Anger Expression Inventory-2, the Maslach Burnout Inventory, the Multidimensional Scale of Perceived Social Support, and the Brief Cope. Results: Higher levels of worry, worse working conditions, a previous history of psychiatric illness, being a nurse, older age, and avoidant and emotion-focused coping strategies seem to be risk factors for healthcare workers' mental health. High levels of perceived social support, the attendance of emergency training, and problem-focused coping strategies play a protective role. Conclusions: An innovative, and more flexible, data mining statistical approach (i.e., a regression trees approach for repeated measures data) allowed us to identify risk factors and derive classification rules that could be helpful to implement targeted interventions for healthcare workers.

Keywords: COVID-19; healthcare workers; mental health; mixed effects model; Random Effects/Expectation Maximization (RE-EM) Tree

Citation: Perego, G.; Cugnata, F.; Brombin, C.; Milano, F.; Preti, E.; Di Pierro, R.; De Panfilis, C.; Madeddu, F.; Di Mattei, V.E. The "Healthcare Workers' Wellbeing [Benessere Operatori]" Project: A Longitudinal Evaluation of Psychological Responses of Italian Healthcare Workers during the COVID-19 Pandemic. *J. Clin. Med.* **2022**, *11*, 2317. https://doi.org/10.3390/jcm11092317

Academic Editor: Alfonso Troisi

Received: 16 March 2022
Accepted: 19 April 2022
Published: 21 April 2022

1. Introduction

Healthcare settings may represent a challenging workplace, characterized by long and undefined working hours, excessive workloads, competitiveness of training, high responsibility, and constant exposure to suffering, illness, and mourning [1,2]. However, lack of time, stigma, and concerns around confidentiality may prevent seeking psychological support [2,3].

Consistently, increasing evidence shows that healthcare workers around the world report high levels of depression, anxiety, stress, burnout, and post-traumatic stress disorder (PTSD) [1,4]. However, the literature is limited, and the samples analyzed are heterogeneous, resulting in a prevalence of psychiatric symptoms ranging from 30% to 60% for physicians [5–7] and from 11% to 73% for nurses [8].

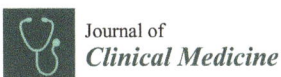

In turn, neglected mental health issues in healthcare workers can affect both team and individual work performance, resulting in a reduced quality of care [9], lower patient satisfaction, and higher rates of medical errors and staff turnover [1,9,10], with a remarkable impact on the healthcare economy [1,10,11].

This topic is currently of critical importance, given the detrimental consequences of the COVID-19 pandemic on the entire population, e.g., ref. [12] and healthcare workers in particular [13], as shown in previous epidemics [14], worsening already-problematic and stressful workplace conditions. Indeed, frontline healthcare workers have been working for more than a year in unprecedented and critical circumstances to cope with the COVID-19 pandemic, while being exposed to potentially traumatic or stressful factors such as fear of contagion, a lack of personal protection equipment, longer working hours, countless patient deaths and numerous critical patients, and continuous updates to hospital procedures [10,15].

Although healthcare workers faced the second wave of the pandemic with more therapeutic knowledge than the first, they still had limited resources to care for COVID-19 patients. In fact, the unpredictability of the disease and the pandemic's course, the extremely high number of deaths and critical patients, and the necessity to make difficult choices about prioritizing care remained serious concerns about COVID-19 [15].

Several reviews and meta-analyses show that working in COVID-19 wards affected healthcare workers' mental health in terms of high rates of depression, anxiety, insomnia, burnout, and PTSD symptoms [13,15–18]. A recent meta-analysis [10] found the following pooled prevalence of psychiatric outcomes among healthcare workers: 30% for anxiety, 31.1% for depression, 56.5% for acute stress, 20.2% for post-traumatic stress, and 44% for sleep disorders. However, as other two meta-analyses pointed out [19,20], most healthcare workers actually experienced mild psychiatric symptoms, with moderate and severe symptoms being less common.

This is in line with our baseline findings, which point to low or mild mental health issues among healthcare workers after the main peak of the outbreak's first phase [21]. Notwithstanding, the pandemic has evolved quickly, and early studies were unable to capture post-traumatic stress disorders and the mental health outcomes associated with a state of prolonged stress. Longitudinal studies are, thus, required to analyze the effect of time on these psychiatric outcomes [10] and to differentiate the effect of the pandemic from all other pre-existing stressors in the hospital work environment [22].

In this contribution, we present findings of the "Healthcare workers' wellbeing [Benessere Operatori]" project, which aims at evaluating psychological distress, as well as socio-demographic, situational, and personal factors that may affect individuals' psychological responses to the COVID-19 pandemic. All these factors have been assessed twice: at baseline (between 9 May and 13 July 2020, after the main peak of the COVID-19 outbreak in Italy) and during the second wave (between 5 and 30 December 2020). Along with more traditional mixed effects modelling approaches, an alternative advanced data mining approach, extending regression trees methodology to repeated measures data, has been applied. The applied procedure is extremely flexible and appealing since it allows for the identification of the best variables with the best cut-off values for discriminating among different outcome responses, while uncovering complex relationships among predictors. It thus provides an effective tool to be used in clinical practice to support decision making process.

2. Materials and Methods

2.1. Participants and Procedure

The study was conducted according to the guidelines of the Declaration of Helsinki and approved by the Ethics Committee of the University of Milano-Bicocca (protocol n. 0024531/20), the Ethics Committee of the IRCCS San Raffaele Scientific Institute (protocol n. 109/2020), and the Ethics Committee of the Parma Local Health Authority (protocol n. PG0019826_2020).

This study is part of a web-based longitudinal project to examine the psychological impact of COVID-19 on a sample of Italian healthcare workers involved in the management of the pandemic. After reading the informed consent, participants voluntarily completed an online survey, administered through Qualtrics and sent to the e-mail address provided, during the baseline assessment. We assessed participants' working conditions, individual perception of the COVID-19 situation, anxiety, depression, and insomnia symptoms, post-traumatic stress, state anger, and burnout levels. In the present study, we will also analyze the coping strategies and perceived social support measured during the baseline study.

In total, 344 healthcare workers participated in the second survey, ten of whom stated that they had not worked in the previous three months and were thus excluded from the analysis. Finally, statistical analyses have been carried out on a sample of 291 respondents with complete records on both demographic and psychological variables.

2.2. Measures

A self-report questionnaire was used to collect socio-demographic and work-related information from participants, including their age, gender, psychological/psychiatric history, ward in which they worked, and whether they had received emergency training.

The Depression Anxiety Stress Scale (DASS-21) [23,24] is a 21-item scale that assesses general distress using a tripartite model of psychopathology. This questionnaire includes three subscales: depression, anxiety, and stress. Each item is rated on a four-level Likert scale (0 = never; 3 = almost always). The total score is calculated by adding together the response values for each item. Higher scores suggest severe levels of depressive, anxiety, and stress symptoms. The original version of the questionnaire showed an internal reliability with Cronbach's alpha coefficient of 0.91 for the depression scale, 0.84 for the anxiety scale, and 0.90 for the stress scale [24]. The total score of the Italian version reported a Cronbach's alpha value of 0.90, with subscale values ranging from 0.74 to 0.85 [23].

The Insomnia Severity Index (ISI) [25,26] is a self-report questionnaire that assesses the nature, severity, and impact of insomnia using seven items rated on a five-level Likert scale (0 = "no problem"; 4 = "very severe problem"), with scores ranging from 0 to 28. The dimensions evaluated are severity of sleep onset, sleep maintenance, early morning awakening problems, sleep dissatisfaction, interference of sleep difficulties with daytime functioning, noticeability of sleep problems by others, and distress caused by the sleep difficulties. The original version of the ISI reported a Cronbach's alpha coefficient of 0.74 [26]. The Italian version showed a Cronbach's alpha coefficient of 0.75 [25].

The Impact of Event Scale-Revised (IES-R) [27,28] is a 22-item self-report questionnaire for evaluating the frequency of intrusive and avoidant thoughts and behaviors associated with a traumatic event. Items are rated on a five-point Likert scale (0 = "not at all"; 4 = "extremely"). The IES-R is divided into three subscales. Intrusion (8 items) assesses intrusive thoughts, nightmares, intrusive feelings, and imagery related to the traumatic event; Avoidance (8 items) evaluates avoidance of feelings, situations, and ideas; Hyperarousal (6 items) measures difficulty in concentrating, anger and irritability, psychophysiological arousal in response to reminders, and hypervigilance. The original version showed high levels of internal consistency (Intrusion: α = 0.87–0.94, Avoidance: α = 0.84–0.87, Hyperarousal: α = 0.79–0.91) [28]. The Italian version shows good (0.84) and acceptable (0.71) internal consistency for the intrusion subscale and the avoidance subscale, respectively [27].

The State-Trait Anger Expression Inventory-2 (STAXI-2) [29] is a 57-item self-report questionnaire that measures five domains of anger: State-Anger, Trait-Anger, Anger Expression-In, Anger Expression-Out, and Anger-Control. Responses are rated on a four-point Likert scale, ranging from 1 (not at all) to 4 (almost always). Cronbach's α coefficients range from 0.73 to 0.76, indicating high internal reliability for all the subscales except for the Trait Anger Scale/Angry Reaction [29]. In the present study, we only used the State-Anger subscale to assess healthcare workers' acute reaction to the pandemic.

The Maslach Burnout Inventory (MBI) [30,31] consists of 22 items, divided into three subscales, that assess the three components of the burnout syndrome: emotional exhaustion

(9 items), depersonalization (5 items), and professional realization (8 items). Each item is rated on a seven-point Likert scale (0 = "never"; 6 = "every day"). The subscales showed good internal consistency both for the original version (α = 0.71–0.90) [30] and for the Italian version (α = 0.68–0.87) [31].

The Brief Cope [32,33] is a 28-item questionnaire, divided into 14 subscales, measuring coping responses. Each item is rated on a four-level Likert scale (0 = "I have not been doing this at all"; 3 = "I have been doing this a lot"). Coping strategies can be grouped into problem-focused (strategies aimed at changing a stressful situation: active coping, use of instrumental support, positive reframing, and planning), emotion-focused (strategies to regulate emotions associated with a stressful situation: use of emotional support, venting, humor, acceptance, self-blame, religion), and avoidance coping strategies (physical or cognitive efforts to disengage from the stressor: self-distraction, denial, substance use, behavioral disengagement) [34,35]. The original version of the questionnaire showed Cronbach's alpha coefficients, ranging from 0.50 to 0.90 [32], while the Italian version of the questionnaire revealed omega coefficients for reliability, ranging from 0.439 to 0.959 [33].

The Multidimensional Scale of Perceived Social Support (MSPSS) [36,37] is a 12-item self-administered questionnaire evaluating social support perceived by family, friends, and significant others, rated on a 7-point Likert scale (1 = "very strongly disagree"; 7 = "very strongly agree"). Higher scores indicate higher perceived social support. The internal reliability of the questionnaire is good, with Cronbach's alpha coefficients ranging from 0.85 to 0.91 [38]. The Italian version shows good indices of reliability with Cronbach's alpha coefficients ranging from 0.81 to 0.98 [36].

Furthermore, we assessed how worried participants were about the possibility that themselves, their relatives, their friends, and their colleagues could contract COVID-19. Four items were rated on a five-point Likert scale (1 = "not at all"; 5 = "extremely"). A total score of worry was obtained by averaging items scores.

Finally, we evaluated participants' working conditions over the previous three months in several areas, including eating, sleeping, working shifts, isolation, and wearing appropriate protective equipment. Seven items were rated on a five-point Likert scale (1 = "not at all"; 5 = "very much"). A total score of working conditions was obtained by averaging item scores. Higher scores indicate worse working conditions.

2.3. Statistical Analysis

Median and interquartile range (IQR) were used as summary statistics to describe continuous variables, while categorical variables were expressed as frequencies and percentages. Radar plots were used to visualize differences between measurements collected during the two evaluations in the different healthcare worker categories.

Linear mixed-effects (LME) models [39] were applied to evaluate the changes in the psychological outcomes over time while accounting for respondent-specific heterogeneity through random effects specification. The variables included in the models were: time (categorical with two levels, T0 and T1, respectively, at baseline and during the second wave), gender, occupation, working or having worked in COVID-19 wards (time dependent variable), worry scores and the evaluation of working conditions, the presence of psychological or psychiatric symptoms in the past, having attended emergency training, perceived social support as measured by the MSPSS, and the three Brief COPE subscales. To highlight specific differences in the outcome variables over time for the different healthcare workers categories, we also entered in the model the interaction between occupation and time.

Standard transformations (square root, power, ordered quantile normalization) were applied to outcome variables to satisfy model regression assumptions.

To examine psychological measure dynamics over time, within a data mining framework, an extension of regression trees methodology accounting for correlation structure among observations was considered. This approach is suited for studies with repeated measures and longitudinal data. The tree-based estimation method, proposed and implemented in the R RE-EM tree package by Sela and Simonoff [40], was considered.

A regression tree [41] implements a binary recursive partitioning in which predictor variables that best discriminate among response profiles, along with the optimal cut-points, are automatically chosen. The splitting criterion is based on maximizing the reduction in the sum of squares, for the node, until convergence is reached. The approach is very flexible in handling missing values and both quantitative and qualitative predictors.

Following the branches of the resulting tree, hence considering rules derived from the variables' best cut-off values, it is possible to derive different patterns of longitudinal responses. Regression trees provide an effective tool for supporting decision-making in clinical practice and identifying relevant variables associated with different outcomes, while uncovering complex relationships among predictors. Trees were estimated using the same covariates included in the mixed models. All the analyses were performed using R statistical software (version 4.1.1, https://cran.r-project.org/index.html, accessed on 10 October 2021). The significance level was set at 0.05.

3. Results

Participants' characteristics are shown in Table 1. The final sample included 291 participants. The median age was 46 years (IQR = [35.00, 54.00]), ranging from 23 to 72 years; 239 (82.1%) were female.

Among the sample, 23% reported having a psychological/psychiatric history, and only 16.8% reported having undergone emergency training.

Concerning their occupation, 31.3% of the participants were physicians, 33.3% were nurses, 27.9% were other healthcare workers, and 7.6% were clerks. At T0, 33.3% of the participants worked in a COVID-19 ward, and 15.5% worked in a COVID-19 ward at T1.

Table 1. Demographic, clinical, and occupational characteristics (n = 291).

Age (median [IQR])—years	46.00 [35.00, 54.00]
Gender = Female—no. (%)	239 (82.1%)
Psych history = Yes—no. (%)	67 (23.0%)
Emergency training = Yes—no. (%)	49 (16.8%)
Occupation	
Physicians—no. (%)	91 (31.3%)
Nurses—no. (%)	97 (33.3%)
Clerks—no. (%)	22 (7.6%)
Other healthcare—no. (%)	81 (27.8%)
T0—Ward COVID-19 = Yes—no. (%)	97 (33.3%)
T1—Ward COVID-19 = Yes—no. (%)	45 (15.5%)

Abbreviation: no., number; Psych History, psychiatric history.

Table 2 shows the characteristics of the participants stratified by occupation, and radar plots in Figure 1 display the average score of the psychological constructs of interest for each occupation group at each time point. Overall clerks reported higher average scores on almost all the scales, and their psychological condition seems to worsen, at least at a descriptive level, at the second time point. State-anger, DASS-21 scales, and emotional exhaustion subscale are, on average, higher for all the healthcare workers at the second time point (complete descriptive statistics are reported in Table S1). Observed ranges for all the psychometric scales are reported in Table S2.

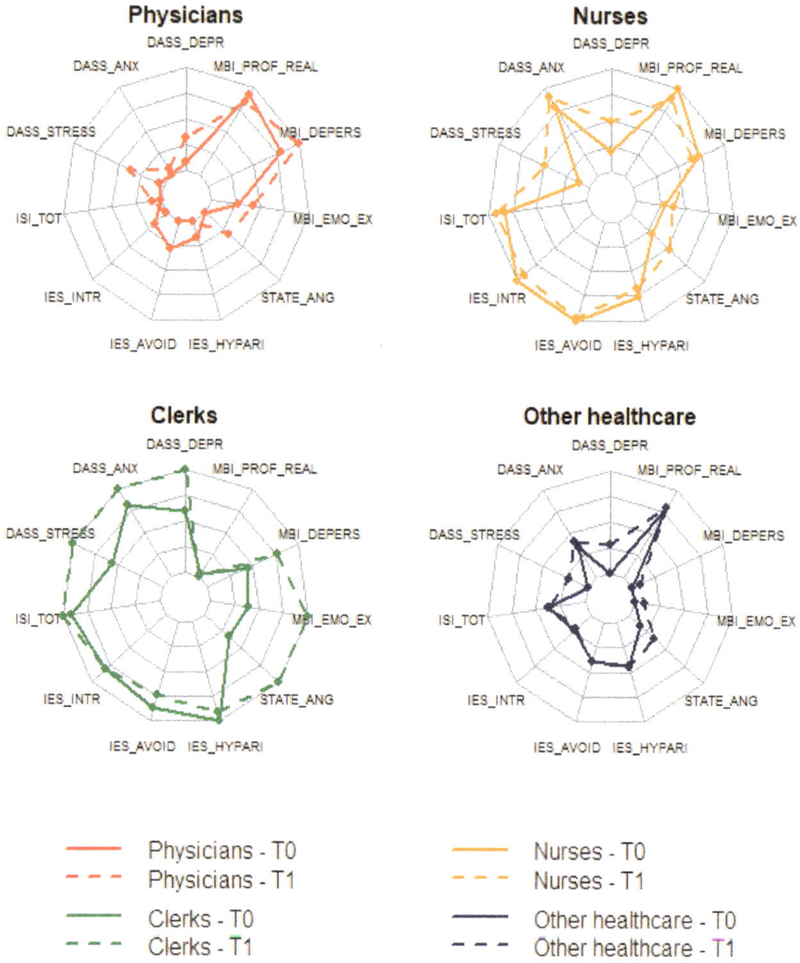

Figure 1. Radar charts displaying average scores of the investigated psychometric variables at T0 and T1, stratified by occupation (Table S1). Out of the 291 participants, 91 were physicians, 97 were nurses, 81 were other healthcare workers, and 22 were clerks. Abbreviation: DASS Depr, Depression Anxiety Stress Scale-Depression; DASS Anx, Depression Anxiety Stress Scale-Anxiety; DASS Stress, Depression Anxiety Stress Scale-Stress; MBI Prof Real, Maslach Burnout Inventory-Professional Realization; MBI Depers, Maslach Burnout Inventory-Depersonalization; MBI Emo Ex, Maslach Burnout Inventory-Emotional Exhaustion; STATE Ang, STATE Anger; IES Hypar, Impact of Event Scale- Hyperarousal; IES Avoid, Impact of Event Scale-Avoidance; IES Intr, Impact of Event Scale-Intrusion; ISI Tot, Insomnia Severity Index Total score.

Table 2. Demographic, clinical, and occupational characteristics stratified by occupation (n = 291).

	Physicians (n = 91)	Nurses (n = 97)	Clerks (n = 22)	Other Healthcare (n = 81)
Age (median [IQR])—years	46.00 [36.00, 56.50]	45.00 [34.00, 51.00]	46.50 [38.00, 53.00]	46.00 [34.00, 54.00]
Gender = Female—no. (%)	60 (65.9%)	88 (90.7%)	17 (77.3%)	74 (91.4%)
Psych history = Yes—no. (%)	28 (30.8%)	15 (15.5%)	4 (18.2%)	20 (24.7%)
Emergency training = Yes—no. (%)	16 (17.6%)	26 (26.8%)	-	7 (8.6%)
T0—Ward COVID-19 = Yes—no. (%)	27 (29.7%)	54 (55.7%)	-	16 (19.8%)
T1—Ward COVID-19 = Yes—no. (%)	13 (14.3%)	24 (24.7%)	-	8 (9.9%)
MSPSS (median [IQR])	72.00 [62.00, 77.00]	71.00 [61.00, 79.00]	67.00 [57.25, 75.75]	71.00 [62.00, 78.00]
COPE—Problem-Focused (median [IQR])	2.88 [2.50, 3.25]	3.00 [2.62, 3.38]	2.94 [2.75, 3.22]	3.00 [2.50, 3.38]
COPE—Emotion-Focused (median [IQR])	2.25 [2.00, 2.50]	2.33 [2.17, 2.67]	2.25 [1.88, 2.40]	2.33 [2.08, 2.58]
COPE—Avoidant (median [IQR])	1.38 [1.19, 1.75]	1.62 [1.38, 1.88]	1.62 [1.38, 1.97]	1.50 [1.38, 1.75]
T0—WORRY (median [IQR])	3.00 [2.50, 3.25]	3.25 [2.75, 3.75]	3.25 [2.81, 4.00]	3.25 [3.00, 3.75]
T0—CONDWORK (median [IQR])	2.71 [2.41, 3.23]	2.86 [2.29, 3.50]	2.90 [2.45, 3.55]	2.43 [2.00, 2.83]
T1—WORRY (median [IQR])	3.25 [3.00, 3.75]	3.25 [3.00, 4.00]	3.50 [3.06, 4.00]	3.25 [3.00, 4.00]
T1—CONDWORK (median [IQR])	2.43 [2.00, 3.07]	2.43 [2.00, 2.86]	2.57 [2.18, 2.86]	2.14 [1.71, 2.57]

Abbreviation: no., number; MSPSS, Multidimensional Scale of Perceived Social Support; COPE, Brief Cope; IQR, InterQuartile Range; Psych History, psychiatric history; CONDWORK, working conditions.

3.1. DASS-21—Depression, Anxiety, and Stress

Table 3 displays the estimated models for the DASS-21 subscales. DASS-21 subscales are not significantly different at T1, with respect to the baseline values (T0). Higher levels of worry, worse working conditions, and having a psychological/psychiatric history significantly increase anxiety, depression, and stress levels. Having undergone emergency training significantly decreases all DASS-21 subscales. Higher levels of perceived social support decrease only participants' depression levels. Considering the effects of coping strategies, we found that the use of problem-focused coping significantly decreases all DASS-21 subscales, avoidant coping significantly increases all DASS-21 subscales, and emotional-focused coping significantly increases only depression and stress levels. Finally, nurses show higher anxiety levels than physicians.

Figure 2 shows the estimated regression trees for the prediction of the DASS-21 subscales scores. For depression, among all the variables, the algorithm selected both avoidant coping and working conditions as the variables best discriminating among participants' response profiles. High levels of avoidant coping and worse working conditions predict the highest levels of depression, whereas low levels of avoidant coping and better working conditions predict lower levels of depression symptoms. For subjects with avoidant coping $\geq$ 2.2, the mean depression level is 4.4. For subjects having a working conditions score < 2.4 and avoidant coping scores lower than 1.7, instead, the predicted depression level is 2.

When anxiety is considered as an outcome, in addition to avoidant coping and working conditions, the algorithm selected the worry scale.

Following the tree branches, participants with higher scores on the worry scale ($\geq$3.4) and avoidant coping scores, greater than or equal to 2.2, show the highest average value equal to 3.9. Conversely, participants with scores on the worry scale lower than 3.4, and showing avoidant coping scores lower than 1.9, show the lowest average value equal to 1.5. In the tree for stress, psychiatric/psychological history and problem-focused coping strategy were selected, in addition to splitting variables characterizing the other two trees, to best discriminate among different response profiles.

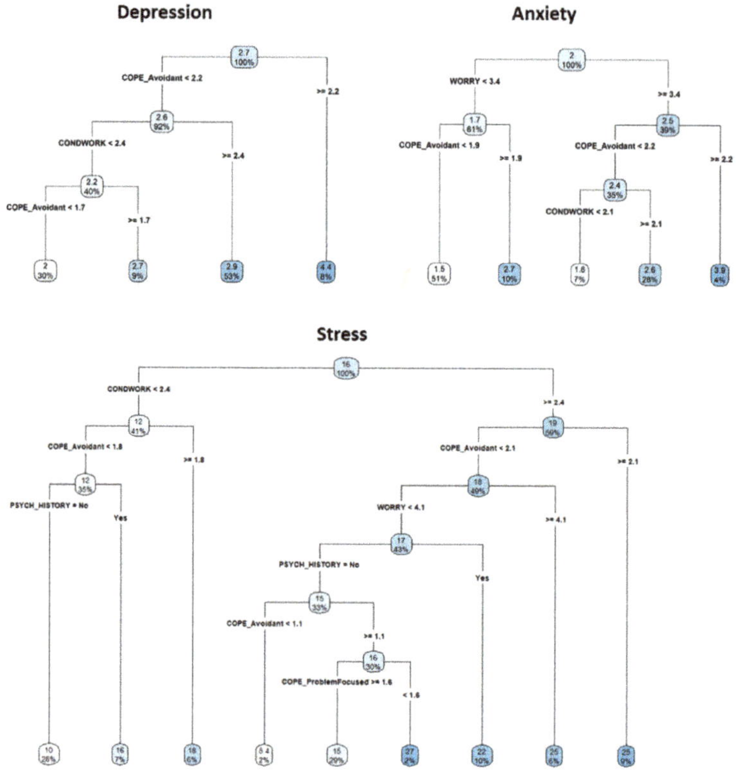

Figure 2. RE-EM tree for the DASS-21 subscales. Depression and anxiety scales were square root transformed. Each tree represents a series of splits starting at the top of the tree. Starting from the top node, a series of questions are presented based on the splitting variables and corresponding cut-off values. Depending on the answer, other branches may appear until the final node, which displays the average predicted outcome value for participants, satisfying all the conditions, leading to that node and the proportion of subjects falling in the node itself. For example, in the first tree for the depression scale, the top split assigns observations having avoidant coping scores greater than or equal to 2.2 to the right branch. The predicted depression level for these subjects is given by the mean response value for the individuals in the data set with avoidant coping $\geq$ 2.2. For such subjects, the mean depression level is 4.4. Among subjects who have avoidant coping scores < 2.2, the working conditions also affect depression level. For subjects with avoidant coping score < 2.2 and working conditions $\geq$ 2.4, the predicted depression level is 2.9. For subjects having working conditions < 2.4 and avoidant coping scores between 1.7 and 2.2, the predicted depression level is 2.7, whereas for subjects having a working conditions score < 2.4 and avoidant coping scores lower than 1.7, the predicted depression level is 2. The same logic applies to all the other trees. Abbreviation: CONDWORK, working conditions; Psych History, psychiatric history.

Table 3. Estimates (standard-errors) of the models for the DASS-21 subscales. Depression and anxiety scales were square root transformed.

Parameter	Depression	Anxiety	Stress
Intercept	−0.69(0.73)	−2.14(0.67) **	−10.96(4.05) **
Time (T1 vs. T0)	0.11(0.15)	−0.1(0.15)	1.68(0.96)
Age	0(0.01)	0(0.01)	−0.03(0.04)
Gender (Female vs. Male)	0.18(0.19)	0.19(0.18)	0.02(1.05)
Occupation (Ref = Physicians)			
Nurses	−0.1(0.21)	0.58(0.2) **	−0.84(1.22)
Clerks	−0.05(0.34)	0.2(0.31)	−0.53(1.92)
Other healthcare	−0.16(0.22)	0.22(0.21)	−0.14(1.26)
Ward COVID (Yes vs. No)	−0.11(0.14)	−0.1(0.14)	−1.6(0.85)
WORRY	0.39(0.09) ***	0.54(0.09) ***	2.41(0.53) ***
CONDWORK	0.51(0.09) ***	0.36(0.08) ***	4.59(0.5) ***
Psych history (Yes vs. No)	0.63(0.17) ***	0.64(0.16) ***	4.88(0.93) ***
Emergency training (Yes vs. No)	−0.44(0.2) *	−0.43(0.18) *	−2.42(1.07) *
MSPSS	−0.02(0.01) **	−0.003(0.005)	−0.05(0.03)
COPE—Problem-Focused	−0.47(0.16) **	−0.34(0.14) *	−2.64(0.85) **
COPE—Emotion-Focused	0.55(0.23) *	0.38(0.21)	3.98(1.24) **
COPE—Avoidant	1.03(0.19) ***	0.93(0.17) ***	5.88(1.02) ***
T1: Occupation = Nurses	0.33(0.21)	0.25(0.2)	1.5(1.29)
T1: Occupation = Clerks	0.56(0.34)	0.37(0.32)	2.78(2.1)
T1: Occupation = Other healthcare	0.19(0.22)	0.14(0.21)	0.06(1.35)

*** $p < 0.0001$; ** $p < 0.01$; * $p < 0.05$. Abbreviation: Ref, reference; CONDWORK, working conditions; Psych History, psychiatric history; MSPSS, Multidimensional Scale of Perceived Social Support, COPE, Brief Cope.

3.2. MBI Emotional Exhaustion, Insomnia, IES-R Intrusion, and State Anger

Table 4 shows the estimated models for the MBI emotional exhaustion scale, the ISI score, the IES-R Intrusion score, and the State anger score. When comparing the two time points, the state anger score significantly increases at T1 with respect to the baseline values (T0). Only for clerks, the MBI emotional exhaustions score also significantly increases at T1 compared to T0. Focusing on the occupation, overall, nurses report higher ISI levels and IES-R Intrusion levels than physicians. Higher levels of worry and worse working conditions significantly increase all of the considered scales. A previous history of psychological or psychiatric symptoms significantly increases the MBI emotional exhaustion score, the ISI score, and the IES-R Intrusion score but not the state anger score. Older age significantly increases the ISI score and the IES-R Intrusion score. Having undergone emergency training significantly decreases the ISI and IES-R Intrusion scores. Higher levels of perceived social support decrease the MBI emotional exhaustion score. Finally, we found that using avoidant coping significantly increases all considered scales, and the use of problem-focused and emotion-focused coping strategies significantly influences the MBI emotional exhaustion scale and state anger scale.

Figure 3 shows the estimated regression trees for the same outcomes.

For emotional exhaustion, the algorithm selected working conditions, avoidant coping strategies, and survey administration time as the best discriminating variables. Worse working conditions and higher use of avoidant coping strategies will lead to the highest predicted levels of emotional exhaustion, whereas the lowest outcome score is predicted for participants with better working conditions (<2.4). Moreover, worse working conditions and avoidant coping scores lower than 2.3, depending on the survey administration time, will lead to different predicted outcome scores, with higher predicted values at the time of the second survey.

For insomnia, the algorithm selected working conditions and the worry scale as the best discriminating variables. Worse working conditions and higher levels of worry will lead to the highest predicted levels of insomnia, whereas the lowest outcome score is predicted for participants with better working conditions (<2.4). Participants with worse working conditions and a level of worry lower than 3.4 will have predicted values lying in the middle and between those found in the previous two scenarios.

With reference to intrusion, working conditions, avoidant coping strategies, and scores on the worry scale are selected as the best splitting variables to identify different response profiles. Higher use of avoidant coping strategies (≥1.8) will lead to higher predicted levels of intrusion.

When avoidant coping strategies are lower than 1.8 and associated with better working conditions and lower levels of worry, the lowest levels of intrusion are predicted.

When avoidant coping strategies are lower than 1.8 and associated with worse working conditions (>2.7), participant profiles, with levels of intrusion lying in the middle, between the best and the worst scenarios, are identified.

For state anger, out of all the variables, only the worry scale plays a role in discriminating among participants' response profiles, with higher levels of worry leading to the highest predicted state anger score.

Estimated LME models for depersonalization and professional realization MBI subscales are reported in Table S3. In Table S4, LME models for the IES-R subscales of avoidance and hyperarousal are reported.

Table 4. Estimates (standard-errors) of the models for the MBI Emotional Exhaustion, ISI total score, IES-R Intrusion, and State Anger. Square root transformation was applied to the MBI Emotional Exhaustion scale, ISI total score, and IES-R Intrusion scale, while ordered quantile normalization was used for the State Anger scale.

Parameter	MBI EMO EX	ISI TOT	IES Intrusion	STATE Anger
Intercept	0.85(0.74)	0.44(0.28)	−1.01(0.19) ***	−2.26(0.44) ***
Time (T1 vs. T0)	0.07(0.13)	0.02(0.06)	−0.02(0.03)	0.3(0.09) **
Age	0.01(0.01)	0.01(0.003) ***	0.005(0.002) *	0.002(0.004)
Gender (Female vs. Male)	0.37(0.2)	0.08(0.08)	0.07(0.05)	−0.21(0.12)
Occupation (Ref = Physicians)				
Nurses	−0.32(0.21)	0.28(0.08) ***	0.16(0.06) **	0.06(0.13)
Clerks	−0.26(0.33)	0.12(0.13)	−0.03(0.09)	0.06(0.2)
Other healthcare	−0.52(0.22)	0.16(0.09)	−0.03(0.06)	0.23(0.13)
Ward COVID (Yes vs. No)	−0.1(0.13)	−0.1(0.05)	−0.02(0.03)	0.16(0.09)
WORRY	0.32(0.09) ***	0.19(0.04) ***	0.13(0.02) ***	0.23(0.06) ***
CONDWORK	0.55(0.08) ***	0.29(0.03) ***	0.15(0.02) ***	0.19(0.05) ***
Psych history (Yes vs. No)	0.74(0.18) ***	0.23(0.07) ***	0.17(0.05) ***	0.2(0.1)
Emergency training (Yes vs. No)	−0.35(0.2)	−0.22(0.08) **	−0.14(0.05) **	−0.15(0.12)
MSPSS	−0.02(0.01) **	−0.002(0.002)	−0.002(0.001)	−0.002(0.003)
COPE—Problem-Focused	−0.51(0.16) **	−0.09(0.06)	−0.02(0.04)	−0.22(0.09) *
COPE—Emotion-Focused	0.79(0.23) ***	0.07(0.09)	0.15(0.06)	0.34(0.14) *
COPE—Avoidant	0.84(0.19) ***	0.35(0.07) ***	0.37(0.05) ***	0.54(0.11) ***
T1: Occupation = Nurses	0.21(0.18)	0.09(0.08)	0.04(0.04)	0.0003(0.12)
T1: Occupation = Clerks	0.74(0.29) *	0.15(0.12)	0.09(0.07)	0.32(0.2)
T1: Occupation = Other healthcare	0.13(0.18)	0.003(0.08)	0.04(0.05)	−0.25(0.13)

*** $p < 0.0001$; ** $p < 0.01$; * $p < 0.05$. Abbreviation: Ref, reference; CONDWORK, working conditions; Psych History, psychiatric history; MSPSS, Multidimensional Scale of Perceived Social Support, COPE, Brief Cope; MBI Emo Ex, Maslach Burnout Inventory-Emotional Exhaustion; ISI TOT, Insomnia Severity Index Total score; IES Intrusion, Impact of Event Scale-Intrusion.

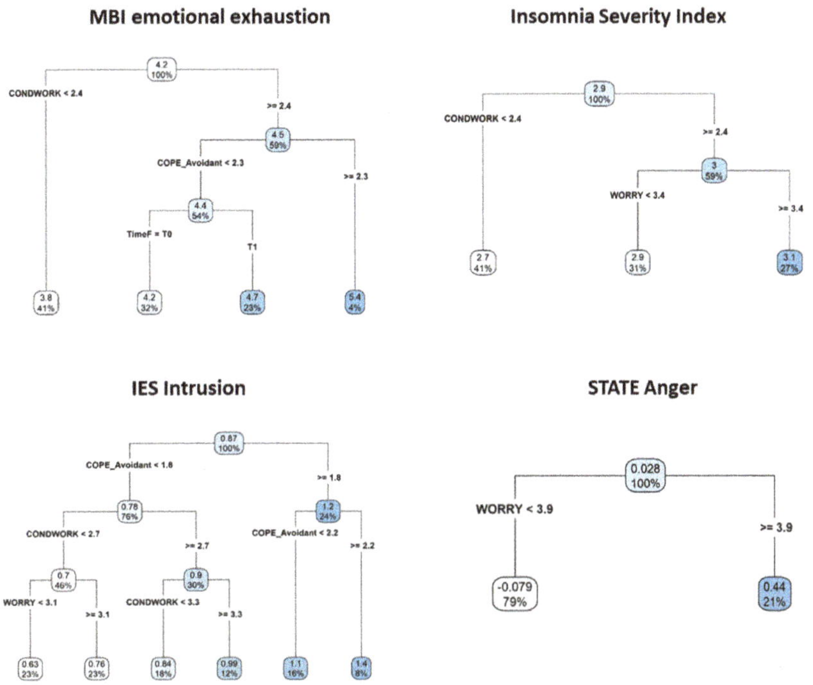

Figure 3. Estimated regression trees for Emotional exhaustion, Insomnia, Intrusion, and State Anger. Square root transformation was applied to the MBI Emotional Exhaustion scale, ISI total score, and IES-R Intrusion scale, while ordered quantile normalization was used for the State Anger scale. Abbreviation: CONDWORK, working conditions.

4. Discussion

The present study is the second phase of a longitudinal study investigating the psychological consequences of the COVID-19 outbreak and their predictive factors in a sample of Italian healthcare workers. To our knowledge, this is one of the few longitudinal studies that monitored the mental health of healthcare workers during the COVID-19 outbreak [22,42,43].

In general, the scores obtained by our sample on the psychological scales during the second phase do not significantly differ from the scores obtained during the first phase. Overall, regardless of the category of healthcare workers, our sample only showed an increase in state anger levels. Furthermore, during the second wave, clerks seemed to experience higher levels of burnout symptoms.

These results are in line with the scant literature, showing a substantial invariance of psychiatric symptoms among healthcare workers throughout the epidemic [22,42,43].

However, working under chronic stress conditions and experiencing a poor quality of sleep both contribute to increased feelings of anger among healthcare workers during the COVID-19 outbreak [44,45]. Moreover, during the second wave of the pandemic, public opinion appears to have shifted, and healthcare workers now feel less support, appreciation, and trust from the general population, and they are viewed less favorably than in the past [22]. Consistently, during previous epidemics, feelings of anger seemed to be frequent among healthcare workers, caused by both long-term stressful working conditions and poor adherence to infection control guidelines, as well as rejection and stigma experienced from relatives and public opinion [46].

Furthermore, the increasing levels of burnout experienced by clerks during the second phase may be explained by the end of smart-working and the subsequent return to work in hospitals.

Concerning predictive factors, our results highlight that higher levels of worry, worse working conditions, a previous history of psychiatric illness, being a nurse, older age, and avoidant and emotion-focused coping strategies seem to be risk factors for healthcare workers' mental health. Conversely, high levels of perceived social support, the attendance of emergency training, and problem-focused coping strategies seem to be protective factors for healthcare workers' mental health.

Specifically, worse working conditions and worry about the infection represent risk factors for higher levels of depression, anxiety, stress, burnout, PTSD, insomnia, and state anger. Considering the regression trees, a score greater than or equal to 2.4 in working conditions is a cut-off for higher depression scores (for participants showing avoidant coping scores lower than 2.2), stress, burnout, and insomnia; a high worry score ($\geq$3.9) is the only factor that distinguishes between the highest and lowest levels of state anger, whereas a score greater than or equal to 3.4 discriminates among participants with more extreme levels of anxiety and insomnia.

These findings are in line with the literature showing that difficult working environments, including poor supervision and organizational support, intense workloads, a lack of personal protective equipment or its continuous use for many hours, and fear and concern about becoming infected or infecting relatives or colleagues, increase the psychological distress' levels of healthcare workers [47–49].

Concerning demographic variables, older age seems a risk factor for higher levels of insomnia and intrusion symptoms. This result is consistent with the literature, which shows an association between increasing age and a physiological decline in sleep quality [50]. Additionally, the literature identifies older age as a risk factor for PTSD symptoms during the COVID-19 pandemic, probably due to the elderly being a high-risk category for infection and death [51,52].

Moreover, a previous history of psychiatric illness seems to be a risk factor for higher levels of depression, anxiety, stress, burnout, PTSD, and insomnia symptoms. The current literature highlights that a history of psychiatric symptoms seems to make healthcare workers more vulnerable and more likely to experience psychological distress during the COVID-19 emergency [53,54].

Furthermore, being a nurse seems to be a risk factor for higher levels of anxiety, PTSD intrusion symptoms, and insomnia. This result is consistent with the literature showing that being a nurse represents a risk factor for worse mental health, which is probably due to the longer time spent with patients in contact with their fears, suffering, and death [18,49,55,56].

Concerning protective factors, having undergone emergency training predicts low levels of depression, anxiety, stress, PTSD, and insomnia symptoms. This result is in line with the literature showing perceived adequacy of training as a protective factor for long-term psychiatric morbidity [57], post-traumatic stress [58,59], and burnout [58] in previous epidemics. This is understandable given that the goal of emergency training is to improve healthcare workers' skills and abilities to increase their sense of control and avoid being overwhelmed during a real emergency [60].

High levels of perceived social support from family and friends seem to be a protective factor for lower depression and burnout symptoms. In line with the literature, high perceived social support from family, colleagues, and friends is helpful to deal with work-related stress and to increase self-confidence [18,47].

Concerning coping strategies, regression trees highlighted that higher avoidant coping scores lead to the highest scores in the depression, anxiety, stress, burnout, and PTSD subscales.

The detrimental role of avoidant coping strategies is consistent with current and past epidemic literature [17,61–63]. Avoidance strategies, such as denial or self-distraction, may be helpful for short periods of time to allow the person to continue with their tasks while also giving them some time to think. However, in the long-term, these coping strategies are dangerous for mental health, provoking dysfunctional detachment and distance from the problem, while changing neither the situation nor the associated psychological distress [64,65].

Conversely, the use of problem-focused coping strategies seems to be a protective factor for lower levels of depression, anxiety, stress, burnout, and state anger. This result is in accordance with the literature, showing that these strategies can increase feelings of autonomy and self-efficacy while reducing psychological distress [17,61,66]. These coping strategies may help in changing the meaning of the event and focusing on a specific goal, thereby increasing the perception of control, and avoiding being overwhelmed by the stressful situation [64,65].

Finally, the use of emotion-focused coping strategies seems to be a risk factor for higher levels of depression, stress, burnout, and state anger. The literature concerning emotion-focused coping strategies is contradictory [17,64], which is probably due to the heterogeneous nature of the strategies included in this subscale (e.g., use of emotional support and self-blaming). Moreover, during an emergency, problem-focused strategies appear more effective and adaptive than emotion-focused strategies [67]. Making difficult decisions in a stressful and extraordinary situation, with little knowledge about the disease and poor support from family and friends due to isolation, may be overwhelming if emotions are prioritized over the problem. Indeed, because of the governments' social restrictions policy in response to the COVID-19 emergency, a typically positive and protective coping strategy, such as the use of emotional support [66,68], could be a risk factor for poor mental health among healthcare workers [63,66,67,69].

In general, our findings align with other Mediterranean studies on the psychological impact of the COVID-19 pandemic on healthcare workers. Indeed, studies conducted in Italy, Greece, Portugal, Spain, and France highlighted a more resilient attitude among healthcare workers compared to studies conducted in China, the United Kingdom, and the Middle East [70]. Moreover, worse working conditions, higher levels of worry about the infection, and a previous history of psychiatric illness seem to be the main risk factors for poor mental health among Mediterranean healthcare workers [71–74].

Limitations and Strengths

Among limitations to be acknowledged, a self-selection bias may have occurred, as only participants experiencing low levels of psychological distress may have taken part in this research. Then, as only a subset of participants completed the assessment twice, the study sample may not be representative of both the healthcare worker population and the initial study sample.

However, this longitudinal study allowed us to monitor the mental health of healthcare workers over time and investigate relationships among variables to identify potential target risk and protective factors. Another strength of our study is the inclusion of healthcare workers from various hospitals located throughout Italy. Finally, the use of an online survey may have encouraged participants to reveal sensitive aspects of their work without worrying about confidentiality [75].

5. Conclusions

Healthcare workers seemed to be resilient in the face of the pandemic. Their mental health and general wellbeing is a complex issue that the government should monitor. In the current context, much can be offered, such as virtual clinics and remotely delivered psychological therapies and psychoeducation. However, it is also necessary to reduce mental health stigma, as physicians appear generally reluctant to disclose their problems, even when they are experiencing significant psychological distress [76]. The proposed data mining approach allowed us to derive classification rules and to identify risk and protective factors for healthcare workers' psychological wellbeing, which should be monitored during emergency situations. The proposed statistical methodology could provide more insight into the psychological aspects which are leveraged when implementing training/intervention programs.

Supplementary Materials: The following supporting information can be downloaded at: https://www.mdpi.com/article/10.3390/jcm11092317/s1, Table S1: Descriptive statistics of investigated psychometric variables; Table S2: Observed ranges of investigated psychometric variables; Table S3: Estimates (standard-errors) of the models. Square root transformation was applied to MBI depersonalization scale, while scores on the MBI professional realization scale were raised to the power of two; Table S4: Estimates (standard-errors) of the models. Square root transformation was applied to scores on both IES-R Avoidance and Hyperarousal scales.

Author Contributions: Conceptualization, G.P., E.P. and V.E.D.M.; Data curation, F.C. and C.B.; Formal analysis, F.C. and C.B.; Investigation, G.P. and C.D.P.; Methodology, G.P.; Project administration, E.P. and V.E.D.M.; Supervision, F.M. (Fabio Madeddu) and V.E.D.M.; Visualization, G.P. and F.M. (Francesca Milano); Writing—original draft, G.P. and F.M. (Francesca Milano); Writing—review & editing, E.P., R.D.P. and V.E.D.M. All authors have read and agreed to the published version of the manuscript.

Funding: This research received no external funding.

Institutional Review Board Statement: The study was conducted in accordance with the Declaration of Helsinki and approved by the Ethics Committee of the University of Milano-Bicocca (protocol n. 0024531/20), the Ethics Committee of the IRCCS San Raffaele Scientific Institute (protocol n. 109/2020), and the Ethics Committee of the Parma Local Health Authority (protocol n. PG0019826_2020).

Informed Consent Statement: Informed consent was obtained from all subjects involved in the study.

Data Availability Statement: Data cannot be shared because participants did not provide written informed consent for it.

Conflicts of Interest: The authors declare no conflict of interest.

References

1. Gray, P.; Senabe, S.; Naicker, N.; Kgalamono, S.; Yassi, A.; Spiegel, J.M. Workplace-Based Organizational Interventions Promoting Mental Health and Happiness among Healthcare Workers: A Realist Review. *Int. J. Environ. Res. Public Health* **2019**, *16*, 4396. [CrossRef] [PubMed]
2. Petrie, K.; Crawford, J.; Baker, S.T.E.; Dean, K.; Robinson, J.; Veness, B.G.; Randall, J.; McGorry, P.; Christensen, H.; Harvey, S.B. Interventions to reduce symptoms of common mental disorders and suicidal ideation in physicians: A systematic review and meta-analysis. *Lancet Psychiatry* **2019**, *6*, 225–234. [CrossRef]
3. Wallace, J.E. Mental health and stigma in the medical profession. *Health Interdiscip. J. Soc. Study Health Illn. Med.* **2012**, *16*, 3–18. [CrossRef] [PubMed]
4. Mark, G.; Smith, A.P. Occupational stress, job characteristics, coping, and the mental health of nurses. *Br. J. Health Psychol.* **2012**, *17*, 505–521. [CrossRef] [PubMed]
5. Lacy, B.E.; Chan, J.L. Physician Burnout: The Hidden Health Care Crisis. *Clin. Gastroenterol. Hepatol.* **2018**, *16*, 311–317. [CrossRef] [PubMed]
6. Mihailescu, M.; Neiterman, E. A scoping review of the literature on the current mental health status of physicians and physicians-in-training in North America. *BMC Public Health* **2019**, *19*, 1363. [CrossRef] [PubMed]
7. West, C.P.; Dyrbye, L.N.; Shanafelt, T.D. Physician burnout: Contributors, consequences and solutions. *J. Intern. Med.* **2018**, *283*, 516–529. [CrossRef]
8. Maharaj, S.; Lees, T.; Lal, S. Prevalence and Risk Factors of Depression, Anxiety, and Stress in a Cohort of Australian Nurses. *Int. J. Environ. Res. Public Health.* **2018**, *16*, 61. [CrossRef]
9. Hall, L.H.; Johnson, J.; Watt, I.; Tsipa, A.; O'Connor, D.B. Healthcare Staff Wellbeing, Burnout, and Patient Safety: A Systematic Review. *PLoS ONE* **2016**, *11*, e0159015. [CrossRef]
10. Marvaldi, M.; Mallet, J.; Dubertret, C.; Moro, M.R.; Guessoum, S.B. Anxiety, depression, trauma-related, and sleep disorders among healthcare workers during the COVID-19 pandemic: A systematic review and meta-analysis. *Neurosci. Biobehav. Rev.* **2021**, *126*, 252–264. [CrossRef]
11. Kim, M.S.; Kim, T.; Lee, D.; Yook, J.H.; Hong, Y.C.; Lee, S.Y.; Yoon, J.H.; Kang, M.Y. Mental disorders among workers in the healthcare industry: 2014 national health insurance data. *Ann. Occup. Environ. Med.* **2018**, *30*, 31. [CrossRef] [PubMed]

12. Xiong, J.; Lipsitz, O.; Nasri, F.; Lui, L.M.W.; Gill, H.; Phan, L.; Chen-Li, D.; Iacobucci, M.; Ho, R.; Majeed, A.; et al. Impact of COVID-19 pandemic on mental health in the general population: A systematic review. *J. Affect. Disord.* **2020**, *277*, 55–64. [CrossRef] [PubMed]
13. da Silva Neto, R.M.; Benjamim, C.J.R.; de Medeiros Carvalho, P.M.; Neto, M.L.R. Psychological effects caused by the COVID-19 pandemic in health professionals: A systematic review with meta-analysis. *Prog. Neuro-Psychopharmacol. Biol. Psychiatry* **2021**, *104*, 110062. [CrossRef] [PubMed]
14. Preti, E.; Di Mattei, V.; Perego, G.; Ferrari, F.; Mazzetti, M.; Taranto, P.; Di Pierro, R.; Madeddu, F.; Calati, R. The Psychological Impact of Epidemic and Pandemic Outbreaks on Healthcare Workers: Rapid Review of the Evidence. *Curr. Psychiatry Rep.* **2020**, *22*, 43. [CrossRef] [PubMed]
15. Sahebi, A.; Nejati, B.; Moayedi, S.; Yousefi, K.; Torres, M.; Golitaleb, M. The prevalence of anxiety and depression among healthcare workers during the COVID-19 pandemic: An umbrella review of meta-analyses. *Prog. Neuro-Psychopharmacol. Biol. Psychiatry* **2021**, *107*, 110247. [CrossRef]
16. d'Ettorre, G.; Ceccarelli, G.; Santinelli, L.; Vassalini, P.; Innocenti, G.P.; Alessandri, F.; Koukopoulos, A.E.; Russo, A.; d'Ettorre, G.; Tarsitani, L. Post-Traumatic Stress Symptoms in Healthcare Workers Dealing with the COVID-19 Pandemic: A Systematic Review. *Int. J. Environ. Res. Public Health* **2021**, *18*, 601. [CrossRef]
17. Labrague, L.J. Psychological resilience, coping behaviours, and social support among healthcare workers during the COVID-19 pandemic: A systematic review of quantitative studies. *J. Nurs. Manag.* **2021**, *29*, 1893–1905. [CrossRef]
18. Sanghera, J.; Pattani, N.; Hashmi, Y.; Varley, K.F.; Cheruvu, M.S.; Bradley, A.; Burke, J.R. The impact of SARS-CoV-2 on the mental health of healthcare workers in a hospital setting—A Systematic Review. *J. Occup. Health* **2020**, *62*, e12175. [CrossRef]
19. Pappa, S.; Ntella, V.; Giannakas, T.; Giannakoulis, V.G.; Papoutsi, E.; Katsaounou, P. Prevalence of depression, anxiety, and insomnia among healthcare workers during the COVID-19 pandemic: A systematic review and meta-analysis. *Brain Behav. Immun.* **2020**, *88*, 901–907. [CrossRef]
20. Sun, P.; Wang, M.; Song, T.; Wu, Y.; Luo, J.; Chen, L.; Yan, L. The Psychological Impact of COVID-19 Pandemic on Health Care Workers: A Systematic Review and Meta-Analysis. *Front. Psychol.* **2021**, *12*, 626547. [CrossRef]
21. Di Mattei, V.E.; Perego, G.; Milano, F.; Mazzetti, M.; Taranto, P.; Di Pierro, R.; De Panfilis, C.; Madeddu, F.; Preti, E. The "Healthcare Workers' Wellbeing (Benessere Operatori)" Project: A Picture of the Mental Health Conditions of Italian Healthcare Workers during the First Wave of the COVID-19 Pandemic. *Int. J. Environ. Res. Public Health* **2021**, *18*, 5267. [CrossRef] [PubMed]
22. Magnavita, N.; Soave, P.M.; Antonelli, M. Prolonged Stress Causes Depression in Frontline Workers Facing the COVID-19 Pandemic. A Repeated Cross-Sectional Study. *Int. J. Environ. Res. Public Health* **2021**, *18*, 7316. [CrossRef] [PubMed]
23. Bottesi, G.; Ghisi, M.; Altoè, G.; Conforti, E.; Melli, G.; Sica, C. The Italian version of the Depression Anxiety Stress Scales-21: Factor structure and psychometric properties on community and clinical samples. *Compr. Psychiatry* **2015**, *60*, 170–181. [CrossRef] [PubMed]
24. Lovibond, P.F.; Lovibond, S.H. The structure of negative emotional states: Comparison of the Depression Anxiety Stress Scales (DASS) with the Beck Depression and Anxiety Inventories. *Behav. Res. Ther.* **1995**, *33*, 335–343. [CrossRef]
25. Castronovo, V.; Galbiati, A.; Marelli, S.; Brombin, C.; Cugnata, F.; Giarolli, L.; Anelli, M.M.; Rinaldi, F.; Ferini-Strambi, L. Validation study of the Italian version of the Insomnia Severity Index (ISI). *Neurol. Sci.* **2016**, *37*, 1517–1524. [CrossRef]
26. Morin, C.M. *Insomnia: Psychological Assessment and Management*; Guilford Press: New York, NY, USA, 1993.
27. Pietrantonio, F.; De Gennaro, L.; Di Paolo, M.C.; Solano, L. The impact of event scale: Validation of an Italian version. *J. Psychosom. Res.* **2003**, *55*, 389–393. [CrossRef]
28. Weiss, D.S.; Marmar, C.R. The Impact of Event Scale-Revised. In *Assessing Psychological Trauma and PTSD—A Practitioner's Handbook*; Guilford Press: New York, NY, USA, 1997; pp. 399–411.
29. Spielberger, C.D. State-Trait Anger Expression Inventory-2 (STAXI-2). In *Professional Manual*; Psychological Assessment Resources: Odessa, FL, USA, 1999.
30. Maslach, C.; Jackson, S.E. The measurement of experienced burnout. *J. Organ. Behav.* **1981**, *2*, 99–113. [CrossRef]
31. Sirigatti, S.; Stefanile, C. Adattamento e Taratura per l'Italia. In *MBI Maslach Burnout Inventory. Manuale*; Organizzazioni Speciali: Florence, Italy, 1993; pp. 33–42.
32. Carver, C.S. You Want to Measure Coping but Your Protocol's Too Long: Consider the Brief COPE. *Int. J. Behav. Med.* **1997**, *4*, 92–100. [CrossRef]
33. Monzani, D.; Steca, P.; Greco, A.; D'Addario, M.; Cappelletti, E.; Pancani, L. The situational version of the Brief COPE: Dimensionality and relationships with goal-related variables. *Eur. J. Psychol.* **2015**, *11*, 295. [CrossRef]
34. Dias, C.; Cruz, J.F.; Fonseca, A.M. The relationship between multidimensional competitive anxiety, cognitive threat appraisal, and coping strategies: A multi-sport study. *Int. J. Sport Exerc. Psychol.* **2012**, *10*, 52–65. [CrossRef]
35. Poulus, D.; Coulter, T.J.; Trotter, M.G.; Polman, R. Stress and coping in esports and the influence of mental toughness. *Front. Psychol.* **2020**, *11*, 628. [CrossRef] [PubMed]
36. Di Fabio, A.; Busoni, L. Misurare il supporto sociale percepito: Proprietà psicometriche della Multidimensional Scale of Perceived Social Support (MSPSS) in un campione di studenti universitari. *Risorsa Uomo. Riv. Psicol. Lav. E Organ.* **2008**, *14*, 339–350.
37. Zimet, G.D.; Dahlem, N.W.; Zimet, S.G.; Farley, G.K. The Multidimensional Scale of Perceived Social Support. *J. Pers. Assess.* **1988**, *52*, 30–41. [CrossRef]

38. Zimet, G.D.; Powell, S.S.; Farley, G.K.; Werkman, S.; Berkoff, K.A. Psychometric characteristics of the multidimensional scale of perceived social support. *J. Pers. Assess.* **1990**, *55*, 610–617.
39. Pinheiro, J.C.; Bates, D.M. Linear mixed-effects models: Basic concepts and examples. In *Mixed-Effects Models in S and S-Plus*; Springer: Berlin/Heidelberg, Germany, 2000; pp. 3–56.
40. Sela, R.J.; Simonoff, J.S. RE-EM trees: A data mining approach for longitudinal and clustered data. *Mach. Learn.* **2012**, *86*, 169–207. [CrossRef]
41. Breiman, L.; Friedman, J.H.; Olshen, R.A.; Stone, C.J. *Classification and Regression Trees, the Wadsworth Statistics and Probability Series*; Wadsworth International Group: Belmont, CA, USA, 1984.
42. Dufour, M.M.; Bergeron, N.; Rabasa, A.; Guay, S.; Geoffrion, S. Assessment of Psychological Distress in Health-care Workers during and after the First Wave of COVID-19: A Canadian Longitudinal Study: Évaluation de la Détresse Psychologique Chez Les Travailleurs de la Santé Durant et Après la Première Vague de la COVID-19: Une étude longitudinale canadienne. *Can. J. Psychiatry* **2021**, *66*, 07067437211025217.
43. Sasaki, N.; Asaoka, H.; Kuroda, R.; Tsuno, K.; Imamura, K.; Kawakami, N. Sustained poor mental health among healthcare workers in COVID-19 pandemic: A longitudinal analysis of the four-wave panel survey over 8 months in Japan. *J. Occup. Health* **2021**, *63*, e12227. [CrossRef]
44. Albott, C.S.; Wozniak, J.R.; McGlinch, B.P.; Wall, M.H.; Gold, B.S.; Vinogradov, S. Battle Buddies: Rapid Deployment of a Psychological Resilience Intervention for Health Care Workers during the COVID-19 Pandemic. *Anesth. Analg.* **2020**, *131*, 43–54. [CrossRef]
45. Lee, H.Y.; Jang, M.H.; Jeong, Y.M.; Sok, S.R.; Kim, A.S. Mediating effects of anger expression in the relationship of work stress with burnout among hospital nurses depending on career experience. *J. Nurs. Scholarsh.* **2021**, *53*, 227–236. [CrossRef]
46. Chew, Q.H.; Wei, K.C.; Vasoo, S.; Sim, K. Psychological and Coping Responses of Health Care Workers Toward Emerging Infectious Disease Outbreaks: A Rapid Review and Practical Implications for the COVID-19 Pandemic. *J. Clin. Psychiatry* **2020**, *81*, 20r13450. [CrossRef]
47. Muller, A.E.; Hafstad, E.V.; Himmels, J.; Smedslund, G.; Flottorp, S.; Stensland, S.Ø.; Stroobants, S.; Van de Velde, S.; Vist, G.E. The mental health impact of the COVID-19 pandemic on healthcare workers, and interventions to help them: A rapid systematic review. *Psychiatry Res.* **2020**, *293*, 113441. [CrossRef] [PubMed]
48. Varghese, A.; George, G.; Kondaguli, S.V.; Naser, A.Y.; Khakha, D.C.; Chatterji, R. Decline in the mental health of nurses across the globe during COVID-19: A systematic review and meta-analysis. *J. Glob. Health* **2021**, *11*, 05009. [CrossRef] [PubMed]
49. Yuan, K.; Gong, Y.M.; Liu, L.; Sun, Y.K.; Tian, S.S.; Wang, Y.J.; Zhong, Y.; Zhang, A.Y.; Su, S.Z.; Liu, X.X.; et al. Prevalence of posttraumatic stress disorder after infectious disease pandemics in the twenty-first century, including COVID-19: A meta-analysis and systematic review. *Mol. Psychiatry* **2021**, *26*, 4982–4998. [CrossRef] [PubMed]
50. Dzierzewski, J.M.; Dautovich, N.; Ravyts, S. Sleep and Cognition in Older Adults. *Sleep Med. Clin.* **2018**, *13*, 93–106. [CrossRef] [PubMed]
51. Li, X.; Li, S.; Xiang, M.; Fang, Y.; Qian, K.; Xu, J.; Li, J.; Zhang, Z.; Wang, B. The prevalence and risk factors of PTSD symptoms among medical assistance workers during the COVID-19 pandemic. *J. Psychosom. Res.* **2020**, *139*, 110270. [CrossRef] [PubMed]
52. Qiu, J.; Shen, B.; Zhao, M.; Wang, Z.; Xie, B.; Xu, Y. A nationwide survey of psychological distress among Chinese people in the COVID-19 epidemic: Implications and policy recommendations. *Gen. Psychiatry* **2020**, *33*, e100213. [CrossRef]
53. Dobson, H.; Malpas, C.B.; Burrell, A.J.; Gurvich, C.; Chen, L.; Kulkarni, J.; Winton-Brown, T. Burnout and psychological distress amongst Australian healthcare workers during the COVID-19 pandemic. *Australas. Psychiatry* **2021**, *29*, 26–30. [CrossRef]
54. Şahin, M.K.; Aker, S.; Şahin, G.; Karabekiroğlu, A. Prevalence of depression, anxiety, distress and insomnia and related factors in healthcare workers during COVID-19 pandemic in Turkey. *J. Community Health* **2020**, *45*, 1168–1177. [CrossRef]
55. Shaukat, N.; Ali, D.M.; Razzak, J. Physical and mental health impacts of COVID-19 on healthcare workers: A scoping review. *Int. J. Emerg. Med.* **2020**, *13*, 40. [CrossRef]
56. Vizheh, M.; Qorbani, M.; Arzaghi, S.M.; Muhidin, S.; Javanmard, Z.; Esmaeili, M. The mental health of healthcare workers in the COVID-19 pandemic: A systematic review. *J. Diabetes Metab. Disord.* **2020**, *19*, 1967–1978. [CrossRef]
57. Lancee, W.J.; Maunder, R.G.; Goldbloom, D.S. Prevalence of psychiatric disorders among Toronto hospital workers one to two years after the SARS outbreak. *Psychiatr. Serv.* **2008**, *59*, 91–95. [CrossRef] [PubMed]
58. Maunder, R.G.; Lancee, W.J.; Balderson, K.E.; Bennett, J.P.; Borgundvaag, B.; Evans, S.; Fernandes, C.M.B.; Goldbloom, D.S.; Gupta, M.; Hunter, J.J.; et al. Long-term psychological and occupational effects of providing hospital healthcare during SARS outbreak. *Emerg. Infect. Dis.* **2006**, *12*, 1924. [CrossRef] [PubMed]
59. Tang, L.; Pan, L.; Yuan, L.; Zha, L. Prevalence and related factors of post-traumatic stress disorder among medical staff members exposed to H7N9 patients. *Int. J. Nurs. Sci.* **2017**, *4*, 63–67. [CrossRef] [PubMed]
60. World Health Organization. WHE Learning Strategy. WHO Health Emergencies October 2018 Programme Learning Strategy. 31 October 2018. Available online: https://www.who.int/emergencies/training (accessed on 30 November 2021).
61. Besirli, A.; Erden, S.C.; Atilgan, M.; Varlihan, A.; Habaci, M.F.; Yeniceri, T.; Ozdemir, H.M. The Relationship between Anxiety and Depression Levels with Perceived Stress and Coping Strategies in Health Care Workers during the COVID-19 Pandemic. *Med. Bull. Sisli Etfal Hosp.* **2021**, *55*, 1–11. [CrossRef] [PubMed]

62. Marjanovic, Z.; Greenglass, E.R.; Coffey, S. The relevance of psychosocial variables and working conditions in predicting nurses' coping strategies during the SARS crisis: An online questionnaire survey. *Int. J. Nurs. Stud.* **2007**, *44*, 991–998. [CrossRef] [PubMed]
63. Tahara, M.; Mashizume, Y.; Takahashi, K. Coping Mechanisms: Exploring Strategies Utilized by Japanese Healthcare Workers to Reduce Stress and Improve Mental Health during the COVID-19 Pandemic. *Int. J. Environ. Res. Public Health* **2020**, *18*, 131. [CrossRef] [PubMed]
64. Ben-Zur, H. Coping styles and affect. *Int. J. Stress Manag.* **2009**, *16*, 87. [CrossRef]
65. Carver, C.S.; Scheier, M.F.; Weintraub, J.K. Assessing coping strategies: A theoretically based approach. *J. Pers. Soc. Psychol.* **1989**, *56*, 267–283. [CrossRef]
66. Chew, Q.H.; Chia, F.L.A.; Ng, W.K.; Lee, W.C.I.; Tan, P.L.L.; Wong, C.S.; Puah, S.H.; Shelat, V.G.; Seah, E.-J.D.; Huey, C.W.T.; et al. Perceived stress, stigma, traumatic stress levels and coping responses amongst residents in training across multiple specialties during COVID-19 pandemic—A longitudinal study. *Int. J. Environ. Res. Public Health* **2020**, *17*, 6572. [CrossRef]
67. Di Monte, C.; Monaco, S.; Mariani, R.; Di Trani, M. From resilience to burnout: Psychological features of Italian general practitioners during COVID-19 emergency. *Front. Psychol.* **2020**, *11*, 2476. [CrossRef]
68. Martínez, J.P.; Méndez, I.; Ruiz-Esteban, C.; Fernández-Sogorb, A.; García-Fernández, J.M. Profiles of burnout, coping strategies and depressive symptomatology. *Front. Psychol.* **2020**, *11*, 591. [CrossRef] [PubMed]
69. Babore, A.; Lombardi, L.; Viceconti, M.L.; Pignataro, S.; Marino, V.; Crudele, M.; Candelori, C.; Bramanti, S.M.; Trumello, C. Psychological effects of the COVID-2019 pandemic: Perceived stress and coping strategies among healthcare professionals. *Psychiatry Res.* **2020**, *293*, 113366. [CrossRef] [PubMed]
70. Chutiyami, M.; Cheong, A.; Salihu, D.; Bello, U.M.; Ndwiga, D.; Maharaj, R.; Naidoo, K.; Kolo, M.A.; Jacob, P.; Chhina, N.; et al. COVID-19 Pandemic and Overall Mental Health of Healthcare Professionals Globally: A Meta-Review of Systematic Reviews. *Front. Psychiatry* **2022**, *12*, 804525. [CrossRef] [PubMed]
71. Cheristanidis, S.; Kavvadas, D.; Moustaklis, D.; Kyriakidou, E.; Batzou, D.; Sidiropoulos, E.; Papazisis, G.; Papamitsou, T. Psychological Distress in Primary Healthcare Workers during the COVID-19 Pandemic in Greece. *Acta Med. Acad.* **2021**, *50*. [CrossRef]
72. Ghaleb, Y.; Lami, F.; Al Nsour, M.; Rashak, H.A.; Samy, S.; Khader, Y.S.; Al Serouri, A.; BahaaEldin, H.; Afifi, S.; Elfadul, M.; et al. Mental health impacts of COVID-19 on healthcare workers in the Eastern Mediterranean Region: A multi-country study. *J. Public Health* **2021**, *43* (Suppl. S3), iii34–iii42. [CrossRef]
73. Prazeres, F.; Passos, L.; Simões, J.A.; Simões, P.; Martins, C.; Teixeira, A. COVID-19-Related fear and anxiety: Spiritual-religious coping in healthcare workers in Portugal. *Int. J. Environ. Res. Public Health* **2021**, *18*, 220. [CrossRef]
74. Romero, C.S.; Delgado, C.; Catalá, J.; Ferrer, C.; Errando, C.; Iftimi, A.; Benito, A.; de Andrés, J.; Otero, M.; The PSIMCOV Group. COVID-19 psychological impact in 3109 healthcare workers in Spain: The PSIMCOV group. *Psychol. Med.* **2022**, *52*, 188–194. [CrossRef]
75. Gnambs, T.; Kaspar, K. Disclosure of sensitive behaviors across self-administered survey modes: A meta-analysis. *Behav. Res. Methods.* **2015**, *47*, 1237–1259. [CrossRef]
76. Galbraith, N.; Boyda, D.; McFeeters, D.; Hassan, T. The mental health of doctors during the COVID-19 pandemic. *BJPsych Bulletin.* **2021**, *45*, 93–97. [CrossRef]

Journal of
Clinical Medicine

MDPI

Article

Fear of COVID-19 among Healthcare Workers: The Role of Neuroticism and Fearful Attachment

Alfonso Troisi [1,*], Roberta Croce Nanni [2], Alessandra Riconi [3], Valeria Carola [4] and David Di Cave [5]

1 Department of Systems Medicine, University of Rome Tor Vergata, Via Montpellier 1, 00133 Rome, Italy
2 Studi Medici Mazzini, Viale Angelico 39, 00195 Rome, Italy; robertacrocenanni@libero.it
3 Psychiatry Residency Program, Medical School, University of Rome Tor Vergata, Via Montpellier 1, 00133 Rome, Italy; alessandrariconi@gmail.com
4 Department of Dynamic and Clinical Psychology, University of Rome La Sapienza, 00143 Rome, Italy; valeria.carola@uniroma1.it
5 Department of Clinical Sciences and Translational Medicine, University of Rome Tor Vergata, Via Montpellier 1, 00133 Rome, Italy; dicave@uniroma2.it
* Correspondence: alfonso.troisi@uniroma2.it

Abstract: Fear of becoming infected is an important factor of the complex suite of emotional reactions triggered by the COVID-19 pandemic. Among healthcare workers (HWs), fear of infection can put at risk their psychological well-being and occupational efficiency. The aim of this study was to analyze the role of personality (i.e., the big five traits) and adult attachment in predicting levels of fear (as measured by the FCV-19S) in 101 HWs employed in a COVID-19 university hospital. The three significant predictors retained by the stepwise regression model were age (beta = 0.26, $t = 2.89$, $p < 0.01$), emotional stability (i.e., the inverse of neuroticism) (beta = −0.26, $t = -2.89$, $p < 0.01$), and fearful attachment (beta = 0.25, $t = 2.75$, $p < 0.01$). Older HWs with higher levels of neuroticism and fearful attachment reported more intense fear of COVID-19. Our results can be useful to identify vulnerable subgroups of HWs and to implement selective programs of prevention based on counseling and psychological support.

Keywords: COVID-19; fear; healthcare workers; neuroticism; insecure attachment

Citation: Troisi, A.; Nanni, R.C.; Riconi, A.; Carola, V.; Di Cave, D. Fear of COVID-19 among Healthcare Workers: The Role of Neuroticism and Fearful Attachment. *J. Clin. Med.* **2021**, *10*, 4358. https://doi.org/10.3390/jcm10194358

Academic Editors: Emmanuel Andrès and Icro Maremmani

Received: 3 September 2021
Accepted: 20 September 2021
Published: 24 September 2021

1. Introduction

COVID-19 has exposed healthcare workers (HWs) and their families to unprecedented levels of risk. While carrying out their duties, HWs face the occupational risk of being infected or unknowingly infecting others. Although HWs represent less than 3% of the population in the large majority of countries and less than 2% in almost all low- and middle-income countries, around 14% of COVID-19 cases reported to WHO is among HWs [1]. As of 1 June 2021, the number of coronavirus cases recorded among medical staff in Italy reached 135,054 [2].

Fear of becoming infected is an important factor of the complex suite of emotional reactions triggered by the COVID-19 pandemic [3]. There is a substantial difference between fear of infection and fear of noninfectious medical conditions (i.e., cancer, Alzheimer's disease, heart disease, stroke, and diabetes) that are feared the most in ordinary times [4]. Fear of these degenerative diseases is largely cognitive and prompted by cultural inputs because their etiology and pathogenesis are largely dependent on risk factors and life habits that are typical of modern environments (e.g., extended longevity, high calories diet, sedentary lifestyle, obesity, smoking, drinking alcohol, pollution, etc.). By contrast, fear of infection is deeply rooted in our emotional brain because it reflects a psychological adaptation evolved to minimize the exposure to a wide and varying array of pathogens that were relatively common throughout the evolutionary history of *Homo sapiens* [5,6].

Studies conducted on the general population during the current pandemic showed that fear of COVID-19 is more intense among women and tends to increase with age [7–10].

Research on the psychological reactions to previous pandemics and epidemics suggests that increased levels of fear of infection are a risk factor for developing depression, hypochondriasis, and post-traumatic stress disorder [3]. A study of 256 adults in the United States found that fear of COVID-19 predicted both depressive symptoms and generalized anxiety [11]. Moreover, fear was also found to be strongly associated with other indicators of emotional distress, such as suicidal ideation, alcohol and drug use, and extreme hopelessness [12].

These findings from the general population gain even greater importance when applied to HWs. Fear of COVID-19 is an expected emotional reaction among HWs because the increased morbidity risk due to their occupational role adds to the natural fear of infection. Previous studies conducted during the current pandemic have confirmed the relevant incidence of fear of infection among HWs and the negative impact on their psychological well-being [13–15]. However, among HWs, fear of infection can put at risk their psychological well-being as well as their occupational efficiency. For example, frontline nurses with greater fear of COVID-19 report less job satisfaction and higher intent to leave the profession [16], and fear of infection has been shown to be a predictor of burnout [17]. Given the strong correlation between fear of infection and the development of negative psychological and occupational outcomes, an enhanced understanding of which HWs are more vulnerable has implications for the treatment and prevention of a broad range of pathologies (e.g., depression and post-traumatic stress disorder) and for the optimization of their professional performance. In addition, the identification of subgroups of HWs with greater levels of fear of infection can allow the implementation of personalized psychological support and programs to facilitate open communication [18,19].

The aim of the present exploratory cross-sectional study was to analyze the role of the big five personality traits and adult attachment style in predicting levels of fear of COVID-19 in a convenience sample of HWs employed in a COVID-19 university hospital. The rationale inspiring the choice of these individual variables was the large body of evidence showing the consistent association between personality traits, attachment style, and vulnerability or resilience to different types of stressful events [20–23], including stress response to COVID-19 pandemic [24,25]. In pre-COVID times, Taylor [26] predicted that individuals high in neuroticism are vulnerable to elevated distress during pandemics because they are sensitive to stress and threats of infection. His prediction has been confirmed by studies conducted during the current pandemic in the general population in the United States [11], Canada [24], and Italy [27]. Similar to neuroticism, insecure attachment has also been linked with enhanced stress sensitivity, emotional dysregulation, and propensity to experience negative affectivity [28,29]. Based on these previous studies, we hypothesized that higher levels of neuroticism and insecure attachment correlated with greater fear of COVID-19.

2. Materials and Methods

2.1. Participants

Participants were 101 healthcare professionals working in a major university hospital that was converted into a COVID hospital in spring 2020. Participants were recruited in the period between June and August 2020 by snowball sampling. In Italy, the COVID-19 pandemic was particularly invasive during the period between March and late April, then decreased in both the number of infections and in the seriousness of the illness throughout the summer of 2020 [30]. The study was conducted when vaccination was not yet available. Thus, all HWs attending the hospital (including the participants of this study) were obliged to adhere to the same strict preventive measures to reduce the risk of infection, independently of their professional roles. Participants' mean age was 39.35 years (SD = 11.52, range: 21–70). In total, 64 were women and 67 were physicians. Other professional roles included nurses and laboratory technicians. Paper questionnaires were used to collect data. Participation was voluntary, and anonymity was guaranteed. To limit the selection biases of snowball sampling, we began with a set of initial informants that were as diverse as possible in terms of age, gender, and professional role followed by respondent-driven sampling method (i.e., weighting the sample in order to compensate for the initial non-random selection). Written informed consent was obtained prior to participation. The study was approved by the Ethical Committee of the Department of Dynamic and Clinical Psychology, Sapienza, University of Rome (Prot. n. 0000453 and Prot. n. 0000112).

2.2. *Psychometric Measures*

2.2.1. Fear of COVID-19

Ahorsu et al. [31] have recently developed a brief and valid scale (FCV-19S) to capture an individual's fear of COVID-19. The FCV-19S is a seven-item scale (e.g., "I am most afraid of COVID-19", "My heart races or palpitates when I think about getting COVID-19"). The participants are asked to indicate their level of agreement with the statements using a five-item Likert-type scale. Answers included "strongly disagree", "disagree", "neither agree nor disagree", "agree", and "strongly agree". The minimum score possible for each question is 1, and the maximum is 5. A total score is calculated by adding up each item score (ranging from 7 to 35). The higher the score, the greater is the fear of COVID-19. The Italian validation of the FCV-19S used in this study [32] showed robust psychometric properties (alpha = 0.82 and ICC = 0.72) and confirmed its stable unidimensional structure.

2.2.2. Big Five Personality Traits

The Ten-Item Personality Inventory (TIPI) [33] is a short scale developed to measure personality traits according to the big five models (also known as the OCEAN model: openness to experience, conscientiousness, extraversion, agreeableness, neuroticism) in working or clinical settings in which assessment time is limited. The TIPI was developed using descriptors from other well-established big five instruments. Each of the 10 items is rated on a 7-point scale ranging from 1 (strongly disagree) to 7 (strongly agree). The version used in this study was the revised Italian version (I-TIPI-R) [34], which showed adequate factor structure, test–retest reliability, self-observer agreement, and convergent and discriminative validity with the Big Five Inventory (BFI). In the I-TIPI-R, the scale measuring neuroticism is inverted and named emotional stability (i.e., people scoring low on emotional stability have high levels of neuroticism). When reporting the results, we refer to emotional stability. Yet, in the discussion, to facilitate the comparison of our findings with those of previous studies, we refer to neuroticism.

2.2.3. Attachment Style

To measure adult attachment style, we used the Italian version [35] of the Relationship Questionnaire (RQ) [36]. The RQ is a single-item measure made up of four short paragraphs, each describing a prototypical attachment pattern as it applies in close adult peer relationships. Participants are asked to rate their degree of correspondence to each prototype on a 7-point scale. The four attachment patterns (i.e., secure, preoccupied, fearful, and dismissing) are defined in terms of two dimensions: anxiety (i.e., a strong need for care and attention from attachment figures coupled with a pervasive uncertainty about the willingness of attachment figures to respond to such needs) and avoidance (i.e., discomfort with psychological intimacy and the desire to maintain psychological independence). The preoccupied, fearful, and dismissing patterns reflect different forms of insecure attachment.

The reliability estimates for the RQ self-ratings are comparable to those for other short questionnaires assessing adult attachment styles (test–retest r's around 0.50) [37]. The RQ shows convergent validity with interview ratings of adult attachment [36]. As for discriminant validity, several studies have demonstrated that the RQ explains individual differences in cognition, emotions, and behaviors even after controlling for the big five personality traits [38].

2.3. Statistical Analysis

Statistical analysis was performed on a personal computer using SPSS for Windows, version 25.0 (SPSS, Inc., Chicago, IL, USA). Spearman's rho was used to calculate bivariate correlations. Stepwise multiple regression analysis was used to identify significant predictors of infection fear. Although the primary aim of our study was to focus on personality traits and attachment as predictors of fear, in the first step of the stepwise multiple regression analysis, we included age, gender, and professional role to control for their possible confounding effects. There were no violations of the assumptions required by multiple regression. In particular, we used the Durbin–Watson statistic (value = 1.481) to check that the values of the residuals were independent, and variation inflation factors (VIF) scores (ranging from 1.012 to 1.033) and tolerances scores (ranging from 0.968 to 0.988) to check that there was no multicollinearity among the independent variables. The software G*Power 3.1.9.7 was used to calculate the minimum sample size for multivariate analysis.

3. Results

Table 1 reports the psychometric data for the entire sample. High levels of fear of infection (FCV-19S score > 18) were reported by 18% of the participants.

Table 1. Psychometric scores for the entire sample (n = 101).

	Mean	SD	Range
FCV-19S	12.89	4.77	7–29
I-TIPI-R EXT	4.32	1.31	1–7
I-TIPI-R AGR	5.33	1.06	2.5–7
I-TIPI-R CON	5.72	1.27	1–7
I-TIPI-R EMS	4.78	1.28	1.5–7
I-TIPI-R OPE	4.84	1.30	1.5–7
RQ SECURE	4.20	1.67	1–7
RQ PREOCCUPIED	2.66	1.47	1–6
RQ FEARFUL	2.78	1.71	1–7
RQ DISMISSING	3.21	1.75	1–7

Legend: FCV-19S, Fear of COVID-19 scale; I-TIPI- R, Ten-Item Personality Inventory, Revised Italian Version; EXT, extraversion; AGR, agreeableness; CON, conscientiousness; EMS, emotional stability (the inverse of neuroticism); OPE, openness to experiences; RQ, Relationship Questionnaire.

Nonparametric bivariate correlations between the I-TIPI-R, the RQ, and the FCV-19S showed higher levels of fear of COVID-19 in participants scoring lower on emotional stability (rho = −0.32, $p < 0.01$) and higher on preoccupied attachment (rho = 0.28, $p < 0.01$) and fearful attachment (rho = 0.27, $p < 0.01$). A stepwise multiple regression was conducted to determine which individual variables were the best predictors of fear of COVID-19, as measured by the FCV-19S. At step 1 of the analysis, age, gender (women vs. men), and professional role (medical doctors vs. other HWs) were entered into the regression model to control for their possible confounding effects. At step 2, the big five dimensions (i.e., extraversion, agreeableness, conscientiousness, emotional stability, and openness to experiences), as measured by the I-TIPI-R scores, were entered into the regression model. In step 3, the RQ scores for the four attachment patterns (i.e., secure, preoccupied, fearful, and dismissing) were entered into the regression model.

The final model explained 24% (R^2) of the variance in the FCV-19S scores. The three significant predictors retained by the final model were age (beta = 0.26, t = 2.89, $p < 0.01$), I-TIPI-R emotional stability (beta = −0.26, t = −2.89, $p < 0.01$), and RQ fearful attachment (beta = 0.25, t = 2.75, $p < 0.01$) (Table 2). Older HWs with lower levels of emotional stability (i.e., higher levels of neuroticism) and higher levels of fearful attachment reported more intense fear of COVID-19.

Table 2. Results of stepwise regression analysis with fear of COVID-19 (FCV-19S) as the dependent variable, and sociodemographic data (step 1), big five personality traits (I-TIPI-R) (step 2), and adult attachment style (RQ) (step 3) as independent variables.

		FCV-19S		
		β	t	*p*
Step 1	Age	0.30	3.13	<0.01
	Model	**R^2 = 0.09**	**F = 9.79**	**<0.01**
Step 2	Age	0.27	2.98	<0.01
	I-TIPI-R EMS	−0.30	−3.25	<0.01
	Model	**ΔR^2 = 0.09**	**ΔF = 10.59**	**<0.01**
Step 3	Age	0.26	2.89	<0.01
	I-TIPI-R EMS	−0.26	−2.89	<0.01
	RQ FEARFUL	0.25	2.75	<0.01
	Model	**ΔR^2 = 0.06**	**ΔF = 7.56**	**<0.01**
		R^2 = 0.24	**F = 10.11**	**<0.01**

Legend: FCV-19S, Fear of COVID-19 scale; I-TIPI- R, Ten-Item Personality Inventory, Revised Italian Version; EMS, emotional stability; RQ, Relationship Questionnaire.

4. Discussion

We found that older age predicted greater fear of infection. One possible explanation is that older HWs knew that they were at higher risk of critical COVID-19 symptoms [39]. In contrast, we found no correlations between gender, professional role, and fear of infection. It is likely that such missing correlations were idiosyncratic to our sample because a recent systematic review of 55 articles found that being a nurse and being female appeared to confer greater risk in terms of fear of infection [14].

We found that two personality traits, neuroticism and fearful attachment, were independent predictors of fear of infection. Neuroticism is a personality trait originally defined to include anxiety, emotional instability, worry, tension, and self-pity. This negative affectivity is accompanied by a pervasive perception that the world is a dangerous and threatening place, along with beliefs about one's inability to manage or cope with challenging events [40]. In accordance with previous studies [11,24,27], our findings confirm the prediction by Taylor [26] that individuals high in neuroticism are vulnerable to elevated distress during pandemics because they are sensitive to stress and threats of infection. The original contribution of our study is that neuroticism is associated with a specific facet of emotional distress (i.e., fear of infection) and that such an association can be found among HWs.

The pattern of insecure attachment that emerged as a significant predictor of fear of COVID-19 over and above the effect of neuroticism was fearful attachment. The finding that fearful attachment was a significant predictor independent of neuroticism was expected because previous studies showed that correlations between attachment patterns and the big five personality traits are weak [41]. The RQ paragraph describing fearful attachment reads as follows: "I am uncomfortable getting close to others. I want emotionally close relationships, but I find it difficult to trust others completely or to depend on them. I worry that I will be hurt if I allow myself to become too close to others".

We hypothesize that the psychological mechanisms linking fearful attachment with fear of infection are mainly related to dysfunctional coping strategies. In general, people with secure attachment tend to appraise stressful events in less threatening ways and to appraise themselves as able to cope effectively. In contrast, insecure attachment (including the fearful pattern) is associated with distress-intensifying appraisals (i.e., appraising threats as extreme and coping resources as deficient). Among people with fearful attachment, there is an additional factor that may increase fear of infection. They have a pervasive uncertainty about the willingness of significant others to respond to their needs for emotional support. Their typical discomfort with psychological intimacy and preference for emotional distance preclude self-disclosure, promote social avoidance, and can also work against attendance at support programs.

The few studies that have analyzed the relationship between adult attachment style and emotional reaction to the COVID-19 pandemic do not allow the assessment of the validity of our hypothesis. The theoretical paper by Rajkumar [42] makes no specific prediction about the pattern of insecure attachment that is expected to correlate with increased stress sensitivity to the COVID-19 outbreak. The report by Moccia et al. [43] on the Italian general population used the Attachment Style Questionnaire (ASQ) which, unlike the RQ used in the present study, does not measure the dimension of fearful attachment. Finally, the study by Lozano and Fraley [44] focused on sentinel behavior (only indirectly related to fear of infection) and found that people higher in attachment avoidance were less likely to protect themselves and protect others. We need further research to ascertain how different patterns of insecure attachment are associated with stress and coping during the current pandemic.

Based on the findings of the present study, neuroticism and fearful attachment may be viewed as vulnerability traits because of their link with fear of infection and the associated higher risk of developing stress-related psychiatric conditions. However, it is worth noting that fear of infection evolved as an adaptation to reduce the risk of contracting deadly diseases and that bold personality traits and lack of fear can lead to underestimating the risk of COVID-19 infection and eluding containment measures [45,46]. It is likely that the most adaptive emotional response to infection risk is to experience intermediate levels of fear (neither too high nor too low).

The main limitations of this study are related to the sampling method. By using snowball sampling, we had no information on how many HWs were approached and declined to participate. In addition, although the inclusion of HWs with different occupations and working in different wards provided a more complete picture of the impact of the pandemic, the limited number of participants and the variety of their duties limit the generalizability of our findings.

5. Conclusions

If confirmed by future studies based on larger samples, our results are relevant for policymakers and mental health professionals engaged to preserve HWs' well-being and professional efficiency. The psychometric battery used in this study includes brief self-report scales that are easy to complete and useful to predict which HWs will be more inclined to react fearfully toward the COVID-19 outbreak. The identification of vulnerable subgroups would allow the selective implementation of prevention programs based on counseling and psychological support [18,19].

Author Contributions: Conceptualization, A.T. and D.D.C.; methodology, R.C.N.; software, V.C.; validation, A.T. and R.C.N.; formal analysis, A.T. and V.C.; investigation, A.R.; resources, A.T. and D.D.C.; data curation, A.R.; original draft preparation, A.T.; review and editing; R.C.N., V.C. and D.D.C.; funding acquisition, not applicable. All authors have read and agreed to the published version of the manuscript.

Funding: This research received no external funding.

Institutional Review Board Statement: The study was conducted according to the guidelines of the Declaration of Helsinki and approved by the Ethical Committee of the Department of Dynamic and Clinical Psychology, Sapienza, the University of Rome (Prot. n. 0000453 and Prot. n. 0000112).

Informed Consent Statement: Informed consent was obtained from all individual participants included in the study.

Data Availability Statement: The data that support the findings of this study are available from the corresponding author upon reasonable request.

Conflicts of Interest: The authors declare no conflict of interest.

References

1. Keep Health Workers Safe to Keep Patients Safe: WHO. Available online: https://www.who.int/news/item/17-09-2020-keep-health-workers-safe-to-keep-patients-safe-w (accessed on 15 June 2021).
2. Available online: https://www.statista.com/statistics/1110950/coronavirus-covid-19-cases-among-medical-staff-italy-as-of-april/ (accessed on 15 June 2021).
3. Coelho, C.M.; Suttiwan, P.; Arato, N.; Zsido, A.N. On the Nature of Fear and Anxiety Triggered by COVID-19. *Front. Psychol.* **2020**, *11*, 581314. [CrossRef]
4. Bystad, M.; Grønli, O.; Lilleeggen, C.; Aslaksen, P.M. Fear of diseases among people over 50 years of age: A survey. *Scand. Psychol.* **2016**, *3*, e19. [CrossRef]
5. Schaller, M.; Murray, D.R.; Bangerter, A. Implications of the behavioural immune system for social behaviour and human health in the modern world. *Philos. Trans. R. Soc. B Biol. Sci.* **2015**, *370*, 20140105. [CrossRef] [PubMed]
6. Troisi, A. Fear of COVID-19: Insights from evolutionary behavioral science. *Clin. Neuropsychiatry* **2020**, *17*, 72–75. [CrossRef]
7. Gritsenko, V.; Skugarevsky, O.; Konstantinov, V.; Khamenka, N.; Marinova, T.; Reznik, A.; Isralowitz, R. COVID 19 Fear, Stress, Anxiety, and Substance Use Among Russian and Belarusian University Students. *Int. J. Ment. Health Addict.* **2020**, 1–7. [CrossRef] [PubMed]
8. Zolotov, Y.; Reznik, A.; Bender, S.; Isralowitz, R. COVID-19 Fear, Mental Health, and Substance Use Among Israeli University Students. *Int. J. Ment. Health Addict.* **2020**, 1–7. [CrossRef] [PubMed]
9. Masuyama, A.; Shinkawa, H.; Kubo, T. Validation and Psychometric Properties of the Japanese Version of the Fear of COVID-19 Scale Among Adolescents. *Int. J. Ment. Health Addict.* **2020**, 1–11. [CrossRef]
10. Winter, T.; Riordan, B.C.; Pakpour, A.H.; Griffiths, M.D.; Mason, A.; Poulgrain, J.W.; Scarf, D. Evaluation of the English Version of the Fear of COVID-19 Scale and Its Relationship with Behavior Change and Political Beliefs. *Int. J. Ment. Health Addict.* **2020**, 1–11. [CrossRef]
11. Lee, S.A.; Crunk, E.A. Fear and Psychopathology During the COVID-19 Crisis: Neuroticism, Hypochondriasis, Reassurance-Seeking, and Coronaphobia as Fear Factors. *Omega* **2020**. [CrossRef] [PubMed]
12. Lee, S.A. Coronavirus Anxiety Scale: A brief mental health screener for COVID-19 related anxiety. *Death Studies* **2020**, *44*, 393–401. [CrossRef]
13. Cawcutt, K.A.; Starlin, R.; Rupp, M.E. Fighting fear in healthcare workers during the COVID-19 pandemic. *Infect. Control Hosp. Epidemiol.* **2020**, *41*, 1192–1193. [CrossRef]
14. Cabarkapa, S.; Nadjidai, S.E.; Murgier, J.; Ng, C.H. The psychological impact of COVID-19 and other viral epidemics on frontline HWS and ways to address it: A rapid systematic review. *Brain Behav. Immun.-Health* **2020**, *8*, 100144. [CrossRef]
15. Vanhaecht, K.; Seys, D.; Bruyneel, L.; Cox, B.; Kaesemans, G.; Cloet, M.; Van Den Broeck, K.; Cools, O.; De Witte, A.; Lowet, K.; et al. COVID-19 is having a destructive impact on health-care workers' mental well-being. *Int. J. Qual. Health Care J. Int. Soc. Qual. Health Care* **2021**, *33*, mzaa158. [CrossRef]
16. Labrague, L.J.; de Los Santos, J. Fear of COVID-19, psychological distress, work satisfaction and turnover intention among frontline nurses. *J. Nurs. Manag.* **2020**, *29*, 395–403. [CrossRef]
17. Giusti, E.M.; Pedroli, E.; D'Aniello, G.E.; Stramba Badiale, C.; Pietrabissa, G.; Manna, C.; Stramba Badiale, M.; Riva, G.; Castelnuovo, G.; Molinari, E. The Psychological Impact of the COVID-19 Outbreak on Health Professionals: A Cross-Sectional Study. *Front. Psychol.* **2020**, *11*, 1684. [CrossRef] [PubMed]
18. Kinman, G.; Teoh, K.; Harriss, A. Supporting the well-being of HWS during and after COVID-19. *Occup. Med.* **2020**, *70*, 294–296. [CrossRef] [PubMed]
19. Wu, A.W.; Connors, C.; Everly, G.S., Jr. COVID-19: Peer Support and Crisis Communication Strategies to Promote Institutional Resilience. *Ann. Intern. Med.* **2020**, *172*, 822–823. [CrossRef] [PubMed]
20. Mohiyeddini, C.; Bauer, S.; Semple, S. Neuroticism and stress: The role of displacement behavior. *Anxiety Stress Coping* **2015**, *28*, 391–407. [CrossRef]
21. Xin, Y.; Wu, J.; Yao, Z.; Guan, Q.; Aleman, A.; Luo, Y. The relationship between personality and the response to acute psychological stress. *Sci. Rep.* **2017**, *7*, 16906. [CrossRef] [PubMed]
22. Mason, R.; Roodenburg, J.; Williams, B. What personality types dominate among nurses and paramedics: A scoping review? *Australas. Emerg. Care* **2020**, *23*, 281–290. [CrossRef]
23. Maunder, R.G.; Lancee, W.J.; Nolan, R.P.; Hunter, J.J.; Tannenbaum, D.W. The relationship of attachment insecurity to subjective stress and autonomic function during standardized acute stress in healthy adults. *J. Psychosom. Res.* **2006**, *60*, 283–290. [CrossRef]
24. Liu, S.; Lithopoulos, A.; Zhang, C.Q.; Garcia-Barrera, M.A.; Rhodes, R.E. Personality and perceived stress during COVID-19 pandemic: Testing the mediating role of perceived threat and efficacy. *Personal. Individ. Differ.* **2021**, *168*, 110351. [CrossRef]
25. Mazza, C.; Ricci, E.; Biondi, S.; Colasanti, M.; Ferracuti, S.; Napoli, C.; Roma, P. A Nationwide Survey of Psychological Distress among Italian People during the COVID-19 Pandemic: Immediate Psychological Responses and Associated Factors. *Int. J. Environ. Res. Public Health* **2020**, *17*, 3165. [CrossRef]
26. Taylor, S. *The Psychology of Pandemics. Preparing for the Next Global Outbreak of Infectious Disease*; Cambridge Scholars Publishing: Newcastle upon Tyne, UK, 2019.
27. Caci, B.; Miceli, S.; Scrima, F.; Cardaci, M. Neuroticism and Fear of COVID-19. The Interplay Between Boredom, Fantasy Engagement, and Perceived Control Over Time. *Front. Psychol.* **2020**, *11*, 574393. [CrossRef] [PubMed]

28. Maunder, R.G.; Hunter, J.J.; Lancee, W.J. The impact of attachment insecurity and sleep disturbance on symptoms and sick days in hospital-based health-care workers. *J. Psychosom. Res.* **2011**, *70*, 11–17. [CrossRef] [PubMed]
29. Halpern, J.; Maunder, R.G.; ScHWsartz, B.; Gurevich, M. Attachment insecurity, responses to critical incident distress, and current emotional symptoms in ambulance workers. *Stress Health J. Int. Soc. Investig. Stress* **2012**, *28*, 51–60. [CrossRef] [PubMed]
30. De Natale, G.; De Natale, L.; Troise, C.; Marchitelli, V.; Coviello, A.; Holmberg, K.G.; Somma, R. The Evolution of Covid-19 in Italy after the Spring of 2020: An Unpredicted Summer Respite Followed by a Second Wave. *Int. J. Environ. Res. Public Health* **2020**, *17*, 8708. [CrossRef]
31. Ahorsu, D.K.; Lin, C.Y.; Imani, V.; Saffari, M.; Griffiths, M.D.; Pakpour, A.H. The Fear of COVID-19 Scale: Development and Initial Validation. *Int. J. Ment. Health Addict.* **2020**, 1–9. [CrossRef]
32. Soraci, P.; Ferrari, A.; Abbiati, F.A.; Del Fante, E.; De Pace, R.; Urso, A.; Griffiths, M.D. Validation and Psychometric Evaluation of the Italian Version of the Fear of COVID-19 Scale. *Int. J. Ment. Health Addict.* **2020**, 1–10. [CrossRef]
33. Gosling, S.D.; Rentfrow, P.J.; Swann, W.B., Jr. A Very Brief Measure of the Big Five Personality Domains. *J. Res. Personal.* **2003**, *37*, 504–528. [CrossRef]
34. Chiorri, C.; Bracco, F.; Piccinno, T.; Modafferi, C.; Battini, V. Psychometric properties of a revised version of the Ten Item Personality Inventory. *Eur. J. Psychol. Assess.* **2015**, *31*, 109–119. [CrossRef]
35. Troisi, A.; D'Argenio, A.; Peracchio, F.; Petti, P. Insecure attachment and alexithymia in young men with mood symptoms. *J. Nerv. Ment. Dis.* **2001**, *189*, 311–316. [CrossRef]
36. Bartholomew, K.; Horowitz, L.M. Attachment styles among young adults: A test of a four-category model. *J. Personal. Soc. Psychol.* **1991**, *61*, 226–244. [CrossRef]
37. Scharfe, E.; Bartholomew, K. Reliability and stability of adult attachment patterns. *Pers. Relatsh.* **1994**, *1*, 23–43. [CrossRef]
38. Mikulincer, M.; Shaver, P.R. *Attachment in Adulthood: Structure, Dynamics, and Change*; Guilford: New York, NY, USA, 2007.
39. Galloway, J.B.; Norton, S.; Barker, R.D.; Brookes, A.; Carey, I.; Clarke, B.D.; Jina, R.; Reid, C.; Russell, M.D.; Sneep, R.; et al. A clinical risk score to identify patients with COVID-19 at high risk of critical care admission or death: An observational cohort study. *J. Infect.* **2020**, *81*, 282–288. [CrossRef]
40. Barlow, D.H.; Ellard, K.K.; Sauer-Zavala, S.; Bullis, J.R.; Carl, J.R. The Origins of Neuroticism. *Perspect. Psychol. Sci. A J. Assoc. Psychol. Sci.* **2014**, *9*, 481–496. [CrossRef] [PubMed]
41. Noftle, E.E.; Shaver, P.R. Attachment dimensions and the big five personality traits: Associations and comparative ability to predict relationship quality. *J. Res. Personal.* **2006**, *40*, 179–208. [CrossRef]
42. Rajkumar, R.P. Attachment Theory and Psychological Responses to the COVID-19 Pandemic: A Narrative Review. *Psychiatr. Danub.* **2020**, *32*, 256–261. [CrossRef] [PubMed]
43. Moccia, L.; Janiri, D.; Pepe, M.; Dattoli, L.; Molinaro, M.; De Martin, V.; Chieffo, D.; Janiri, L.; Fiorillo, A.; Sani, G.; et al. Affective temperament, attachment style, and the psychological impact of the COVID-19 outbreak: An early report on the Italian general population. *Brain Behav. Immun.* **2020**, *87*, 75–79. [CrossRef]
44. Lozano, E.B.; Fraley, R.C. Put your mask on first to help others: Attachment and sentinel behavior during the COVID-19 pandemic. *Personal. Individ. Differ.* **2021**, *171*, 110487. [CrossRef]
45. Paiva, T.O.; Cruz-Martins, N.; Pasion, R.; Almeida, P.R.; Barbosa, F. Boldness Personality Traits Are Associated With Reduced Risk Perceptions and Adoption of Protective Behaviors during the First COVID-19 Outbreak. *Front. Psychol.* **2021**, *12*, 633555. [CrossRef] [PubMed]
46. Rolón, V.; Geher, G.; Link, J.; Mackiel, A. Personality correlates of COVID-19 infection proclivity: Extraversion kills. *Personal. Individ. Differ.* **2021**, *180*, 110994. [CrossRef] [PubMed]

Journal of
Clinical Medicine

MDPI

Article

Can Psychological Empowerment Prevent Emotional Disorders in Presence of Fear of COVID-19 in Health Workers? A Cross-Sectional Validation Study

Marta Llorente-Alonso [1,2,*], Cristina García-Ael [3], Gabriela Topa [3], María Luisa Sanz-Muñoz [2], Irene Muñoz-Alcalde [2] and Beatriz Cortés-Abejer [2]

1 Health Psychology Program, International School of Doctorate, National Distance Education University (UNED), C/Bravo Murillo, 38, 3ª, 28015 Madrid, Spain
2 Gerencia de Asistencia Sanitaria del Área de Salud de Soria, Complejo Hospitalario de Soria, Gerencia Regional de Salud de Castilla y León (Sacyl), Pº Santa Bárbara s/n, 42005 Soria, Spain; mlsanzm@saludcastillayleon.es (M.L.S.-M.); ima87312@gmail.com (I.M.-A.); becorabe@gmail.com (B.C.-A.)
3 Department of Social and Organizational Psychology, Faculty of Psychology, National Distance Education University (UNED), C/ Juan del Rosal, 10, 28040 Madrid, Spain; cgarciaael@psi.uned.es (C.G.-A.); gtopa@psi.uned.es (G.T.)
* Correspondence: martallorentealonso@gmail.com; Tel.: +34-636-85-78-12

Abstract: The global emergency produced by COVID-19 has been a turning point for health organizations. Healthcare professionals have been exposed to high levels of stress and workload. Close contact with infected patients and the infectious capacity of COVID-19 mean that this group is especially vulnerable to contagion. In various countries, the Fear of COVID-19 Scale has been shown to be a fast and reliable tool. Early detection of fear complements clinical efforts to prevent emotional disorders. Thus, concepts focused on positive occupational health, such as Job Crafting or psychological empowerment (PE), have been examined as a tool to prevent mental health problems at work. In this work, we intended to adapt and validate the 7-item Fear of COVID-19 Scale in health workers ($N = 194$). The interpretation of the measurement model indicates adequate values of internal consistency reliability, and convergent and discriminant validity. The overall goodness of fit of the model was also adequate. The structural model indicates that the implementation of job crafting measures in health services leads to workers' greater PE. High levels of anxiety and depression prevent health professionals from psychologically detaching from work. In turn, PE can reduce the emotional disorders caused by the fear of COVID-19.

Keywords: psychological empowerment; fear of COVID-19; collaborative crafting; job crafting; emotional disorders; psychological detachment

Citation: Llorente-Alonso, M.; García-Ael, C.; Topa, G.; Sanz-Muñoz, M.L.; Muñoz-Alcalde, I.; Cortés-Abejer, B. Can Psychological Empowerment Prevent Emotional Disorders in Presence of Fear of COVID-19 in Health Workers? A Cross-Sectional Validation Study. *J. Clin. Med.* **2021**, *10*, 1614. https://doi.org/10.3390/jcm10081614

Academic Editor: Alfonso Troisi

Received: 21 March 2021
Accepted: 7 April 2021
Published: 10 April 2021

1. Introduction

The health emergency caused by the SARS-COV-2 virus has led to serious physical and psychological problems worldwide [1,2]. In Spain, the "Center for Sociological Research" (October 2020) [3] reports that 79.3% of the Spanish population considers that the pandemic has affected the emotional health of the entire population. This survey was conducted on 2861 people and it values the effects and consequences of the Coronavirus in the Spanish population. Of the participants, 50.6% expressed anxiety during the health crisis, 29.3% felt depressed, and 57.5% were afraid of getting sick. In addition, subsequent surveys have shown that the pandemic has changed the way a large part of Spanish society thinks. In fact, 12.3% of the respondents consider that they live in fear, unease, or apprehension of the pandemic (CIS, December 2020) [4].

The high contagion rate and increased mortality of the SARS-COV-2 virus compared with other respiratory pathologies [5] have caused feelings of fear and uncertainty about the future in part of the population [4]. Fear consists of anguish over a real or imaginary risk or harm [6]. Extreme fear has even led to cases of suicide in people not diagnosed with COVID-19 [7,8]. Gunnell et al. suggest that the COVID-19 pandemic can trigger profound effects on mental health, and that suicide rates may increase, given the increase in the number of suicides in previous epidemics (in the USA during the 1918–1919 flu and among older people, in Hong Kong during the 2003 Severe Acute Respiratory Syndrome (SARS) epidemic) [9]. Therefore, fear assessment can be an important mechanism for preventing emotional or mental health disorders.

The general objective of this study is to adapt and validate the Fear of COVID-19 Scale of Ahorsu et al. [10], made up of 7 items, in health workers. This research also comprises several specific objectives. First, we aim to examine the role that fear of COVID-19 plays in emotional disorders and, in turn, in psychological detachment. Second, we will assess whether positive occupational health, through collaborative crafting and psychological empowerment (PE), can act as a relevant factor in preventing emotional disorders and lead to better recovery experiences after the workday. Finally, we intend to determine whether the fear of COVID-19 has any negative effect on PE and, in turn, whether it affects how healthcare professionals' distance themselves from work.

1.1. Current Situation of the Fear of COVID-19

Ahorsu et al. developed a brief instrument to detect fear of COVID-19 in the general population [10]. As these authors explained, fear is directly associated with the transmission rate and morbidity. This scale has been adapted to other cultures in general population [11–19]. However, no psychometric adaptations and assessments of the Fear of COVID-19 Scale in health workers were found in the literature. The assessment of fear of COVID-19 levels in different sociodemographic groups is relevant for the implementation of specific prevention programs [8]. We also consider it especially important to know whether there is fear in professional sectors that are in direct contact with the virus and that have a high risk of exposure contagion. Early detection of fear of COVID-19 can act as an alarm signal to health workers to prevent the development of emotional disorders and, therefore, be able to recover from stressful work situations.

On the other hand, a recent meta-analysis showed that health professionals working to combat COVID-19 are more affected by psychiatric disorders, sleep disorders, stress, and indirect trauma than other occupational groups [20]. Pappa et al. Additionally suggested that a significant proportion of health workers have experienced mood and sleep disorders [21]. De Brier et al. stated that the level of exposure to the disease and fear for health were significantly associated with worse mental health outcomes [2]. Additionally, finding oneself in stressful, scary situations can lead to emotional disorders that, in turn, can prevent proper psychological detachment from work. This detachment is part of a process called recovery, through which people stop facing a demanding situation to regain energy to continue and renew the resources invested in that situation [22]. Stressful experiences are considered the opposite process of recovery [22]. Sonnentag et al. reported that employees who felt exhausted found it more difficult to disconnect psychologically from work [23]. They also stressed the importance of time pressure in the increase of the association between exhaustion and lower psychological detachment. In this sense, the duration of stressful experiences and feelings of fear during the COVID-19 pandemic can contribute to health workers' being unable to disconnect from work, thus preventing adequate recovery experiences.

1.2. Job Crafting and Psychological Empowerment

Job crafting is defined as employee's proactive behavior aiming to modify the relational, cognitive, or task limits to shape or redesign a job [24]. Most research has studied job crafting on an individual level. However, Leana et al. consider job crafting not only to consist of an individual employee's activity, but of the fact that workers participate in similar work processes, relate to each other, and experience common events [25]. This refers to collaborative crafting, whereby employees can team up and decide how to modify tasks to achieve their goals. Moreover, in certain professions, such as in health care or education, it is difficult to adapt individual work due to the high degree of interdependence between groups [26]. Research linking job crafting to PE is still scarce. However, several authors have shown that job crafting is strongly related to PE [27,28]. Specifically, Harbridge conducted a study on registered nurses and highlighted job crafting as an important predictor of PE [28]. Demerouti proposed that job crafting may lead to greater motivation, performance, or engagement [29].

On the other hand, PE consists of a subjective, cognitive, and attitudinal process through which the individual feels effective, competent, and authorized to perform tasks. Spreitzer considers that PE reflects an active orientation and self-perception of the ability to shape one's working role [30]. While PE is not synonymous with intrinsic motivation, it can be considered a predictor of it [31], and therefore a motivational factor. The four components of PE are a proximal cause of intrinsic task motivation and satisfaction [31]. Schermuly and Meyer showed that PE leads to less emotional fatigue and depression [32]. It also strongly influences the degree of work stress experienced by workers [33]. Petersen et al. found evidence that self-efficacy is amendable to change and exerts an effect on protective behavior. The effects of fear were small among those who felt efficacious [34].

On the other hand, Ghosh et al. found that psychological detachment acts as a moderator between intrinsic motivation and engagement [35]. Employees who feel motivated and psychologically detached from work in their free time are also more creative [35].

Thirdly, to test the last specific objective, we aim to determine whether fear of COVID-19 has any negative effect on psychological detachment, through the mediation of PE. There is no literature linking the fear of COVID-19 to organizational variables such as PE. However, other types of fear, such as fear of success, have been linked to self-efficacy and intrinsic motivation. Specifically, both of them can be used to mitigate the potentially adverse effects of this type of fear [36]. In this sense, in a situation of fear of COVID-19, workers are expected to have reduced PE and be incapable of activating the cognitive processes that enable them to perform tasks effectively and competently. In this way, they will not be able to distance themselves from their work in their free time.

Hypothesis 1. *Emotional disorders will play a mediating role in the relationship between the fear of COVID-19 and psychological detachment.*

Hypothesis 2. *PE will mediate the relationship between collaborative crafting and emotional disorders.*

Hypothesis 3. *Emotional disorders will mediate between PE and psychological detachment.*

Hypothesis 4. *PE will mediate the relationship between fear of COVID-19 and the psychological detachment of health professionals.*

2. Materials and Methods

2.1. Participants and Procedure

The sample was made up of a total of 194 workers from the health centers of the province of Soria belonging to the Health Service of Castilla y León (Sacyl) in Spain. Permission was requested from the organization's Ethics Committee, and the questionnaires were forwarded to a total of 1056 workers, obtaining a response rate of 18.37%. Data collection took place in July 2020 via email. Through this means, participants accessed a link in Google Forms by which, after providing their informed consent, access was given to fill out the questionnaire. The final sample consisted of 162 women and 32 men, with an average age of 45.94 (SD = 12.39). Of the sample, 28.4% had been diagnosed with COVID-19 or had been detected to have antibodies after a test. Concerning their employment status, 50.5% of the participants were nurses or specialist nurses, 26.3% were specialized graduates, and 12.4% were assistant nursing technicians. Hence, most of the participants were healthcare professionals. Additionally, 45.9% of the sample considered that their tasks or work activities during the COVID-19 pandemic had changed compared with those they had performed previously. (see Table 1).

Table 1. Demographics.

	N	%	*M*	*SD*
Age	194		45.94	12.39
Gender				
Female	162	83.5		
Male	32	16.5		
Professional category				
TCAE (nursing assistant)	24	12.4		
Nurse/Specialist Nurse	98	50.5		
Specialist graduate	51	26.3		
Administration	6	3.1		
Physiotherapy	7	3.6		
Social work	3	1.5		
Higher technician	5	2.6		
Organizational rank				
Intermediate or higher posts	46	23.7		
Workers without people in their care	148	76.3		
Job tenure in the current contract			12.20	12.97
Changing tasks or activities during the pandemic:				
Changes	89	45.9		
No changes	105	54.1		
COVID-19 diagnosis				
Yes	55	28.4		
No	139	71.6		
Type of contract				
Permanent	101	52.1		
Temporary	93	47.9		
Workplace during the pandemic				
COVID Floor or Team	83	42.8		
Non-COVID Service	46	23.7		
Health Center	57	29.4		
Telework/union release/administration	8	4.1		

Note: *N*, Sample Size; M, Mean; SD, Standard Deviation; TCAE, Technician in Auxiliary Nursing Care.

2.2. Instrument

To assess fear of COVID-19, the Fear of COVID-19 Scale was used [10]. As a preliminary step, the questionnaire was translated into Spanish by a blind back-translation process [37]. Two methodology experts compared the original scale and the final Spanish version [38]. The questionnaire is a one-dimensional scale consisting of seven items measured on a Likert-like response scale ranging from 1 (Totally Disagree) to 5 (Totally Agree). The internal consistency index of the scale ($\alpha = 0.90$) was higher than that obtained for the original scale ($\alpha = 0.82$) [10].

As mentioned above, PE refers to several cognitive processes that modify the subjective self-perception, by which the worker feels intrinsically motivated and effective to perform tasks [30]. In this study, PE was evaluated using the Psychological Empowerment Scale [30], adapted to Spanish [39] consisting of four subscales: (a) Meaning (three items, e.g., "My work activities have been personally valuable"); (b) Competence (three items, e.g., "I trust my ability to get the job done"); (c) Self-determination (three items, e.g., "I have had the autonomy to determine how to do my job"); and (d) Impact (three items, e.g., "I've had enough influence on what was going on in my work"). The Likert-type response scale ranged from 1 (Totally Disagree) to 5 (Totally Agree). High scores indicate greater PE. The reliability coefficient was high ($\alpha = 0.84$).

To assess participants' anxiety and depression, we used the Hospital Scale of Anxiety and Depression (HADS) [40], consisting of two subscales of seven items each. Items in the Anxiety subscale aim to detect generalized anxiety ("I feel tense or nervous"), and the subscale of Depression primarily assesses the state of anhedonia ("I feel like I'm slowing down every day"). The response range ranged from 1 (Totally Disagree) to 5 (Totally Agree). The internal consistency in this study was high for both the total scale ($\alpha = 0.92$), the Anxiety subscale ($\alpha = 0.91$), and the Depression subscale ($\alpha = 0.87$).

To evaluate collaborative crafting, the two-dimensional Spanish-validated Job Crafting Questionnaire [25,26] was used. In the study, we used the 6-item Collaborative Crafting Subscale, of which only five items were used (e.g., "You work together with your peers to introduce new approaches to improving your work"). Specifically, the item that refers to celebrations or events at work was removed, as it was deemed inappropriate in the pandemic situation. The response scale ranged from 1 (Totally Disagree) to 5 (Totally Agree). The reliability coefficient was high ($\alpha = 0.91$).

To measure psychological detachment, we used the Recovery Experience Questionnaire [41] validated in Spanish [22], which presents four subdimensions: Psychological Detachment, Relaxation, Challenge-Seeking, and Control. For the study, three items of the Psychological Detachment subscale were used (e.g., "After work, I can disconnect) measured on a Likert-type scale ranging from 1 (Totally disagree) to 5 (Totally agree). The reliability coefficient was high ($\alpha = 0.95$).

Finally, the following demographic data were collected: age, gender, professional category, organizational rank, job tenure in the current contract, diagnosis of Covid, place of work, type of contract, and modification of tasks or activities during the pandemic.

2.3. Data Analysis

To evaluate the descriptive statistics and bivariate correlations of the study variables, we used the IBM SPSS Statistics 26 program [42]. The data was then analyzed using a structural equations model (SEM) based on the variance, with the method of partial least squares (PLS) [43]. This procedure allows simultaneously assessing the reliability and validity of the measures of the theoretical construct (measurement model) and estimating the relationships between constructs (structural model) [44]. A new approach called consistent PLS was used because, if the common factor model is retained, consistent PLS or covariance-based SEM should be the first choice of researchers over traditional PLS [45]. Additionally, when comparing PLS-SEM with CB-SEM, PLS can handle small sample sizes and discard the assumption of normality, so it is recommended for social science research [46]. Thus, in the present investigation the method of choice is PLS-SEM, which is considered a more robust method when the sample size is reduced. The data were analyzed with the statistical software SmartPLS (v.3.3.2) [47].

3. Results

The mean, standard deviations, and correlations of the study variables are presented in Table 2.

Table 2. Bivariate correlations, means, and standard deviations.

Variables	*M*	*SD*	1	2	3	4
Collaborative Crafting	3.63	0.97	-			
Psychological Empowerment	3.90	0.70	0.48 **	-		
Fear of COVID-19	2.38	0.90	−0.12	−0.16 *	-	
Emotional disorders	2.36	0.83	−0.17 *	−0.26 **	0.77 **	-
Psychological Detachment	2.92	1.20	0.16 *	0.20 **	−0.43 **	−0.59 **

Note: $N = 302$. * $p < 0.05$, ** $p < 0.01$. - indicates a blank space.

Before analyzing the data for the adaptation of the Fear to COVID-19 scale, we examined skewness and kurtosis to verify that the data did not stray excessively from a normal distribution. PLS-SEM is a non-parametric statistical method [48]. Although the data are not required to have a normal distribution, if extremely non-normal data were present, the standard errors obtained through bootstrapping could be inflated, and the probability of finding significant relationships between variables would decrease [48]. These authors recommend examining two distribution measures, skewness and kurtosis. In most indicators, values between −0.99 and +0.98 were obtained, so we decided not to eliminate any of them, as there was no problem of non-normality.

The interpretation of the PLS model comprises three phases: (a) evaluation of the global model, (b) measurement model (external model), and (c) structural model (internal model). We also performed an analysis of the invariance of the measurement model to determine whether similar measures were obtained in different groups.

3.1. Global Model

To evaluate the global model, the Standardized Root Mean Square Residual (SRMR) parameter was used, which measures the difference between the observed correlation matrix and the correlation matrix implied by the model. Hu and Bentler proposed values of SRMR < 0.08 to achieve a good fit of the data [49]. Ringle proposed a more flexible option (SRMR < 0.10) [50]. In this study, we obtained an SRMR of 0.077 both in the saturated and estimated models.

3.2. Measurement Model

The evaluation of the reflective measurement models includes composite reliability (to assess internal consistency), the reliability of the individual indicator, and the mean-variance extracted (AVE) to assess convergent validity [48]. In addition, such measurement models also assess discriminant validity.

First, the internal consistency reliability of the Fear of COVID-19 Scale was tested. Cronbach's alpha coefficient obtained a high value of 0.90. Composite reliability and reliability rho_A obtained values of 0.89 and 0.90, respectively. These composite reliability values are considered satisfactory. Values greater than 0.95 are not adequate because they could suggest that all indicators are measuring the same phenomenon [48]. The rest of the variables also obtained high levels of internal consistency.

Second, convergent validity was assessed, examining the loadings or simple correlations of indicators with their construct. The external loadings of the indicator should be greater than 0.707 [51]. In the case of our Fear of COVID-19 Scale, items 5, 6, and 7 exceeded the value of 0.707, whereas the rest obtained values between 0.58 and 0.67. Indicators with loadings between 0.40 and 0.70 should be removed if there is an increase in composite reliability [52]. After performing the analyses without these items, the composite reliability only decreased from 0.89 to 0.84, so we decided to maintain them. For all other variables, several analyses were performed, eliminating indicators with values between 0.40 and 0.70. In the case of emotional disorders, there was an increase in composite reliability (0.92) and AVE (0.50), so item 4 was removed from the Anxiety scale and item 4 from the Depression scale. On the PE scale, items 1 and 2 (Meaning subscale), 5 (Competency subscale), 7 (Self-Determination subscale), and 10 (Impact subscale) were also removed. Thus, a high composite reliability value (0.84) was obtained.

Convergent validity was evaluated through AVE. The Fear of COVID-19 Scale obtained a value of 0.55, above the recommended value of 0.50. This indicates that the construct explains more than half of the variance of its indicators. The rest of the variables, except for PE, achieved values greater than 0.50.

Finally, discriminant validity was assessed through the cross-loads, following the criterion of Fornell and Larcker and the Heterotrait-Monotrait ratio (HTMT). The load of the indicators on the Fear of COVID-19 Scale was higher than their cross-loads with other constructs, indicating discriminant validity. Concerning the Fornell criterion, the square root of the AVE of the Fear of COVID-19 (0.75) was not higher than the correlation between fear and emotional disorders (0.87). However, given the absence of discrepancies between the two criteria, we valued the HTMT. The Fornell and Larcker criterion is not appropriate when the loadings of the indicators of the constructs differ only slightly [48]. HTMT should be lower than 0.85. All the variables had lower values, so discriminant validity was achieved (see Table 3) [53].

Table 3. Measurement model: loads, construct reliability, and convergent validity.

Latent Variable	Item	λ	CR	α	Rho_A	AVE
Collaborative Crafting	CC1	0.71	0.91	0.91	0.91	0.66
	CC2	0.84				
	CC3	0.68				
	CC4	0.86				
	CC5	0.94				
Psychological empowerment	PE3	0.51	0.84	0.84	0.85	0.44
	PE4	0.56				
	PE6	0.56				
	PE8	0.71				
	PE9	0.70				
	PE11	0.73				
	PE12	0.77				
Fear of COVID-19	F1	0.67	0.89	0.90	0.90	0.55
	F2	0.58				
	F3	0.66				
	F4	0.67				
	F5	0.89				
	F6	0.88				
	F7	0.81				
Psychological detachment	PD1	0.98	0.95	0.95	0.95	0.86
	PD2	0.91				
	PD3	0.88				
Emotional disorders	ED1	0.81	0.92	0.92	0.92	0.50
	ED2	0.84				
	ED3	0.74				
	ED5	0.77				
	ED6	0.71				
	ED7	0.82				
	ED8	0.62				
	ED9	0.63				
	ED10	0.67				
	ED12	0.63				
	ED13	0.57				
	ED14	0.60				

Note: λ = Loadings. CR = Composite reliability. Rho_A = Dijkstra-Henseler's rho (ρA). AVE = Average variance extracted. A = Cronbach's alpha. Items removed: Psychological empowerment 1, 2, 5, 7, and 10; Emotional disorders 4 and 11.

3.3. Structural Model

Having verified that the measures of the constructs are reliable and valid, we valued the structural model. First, we evaluated the collinearity of the structural model, using the variance inflation factor (VIF) whose value must be 5 or less [52]. The results showed that all VIF values were below 5, indicating the absence of collinearity between predictors. Specifically, the VIF value between EP and Collaborative Crafting, and between EP and fear of COVID-19 was 1.01. Between emotional disorders and PE, and emotional disorders and fear, the VIF was 1.05, whereas between PE and psychological detachment, it was 1.12. The highest values of VIF were 4.53 and 4.30, between detachment and emotional disorders, and detachment and fear, respectively.

The algebraic sign, magnitude, and statistical significance of the path coefficients were also evaluated. The signs of the path coefficients matched the hypotheses raised. The highest values of the standardized beta coefficients (β) were between fear of COVID-19 and emotional disorders ($\beta = 0.85$, $p < 0.001$) and between emotional disorders and psychological detachment ($\beta = -0.82$, $p < 0.001$).

Bootstrapping was used for consistent PLS (10,000 subsamples) to assess the meaning of the path coefficients. The relationships between Collaborative Crafting and PE ($t = 7.90$, $p < 0.001$), between PE and emotional disorders ($t = 2.28$, $p = 0.023$), between fear of COVID-19 and emotional disorders ($t = 24.01$, $p < 0.001$), and between emotional disorders and psychological detachment ($t = 3.95$, $p < 0.001$) were significant. In contrast, fear of COVID-19 was not directly related to psychological detachment ($t = 1.24$, $p = 0.21$), or to PE ($t = 1.90$, $p = 0.05$).

On the other hand, we calculated the indirect effects between the variables. The indirect effect of fear of COVID-19 on psychological detachment ($\beta = -0.69$, $p < 0.001$), through the mediation of emotional disorders, was significant. The indirect effect of collaborative crafting on emotional disorders was also significant, through the mediation of PE ($\beta = -0.06$, $p = 0.033$). Additionally, the mediation of emotional disorders in the relationship between PE and psychological detachment was significant ($\beta = 0.10$, $p < 0.001$). These results support Hypotheses 1, 2, and 3. However, Hypothesis 4 could not be confirmed. In Figure 1, we specify the structural model. In Table 4, we specify the total effects of the model.

Table 4. Total effects.

	Beta Coefficients	*t* Statistics	*p* Value
Crafting -> Detachment	0.091	2.228	0.026
Crafting -> Emocional Disorders	−0.064	2.132	0.033
Crafting -> Empowerment	0.513	7.863	0.001
Emocional Disorders -> Detachment	−0.822	3.975	0.001
Empowerment -> Detachment	0.177	2.404	0.016
Empowerment -> Emocional Disorders	−0.125	2.297	0.023
Fear -> Detachment	−0.468	8.114	0.001
Fear -> Emocional Disorders	0.866	27.97	0.001
Fear -> Empowerment	−0.152	1.912	0.056

With regard to the coefficient of determination, the model explained 40.9% of the variance of psychological detachment, 77.9% of the variance of emotional disorders, and 30.6% of PE.

3.4. MICOM Model: Analysis of the Invariance of the Measurement Model

Measurement invariance, or measure equivalence, means that group differences in model estimates are not due to the different content or meaning of the latent variables between groups [48], but as to whether, under different conditions of observation and study of the phenomena, the measurement operations produce measurements of the same attribute [54]. Henseler et al. developed a procedure for calculating the measurement invariance of composite models (MICOM) [55]. This method is developed in three hierarchically interrelated stages. As Henseler et al. explain, variance-based SEM techniques model latent variables as composite variables, so this procedure is considered appropriate for assessing common factor models, such as the one presented in this study [55].

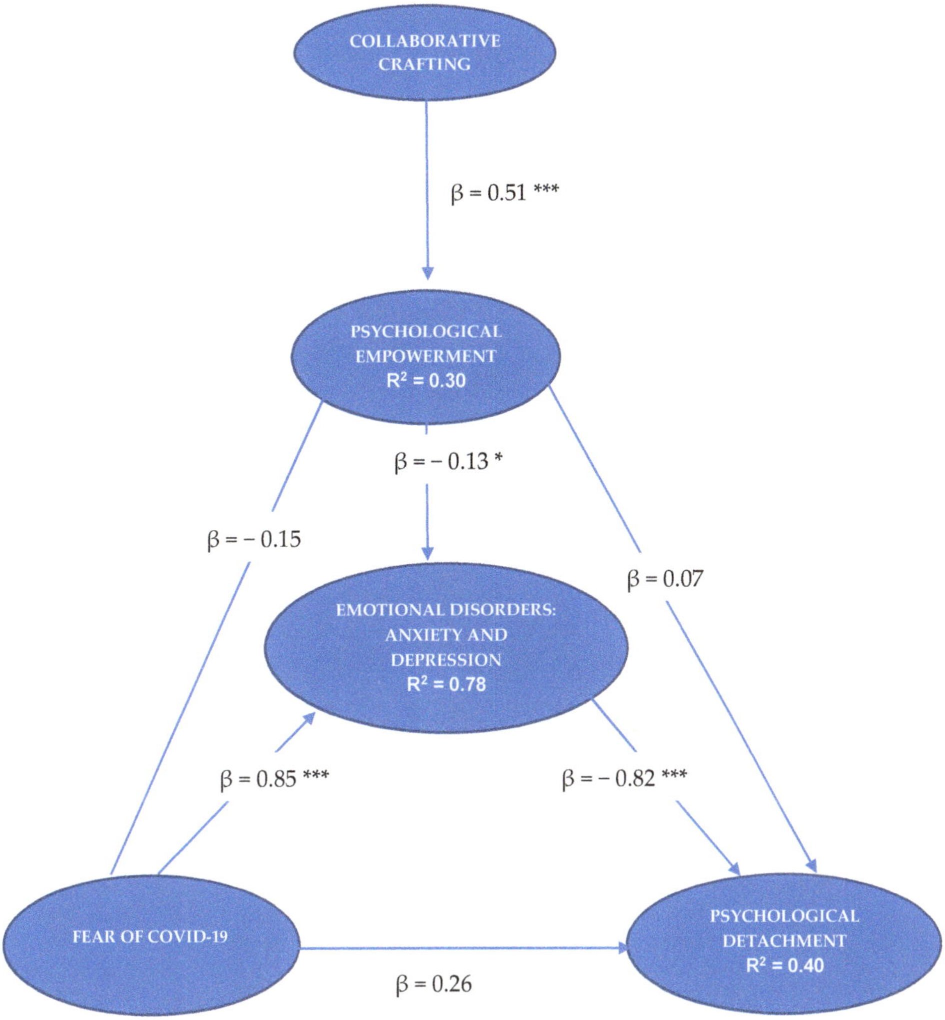

Figure 1. Structural model. * $p < 0.05$. *** $p < 0.001$.

3.4.1. First Stage: Configuration Invariance

This determines whether a composite has been specified equally in all groups and whether it emerges as a one-dimensional entity in the same nomological network for all groups [55]. In this study, the initial qualitative evaluation ensures that the same indicators are used in each measurement model, the data are processed in the same way, and the algorithm is also configured identically.

3.4.2. Second Stage: Composite Invariance

It analyzes whether a composite is formed in the same way in all groups [55]. To evaluate composite invariance, we performed a permutation algorithm with PLS (5000 permutations), in which the selected groups were, on the one hand, the participants whose work tasks or activities had been changed during the COVID-19 pandemic, and on the other hand, those whose activity was similar to before the health emergency. To test composite invariance, the original correlation must be greater than or equal to the 5% quantile.

In Table 5, MICOM results show that the composite scores did not differ between the two groups.

Table 5. MICOM. Stage 2 results.

	Original Correlation	Correlation of Permutation Means	5.0%	p-Values of the Permutation
Collaborative Crafting	0.999	0.998	0.995	0.50
Psychological Detachment	1.000	1.000	1.000	0.95
Emotional Disorders	0.999	0.999	0.997	0.25
Psychological Empowerment	0.983	0.986	0.958	0.27
Fear of COVID-19	0.999	0.999	0.997	0.31

3.4.3. Third Stage: Evaluation of Equal Means and Variances of the Composite Variables

In the third step, we determined whether the original differences in means and variances were between 2.5% and 97.5%, and complete invariance was established. If only one of these variances fell between 2.5% and 97.5%, then partial invariance of means and variances would be considered. In Table 6, the results of the third MICOM stage suggest equality of means and variances.

Table 6. MICOM. Stage 3 results. Original differences in mean and variance.

	Mean-Original Differences (Mean-Difference of Permutation Means)	2.5%	97.5%	p-Values of the Permutation	Variance-Original Difference (Variance-Difference of Permutation Means)	2.5%	97.5%	p-Values of the Permutation
Psychological Empowerment	0.18 (0.002)	−0.28	0.28	0.19	−0.18 (−0.004)	−0.42	0.43	0.40
Collaborative Crafting	0.18 (0.002)	−0.27	0.27	0.21	−0.10 (−0.004)	−0.36	0.36	0.61
Emotional Disorders	0.008 (−0.002)	−0.28	0.27	0.95	−0.07 (−0.004)	−0.34	0.32	0.67
Fear of COVID-19	−0.07 (−0.001)	−0.29	0.28	0.58	−0.07 (−0.001)	−0.42	0.39	0.72
Psychological Detachment	−0.18 (0.002)	−0.29	0.28	0.21	−0.02 (−0.002)	−0.27	0.27	0.88

Therefore, after observing that all three stages were met, we performed multigroup analysis based on group data [48]. We ran the multigroup analysis in PLS and analyzed the non-parametric PLS-MGA approach, which compares each bootstrap estimate of a given parameter between each of the groups [48]. Again, we performed the calculation with 5000 subsamples. All values were nonsignificant, indicating that no bootstrap estimate of a parameter differed between groups. As can be seen in Table 7, our results suggest that there are no significant differences between the two groups (changes in work activities vs. no changes in work activities).

Table 7. PLS-MGA (PLS-Multigroup Analysis results).

	Path Coefficients	Original 1-Tail p-Value	New p-Value
Crafting and Empowerment	−0.06	0.71	0.57
Emotional Disorders and Detachment	−0.16	0.78	0.42
Empowerment and Detachment	−0.18	0.94	0.12
Empowerment and Emotional Disorders	0.08	0.18	0.37
Fear and Detachment	0.33	0.05	0.11
Fear and Emotional Disorders	0.06	0.15	0.30
Fear and Empowerment	−0.04	0.61	0.77

Note: The contrasting groups were: Participants with changes in their tasks or work activities during the COVID-19 pandemic vs. participants with no changes in their tasks.

4. Discussion

The main objective of this work was to adapt and validate the Fear of COVID-19 Scale [10], composed of seven items, in health workers. The results show that it is a valid and reliable scale and that its structure consists of a single factor, as other authors have suggested [10,12,13,15,16,18]. First, the evaluation of the overall model based on the SRMR criterion showed adequate goodness of fit, thus indicating that the model is probably appropriate. Second, by rating the external or measurement model, we conclude that both the composite reliability of the scale and the internal consistency reliability are adequate. Appropriate values of convergent and discriminant validity were also obtained. Other authors have found similar results in terms of composite reliability [10], internal consistency [13], convergent validity [10], and discriminant validity [56]. Finally, to ensure that the differences between groups are not due to the content or meaning of the latent variables, we tested the measurement invariance of composite models (MICOM). The results showed that there were no differences between the groups of participants (with and without changes in their tasks or activities), indicating the existence of measurement equivalence between the two groups.

The evaluation of the structural model determines whether the postulated assumptions are met. Concerning the first hypothesis, this research was intended to assess the role of fear of COVID-19 in the development of anxious-depressive disorders, and in health workers' ability to distance themselves psychologically from their work. The results have shown that fear of COVID-19 is a strong predictor of emotional disorders, such that health professionals who score higher in fear of COVID-19 are more likely to develop anxiety and/or depression. Ahorsu et al. also found significant relationships between fear and anxiety or depression, suggesting that people with severe fear may have these emotional disorders [10]. Additionally, in this study, we found that fear determines health workers' inability to distance themselves from work, but only if they suffer some degree of comorbid anxiety and depression. This result is in line with the results of Sonnentag et al., because health workers who feel more exhausted find it more difficult to detach psychologically from work [23].

Concerning the second hypothesis, which sought to test the ability of positive occupational health to prevent mental health problems at work, we found that collaborative crafting behaviors lead to health-care workers' greater PE. In the first months of the pandemic, uncertainty due to the lack of knowledge of the coronavirus disease and the hospital collapse determined the need to work collaboratively and to modify the usual tasks of healthcare professionals (e.g., nurses or technicians who changed their jobs to work on Covid floors or doctors with non-COVID-19 specialties working together with internists or intensive care doctors). These collaborative crafting behaviors have proven to be important predictors of PE. Other authors have shown that PE leads to less emotional fatigue and depression [32]. In this study, we highlight the importance of PE as a mediator in the relationship between collaborative crafting and emotional disorders. These results provide evidence to the literature about the importance of job crafting interventions to enable employees to proactively create a motivating work environment and improve their well-being [57].

Next, we discuss the confirmation of the third hypothesis. We expected that the most empowered workers could psychologically distance more from work than those who are not empowered. In this relationship, we observed the importance of having no emotional disorders for health workers to recover after their working day, as anxiety and depression problems acted as a total mediator. Hochwälder and Brucefors also found that greater PE at work generally corresponds with fewer health problems [58].

Concerning the fourth hypothesis, which tested the role of fear in detachment through the mediation of PE, we found no significant relationships. Faced with a situation of fear of COVID-19, workers' PE is not reduced, but other organizational variables, such as job crafting, activate the cognitive processes that enable them to perform their tasks.

Finally, we consider that one of the strengths of this research has been to relate positive organizational psychology to the prevention of basic emotions such as fear to decrease emotional disorders. Thus, we link lower fear scores with the preventive role of PE (after the development of collaborative crafting interventions) to develop fewer mental health problems and recover psychologically from work.

4.1. Limitations

Firstly, and as the main limitation, we highlight the impossibility of establishing relationships of direct causality. The findings should be interpreted with caution due to the cross-sectional nature of the data and the lack of longitudinal research on COVID-19 fear and emotional disorders. Secondly, the data are self-reported, so they should be treated with caution. Additionally, we consider a possible threat to external validity. When health workers responded to the questionnaire, they could react to the pandemic situation and respond according to the social norm, as a function of what is expected of the group of health professionals. For example, if a healthcare provider verbalizes that he or she is afraid of COVID-19, this may be criticized from the point of view of normative influence. Thirdly, as a threat to internal validity, we highlight the motivation to answer the questionnaire, or self-selection bias. The participants in this study may have had different expectations than those who chose not to participate. In future research focused on health workers, it would be advisable to assess the participants' degree of social desirability.

On the other hand, this study was carried out in a single health institution and in the province with the highest incidence of seroprevalence in Spain [59]. This could pose a problem for the generalization of the results to the rest of health professionals in this country. In addition, another important limitation is the small size of the sample that can cause low representativeness.

In addition, this study was carried out in July 2020, after three months of quarantine in Spain, and Soria was the most affected province, with a 14% seroprevalence of SARS-COV-2 [59]. However, the study was conducted at a time when the hospital situation was adequate. There was no hospital overload or collapse. In the questionnaire, professionals were instructed to evaluate the previous three months. However, these previous circumstances could have altered the answers.

Finally, it should be noted that these results were obtained in an exceptional situation of a global pandemic. Health workers were exposed to contagion due to lack of personal protective equipment, uncertainty, fear of infecting family members, helplessness from lack of knowledge about the disease, etc. Collaborative crafting was analyzed in a situation where health workers performed as a team and collaboratively more than ever. For this reason, we must be cautious and consider the exceptionality of the situation as a limitation of this study and analyze these organizational variables (job crafting and PE) in times of non-pandemic normality.

4.2. Future Lines of Research and Practical Implications

This study has important practical implications. We emphasize the importance of early detection of fear of COVID-19 to prevent emotional disorders, as well as to improve recovery experiences after the workday. Additionally, the Fear of COVID-19 Scale was adapted [10] for health workers, so it can be appropriately used to analyze this emotion in them. We also know the importance of promoting positive occupational health to prevent these anxious-depressive disorders. Through practices that enhance collaborative crafting, health workers can be empowered and thereby, reduce mental health problems.

We found no research papers in the literature that relate positive organizational psychology and the psychology of emotions to mental health problems and recovery experiences. Coelho et al. recommended that future research on fear of COVID-19 and anxiety should focus on pointing to protective and risk factors of psychological well-being [60]. Other authors consider that leaders need to have the appropriate communication that provides up-to-date information and encourages individual empowerment to support their staff [61]. As future lines of research, more studies are proposed that investigate these models and analyze them over time through longitudinal research.

Author Contributions: Writing—Original draft, M.L.-A., C.G.-A. and G.T.; Writing—review and editing, M.L.-A., C.G.-A. and G.T. Resources, M.L.S.-M., I.M.-A., and B.C.-A. All authors have read and agreed to the published version of the manuscript.

Funding: This research received no external funding.

Institutional Review Board Statement: The study was conducted according to the guidelines of the Declaration of Helsinki, and approved by the Ethics Committee of Burgos and Soria health area of Castile and Leon Health Service (Protocol Code REF CEim 2349 and date of approval 12 June 2020).

Informed Consent Statement: Informed consent was obtained from all subjects involved in the study.

Data Availability Statement: The datasets generated and analyzed during the current study are available from the corresponding author on reasonable request.

Conflicts of Interest: The authors declare no conflict of interest.

References

1. Luo, M.; Guo, L.; Yu, M.; Jiang, W.; Wang, H. The psychological and mental impact of coronavirus disease 2019 (COVID-19) on medical staff and general public—A systematic review and meta-analysis. *Psychiatry Res.* **2020**, *291*, 113190. [CrossRef] [PubMed]
2. De Brier, N.; Stroobants, S.; Vandekerckhove, P.; De Buck, E. Factors Affecting Mental Health of Health Care Workers during Coronavirus Disease Outbreaks (SARS, MERS & COVID-19): A Rapid Systematic Review. *PLoS ONE* **2020**, *15*, e0244052.
3. Center for Sociological Research, CIS. Efectos y Consecuencias del Coronavirus (I). Estudio nº 3298. Available online: http://www.cis.es/cis/export/sites/default/-Archivos/Marginales/3280_3299/3298/es3298mar.pdf (accessed on 31 October 2020).
4. Center for Sociological Research, CIS. Efectos y Consecuencias del Coronavirus (III). Estudio nº 3305. Available online: http://datos.cis.es/pdf/Es3305marMT_A.pdf. (accessed on 28 December 2020).
5. Pastor-Barriuso, R.; Pérez-Gómez, B.; Hernán, M.; Pérez-Olmeda, M.; Yotti, R.; Oteo-Iglesias, J.; Sanmartín, J.; León-Gómez, I.; Fernández-García, A.; Fernández-Navarro, P.; et al. Infection fatality risk for SARS-CoV-2 in community dwelling population of Spain: nationwide seroepidemiological study. *BMJ* **2020**, *371*, m4509. [CrossRef] [PubMed]
6. Royal Spanish Academy. *Diccionario de la Lengua Española*, 23th ed.; Version 23.4 Online. Available online: https://dle.rae.es (accessed on 21 February 2021).
7. Goyal, K.; Chauhan, P.; Chhikara, K.; Gupta, P.; Singh, M. Fear of COVID 2019: First Suicidal Case in India. *Asian J. Psychiatr.* **2020**, *49*, 101989. [CrossRef]
8. Pakpour, A.; Griffiths, M. The fear of COVID-19 and its role in preventive behaviors. *J. Concurr. Disord.* **2020**, *2*, 58–63. Available online: http://irep.ntu.ac.uk/id/eprint/39561/ (accessed on 10 March 2021).
9. Gunnell, D.; Appleby, L.; Arensman, E.; Hawton, K.; John, A.; Kapur, N.; Khan, M.; O'Connor, R.; Pirkis, J.; Appleby, L.; et al. Suicide Risk and Prevention during the COVID-19 Pandemic. *Lancet Psychiatry* **2020**, *7*, 468–471. [CrossRef]
10. Ahorsu, D.; Lin, C.; Imani, V.; Saffari, M.; Griffiths, M.; Pakpour, A. The Fear of COVID-19 Scale: Development and Initial Validation. *Int J. Ment Health Addict.* **2020**, *27*, 1–9. [CrossRef]
11. Tzur Bitan, D.; Grossman-Giron, A.; Bloch, Y.; Mayer, Y.; Shiffman, N.; Mendlovic, S. Fear of COVID-19 scale: Psychometric characteristics, reliability and validity in the Israeli population. *Psychiatry Res.* **2020**, *289*, 113100. [CrossRef]
12. Martínez-Lorca, M.; Martínez-Lorca, A.; Criado-Álvarez, J.J.; Armesilla, M.; Latorre, J.M. The fear of COVID-19 scale: Validation in spanish university students. *Psychiatry Res.* **2020**, *293*, 113350. [CrossRef]
13. Soraci, P.; Ferrari, A.; Abbiati, F.A.; Del Fante, E.; De Pace, R.; Urso, A.; Griffiths, M.D. Validation and Psychometric Evaluation of the Italian Version of the Fear of COVID-19 Scale. *Int J. Ment Health Addict.* **2020**, *4*, 1–10. [CrossRef]
14. Reznik, A.; Gritsenko, V.; Konstantinov, V.; Khamenka, N.; Isralowitz, R. COVID-19 Fear in Eastern Europe: Validation of the Fear of COVID-19 Scale. *Int. J. Ment. Health Addict.* **2020**, *12*, 1–6. [CrossRef] [PubMed]
15. Alyami, M.; Henning, M.; Krägeloh, C.U.; Alyami, H. Psychometric Evaluation of the Arabic Version of the Fear of COVID-19 Scale. *Int. J. Ment. Health Addict.* **2020**, 1–14, Advance online publication. [CrossRef]
16. Sakib, N.; Bhuiyan, A.K.M.I.; Hossain, S.; Al Mamun, F.; Hosen, I.; Abdullah, A.H.; Mamun, M.A.; Mohiuddin, M.S.; Rayhan, I.; Hossain, M.; et al. Psychometric Validation of the Bangla Fear of COVID-19 Scale: Confirmatory Factor Analysis and Rasch Analysis. *Int J. Ment Health Addict.* **2020**, *11*, 1–12. [CrossRef] [PubMed]
17. Pang, N.T.P.; Kamu, A.; Hambali, N.L.B.; Mun, H.C.; Kassim, M.A.; Mohamed, N.H.; Ayu, F.; Rahim, S.S.S.A.; Omar, A.; Jeffree, M.S. Malay Version of the Fear of COVID-19 Scale: Validity and Reliability. *Int. J. Ment. Health Addict.* **2020**, *3*, 1–10. [CrossRef]
18. Satici, B.; Gocet-Tekin, E.; Deniz, M.E.; Satici, S.A. Adaptation of the Fear of COVID-19 Scale: Its Association with Psychological Distress and Life Satisfaction in Turkey. *Int. J. Ment. Health Addict.* **2020**, 1–9, Advance online publication. [CrossRef] [PubMed]
19. Chi, X.; Chen, S.; Chen, Y.; Chen, D.; Yu, Q.; Guo, T.; Cao, Q.; Zheng, X.; Huang, S.; Hossain, M.; et al. Psychometric Evaluation of the Fear of COVID-19 Scale Among Chinese Population. *Int J. Ment. Health Addict.* **2020**, *11*, 1–16. [CrossRef]

20. Da Silva, F.; Neto, M. Psychiatric symptomatology associated with depression, anxiety, distress, and insomnia in health professionals working in patients affected by COVID-19: A systematic review with meta-analysis. *Prog. Neuropsychopharmacol. Biol. Psychiatry* **2021**, *104*, 110057. [CrossRef]
21. Pappa, S.; Ntella, V.; Giannakas, T.; Giannakoulis, V.G.; Papoutsi, E.; Katsaounou, P. Prevalence of depression, anxiety, and insomnia among healthcare workers during the COVID-19 pandemic: A systematic review and meta-analysis. *Brain Behav. Immun.* **2020**, *88*, 901–907. [CrossRef]
22. Sanz-Vergel, A.I.; Sebastián, J.; Rodríguez-Muñoz, A.; Garrosa, E.; Moreno-Jiménez, B.; Sonnentag, S. Adaptación del Cuestionario de Experiencias de Recuperación a una muestra española. *Psicothema* **2010**, *22*, 990–996.
23. Sonnentag, S.; Arbeus, H.; Mahn, C.; Fritz, C. Exhaustion and lack of psychological detachment from work during off-job time: Moderator effects of time pressure and leisure experiences. *J. Occup. Health Psychol.* **2014**, *19*, 206–216. [CrossRef]
24. Wrzesniewski, A.; Dutton, J.E. Crafting a job: Revisioning employees as active crafters of their work. *Acad Manag. Rev.* **2001**, *26*, 179–201. [CrossRef]
25. Leana, C.; Appelbaum, E.; Schevchuk, I. Work process and quality of care in early childhood education: The role of job crafting. *Acad Manag. J.* **2009**, *52*, 1169–1192. [CrossRef]
26. Llorente-Alonso, M.; Topa, G. Individual Crafting, Collaborative Crafting, and Job Satisfaction: The Mediator Role of Engagement. *J. Work Organ. Psychol.* **2019**, *35*, 217–226. [CrossRef]
27. Miller, M. Relationships between Job Design, Job Crafting, Idiosyncratic Deals, and Psychological Empowerment. Ph.D.Thesis, Walden University, Minneapolis, MI, USA, 2015. Available online: https://scholarworks.waldenu.edu/cgi/viewcontent.cgi?article=2362&context=dissertations (accessed on 5 February 2021).
28. Harbridge, R.R. Psychological Empowerment and Job Crafting among Registered Nurses Working in Public Health in Ontario, Canada. Ph.D. Thesis, Central Michigan University, Mount Pleasant, MI, USA, 2018. Available online: https://scholarly.cmich.edu/?a=d&d=CMUGR2018-096 (accessed on 23 February 2021).
29. Demerouti, E. Design your own job through job crafting. *Eur. Psychol.* **2014**, *19*, 237–243. [CrossRef]
30. Spreitzer, G.M. Psychological Empowerment in the workplace: Dimensions, measurement, and validation. *Acad Manag. J.* **1995**, *38*, 1442–1465. [CrossRef]
31. Thomas, K.W.; Velthouse, B.A. Cognitive elements of empowerment: an 'interpretative' model of intrinsic task motivation. *Acad Manag. Rev.* **1990**, *15*, 666–681.
32. Schermuly, C.C.; Meyer, B. Good relationships at work: The effects of Leader-Member Exchange and Team-Member Exchange on psychological empowerment, emotional exhaustion, and depression. *J. Organ. Behav.* **2015**, *37*, 673–691. [CrossRef]
33. Laschinger, H.K.S.; Finegan, J.; Shamian, J. Promoting Nurses' Health: Effect of Empowerment on Job Strain and Work Satisfaction. *Nurs. Econ.* **2001**, *19*, 42–52.
34. Petersen, M.B.; Jørgensen, F.J.; Bor, A. Compliance Without Fear: Predictors of Protective Behavior During the First Wave of the COVID-19 Pandemic. *PsyArXiv* **2021**. Available online: osf.io/asczn (accessed on 3 April 2021).
35. Ghosh, D.; Sekiguchi, T.; Fujimoto, Y. Psychological Detachment: A creativity perspective on the link between intrinsic motivation and employee engagement. *Pers. Rev.* **2020**, *49*, 1789–1804. [CrossRef]
36. Sheaffer, Z.; Levy, S.; Navot, E. Fears, discrimination and perceived workplace promotion. *Balt. J. Manag.* **2018**, *13*, 2–19. [CrossRef]
37. Jackson, D.N.; Guthrie, G.M.; Astilla, E.; Elwood, B. The cross-cultural generalizability of personality construct measures. In *Human Assessment and Cultural Factors*; NATO Conference Series; Berry, J.W., Irvine, S.H., Eds.; Springer: Berlin/Heidelberg, Germany, 1983; pp. 365–375.
38. Balluerka, N.; Gorostiaga, A.; Alonso-Arbiol, I.; Haranburu, M. La adaptación de instrumentos de medida de unas culturas a otras: Una perspectiva práctica. *Psicothema* **2007**, *19*, 124–133.
39. Albar, M.-J.; García-Ramírez, M.; López, A.M.; Garrido, R. Spanish Adaptation of the Scale of Psychological Empowerment in the Workplace. *Span. J. Psychol.* **2012**, *15*, 793–800. [CrossRef] [PubMed]
40. Zigmond, A.S.; Snaith, R.P. The hospital anxiety and depression scale. *Acta Psychiatr. Scand.* **1983**, *67*, 361–370. [CrossRef]
41. Sonnentag, S.; Fritz, C. The Recovery Experience Questionnaire: Development and validation of a measure for assessing recuperation and unwinding from work. *J. Occup. Health Psychol.* **2007**, *12*, 204–221. [CrossRef]
42. IBM Corp. *IBM SPSS Statistics for Windows*; Version 26.0; IBM Corp: New York, NY, USA, 2019.
43. Reinartz, W.; Haenlein, M.; Henseler, J. An empirical comparison of the efficacy of covariance-based and variance-based SEM. *Int. J. Res. Mark.* **2009**, *26*, 332–344. [CrossRef]
44. Barroso, C.; Cepeda, G.; Roldán, J.L. Applying maximum likelihood and PLS on different sample sizes: Studies on SERVQUAL model and employee behaviour model. In *Handbook of Partial Least Squares: Concepts, Methods and Applications*; Esposito Vinzi, V., Chin, W.W., Henseler, J., Wang, H., Eds.; Springer-Verlag: Berlin/Heidelberg, Germany, 2010; pp. 427–447.
45. Dijkstra, T.K.; Henseler, J. Consistent Partial Least Squares Path Modeling. *Mis. Q.* **2015**, *39*, 297–316. [CrossRef]
46. Astrachan, C.B.; Patel, V.K.; Wanzenried, G. A comparative study of CB-SEM and PLS-SEM for theory development in family firm research. *J. Fam. Bus. Strategy* **2014**, *5*, 116–128. [CrossRef]
47. Ringle, C.M.; Wende, S.; Becker, J.M. *SmartPLS 3*; SmartPLS GmbH: Boenningstedt, Germany, 2015. Available online: http://www.smartpls.com (accessed on 7 January 2021).

48. Hair, J.F.; Hult, T.M.; Ringle, C.M.; Sarstedt, M.; Castillo, J.; Cepeda, G.; Roldan, J.L. *Manual de Partial Least Squares Structural Equation Modeling (PLS-SEM)*, 2nd ed.; SAGE Publishing: Thousand Oaks, CA, USA, 2019. [CrossRef]
49. Hu, L.T.; Bentler, P.M. Cut-off criteria for fit indexes in covariance structure analysis: conventional criteria versus new alternatives. *Struct. Equ. Model.* **1999**, *6*, 1–55. [CrossRef]
50. Ringle, C.M. *Advanced PLS-SEM Topics: PLS Multigroup Analysis*; Working paper; University of Seville: Seville, Spain, 20 November 2016.
51. Hair, J.F.; Hult, G.T.M.; Ringle, C.; Sarstedt, M. *A Primer on Partial Least Squares Structural Equation Modeling (PLS-SEM)*; SAGE Publications, Inc.: Thousand Oaks, CA, USA, 2014.
52. Hair, J.F.; Ringle, C.M.; Sarstedt, M. PLS-SEM: Indeed, a silver bullet. *J. Mark. Theory Pract.* **2011**, *19*, 139–151. [CrossRef]
53. Kline, R.B. *Principles and Practice of Structural Equation Modeling*; Guilford Press: New York, NY, USA, 2011.
54. Horn, J.L.; McArdle, J.J. A Practical and Theoretical Guide to Measurement Invariance in Aging Research. *Exp. Aging Res.* **1992**, *18*, 117–144. [CrossRef]
55. Henseler, J.; Ringle, C.M.; Sarstedt, M. Testing measurement invariance of composites using partial least squares. *Int. Mark. Rev.* **2016**, *33*, 405–431. [CrossRef]
56. Stănculescu, E. Fear of COVID-19 in Romania: Validation of the Romanian Version of the Fear of COVID-19 Scale Using Graded Response Model Analysis. *Int J. Ment Health Addict.* **2021**, *6*, 1–16. [CrossRef]
57. Van den Heuvel, M.; Demerouti, E.; Peeters, M.C.W. The job crafting intervention: Effects on job resources, self-efficacy, and affective well-being. *J. Occup. Organ. Psychol.* **2015**, *88*, 511–532. [CrossRef]
58. Hochwälder, J.; Brucefors, A.B. Psychological empowerment at the workplace as a predictor of ill health. *Pers. Individ. Differ.* **2005**, *39*, 1237–1248. [CrossRef]
59. Pollán, M.; Pérez-Gómez, B.; Pastor-Barriuso, R.; Oteo, J.; A Hernán, M.; Pérez-Olmeda, M.; Sanmartín, J.L.; Fernández-García, A.; Cruz, I.; de Larrea, N.F.; et al. Prevalence of SARS-CoV-2 in Spain (ENE-COVID): a nationwide, population-based seroepidemiological study. *Lancet* **2020**, *396*, 535–544. [CrossRef]
60. Coelho, C.M.; Suttiwan, P.; Arato, N.; Zsido, A.N. On the Nature of Fear and Anxiety Triggered by COVID-19. *Front. Psychol.* **2020**, *11*, 3109. [CrossRef]
61. Kinman, G.; Teoh, K.; Harriss, A. Supporting the well-being of healthcare workers during and after COVID-19. *Occup. Med.* **2020**, *70*, 294–296. [CrossRef]

Journal of
Clinical Medicine

MDPI

Article

How Did COVID-19 Affect Suicidality? Data from a Multicentric Study in Lombardy

Camilla Gesi [1], Federico Grasso [2,3,*], Filippo Dragogna [1], Marco Vercesi [2,3], Silvia Paletta [2], Pierluigi Politi [3], Claudio Mencacci [1] and Giancarlo Cerveri [2]

1 Department of Mental Health and Addiction, ASST Fatebenefratelli-Sacco, 20157 Milan, Italy; gesi.camilla@asst-fbf-sacco.it (C.G.); filippo.dragogna@asst-fbf-sacco.it (F.D.); claudio.mencacci@gmail.com (C.M.)
2 Department of Mental Health and Addiction, ASST Lodi, 26900 Lodi, Italy; marco.vercesi@asst-lodi.it (M.V.); silvia.paletta@gmail.com (S.P.); giancarlo.cerveri@asst-lodi.it (G.C.)
3 Department of Brain and Behavioral Sciences, University of Pavia, 27100 Pavia, Italy; pierluigi.politi@unipv.it
* Correspondence: federico.grasso@asst-lodi.it; Tel.: +39-0371-372940

Abstract: The aim of the study was to describe the characteristics of subjects accessing the emergency rooms for suicidal behavior during the first epidemic wave of COVID-19 in three Emergency Departments (EDs) in Lombardy (Italy). A retrospective chart review was conducted for the period 8 March–3 June 2020, and during the same time frame in 2019. For all subjects accessing for suicidality, socio-demographic and clinical data were collected and compared between the two years. The proportion of subjects accessing for suicidality was significantly higher in 2020 than in 2019 (13.0 vs. 17.2%, $p = 0.03$). No differences between the two years were found for sex, triage priority level, history of substance abuse, factor triggering suicidality and discharge diagnosis. During 2020 a greater proportion of subjects did not show any mental disorders and were psychotropic drug-free. Women were more likely than men to receive inpatient psychiatric treatment, while men were more likely to be discharged with a diagnosis of acute alcohol/drug intoxication. Our study provides hints for managing suicidal behaviors during the still ongoing emergency and may be primary ground for further studies on suicidality in the course of or after massive infectious outbreaks.

Keywords: COVID-19; SARS-CoV-2; suicidal behavior; first emergency care; multicentric; Lombardy

Citation: Gesi, C.; Grasso, F.; Dragogna, F.; Vercesi, M.; Paletta, S.; Politi, P.; Mencacci, C.; Cerveri, G. How Did COVID-19 Affect Suicidality? Data from a Multicentric Study in Lombardy. *J. Clin. Med.* **2021**, *10*, 2410. https://doi.org/10.3390/jcm10112410

Academic Editor: Laurent Boyer

Received: 25 March 2021
Accepted: 26 May 2021
Published: 29 May 2021

1. Introduction

About 800,000 people worldwide die every year due to suicide and an even greater number attempts suicide or engages in self-injuring behaviors [1]. Up to 90% of suicides around the world are associated with mental disorders and substance abuse, including harmful use of alcohol [2]. However, a broad variety of environmental factors also contribute to suicidal behavior, many of which originate from the concurrent cultural, social and economic context [1]. Suicidal spectrum behaviors include a broad variety of manifestations, from suicidal thoughts and plans, to suicidal self-injuring and suicide attempts, to completed suicide [3,4]. Despite the fact that most subjects with suicidal thoughts do not attempt suicide, suicidal ideation may often precede suicide attempts. However, according to the ideation-to-action framework, the development of suicidal ideation and the progression from ideation to suicide attempts are distinct phenomena with distinct explanations and predictors [5].

Individuals with suicidality often are referred to Emergency Departments (EDs), and EDs also frequently provide care for people with other risk factors for suicide, such as serious mental illness, substance use, and chronic pain. Every month, the number of visits to EDs prompted by suicidality is considerable, accounting for about 4% of accesses yearly in the US [6,7]. In addition, suicidal behaviors may not only represent the overt reason for the access, but also emerge as part of a broader constellation of psychiatric symptoms or be hidden by other complaints, so that the ED consultation itself may end up unraveling a current suicide risk [8,9]. Therefore, the emergency room of the EDs is an especially privileged observatory for the whole spectrum of suicidal behaviors [10].

The effect of natural and man-made disasters on suicidality has been evaluated in previous studies. Despite some inconsistent report, most data indicate a significant impact, either immediate or delayed, of disasters on suicide behaviors [11–14]. This is likely due to the detrimental effect of collective emergencies on mental health and psychosocial well-being, as well as to the socio-economic upheaval brought about by a range of consequences of disasters, such as the death or injury of family members, the loss of employment and properties, and the disruption of community cohesion and support [15,16].

Data focusing on the effect of massive infectious outbreaks on suicide behaviors are sparse, consistently with the relatively rare occurrence of epidemics in the last decades. Only poor evidence is available about the Spanish Flu, infecting 500 million people between 1918 and 1919 and narratively associated with a high risk of enacting suicidal behaviors among survivors [17]. During the more recent outbreak of SARS in Honk-Hong in 2003, rates of suicide were shown to rise compared to the previous year among elderly females, but not among elderly males or younger age groups. A recent nationwide cohort study conducted in Taiwan found significant higher rates of suicide, anxiety, depression, sleep- and trauma-related disorders among SARS survivors compared to non-affected subjects in the five years following the 2003 outbreak [18]. As for referral to EDs for suicidality, a study evaluating accesses to the emergency room in a SARS-dedicated hospital in northern Taiwan during 2003 SARS outbreak found an increased number of suicide attempts from drug overdoses during peak- versus pre-epidemic stages, despite the difference not being statistically significant [19].

The ongoing pandemic due to Sars-Cov-2 has obvious similarities with previous outbreaks, but also bears a few differences. After beginning in China in 2019, the COVID-19 has rapidly spread on a global scale with multiple epidemic waves in 2020. At the time of writing this paper, about 100 million people [20] have contracted the virus globally and more than two million have died. Besides the massive toll in terms of mortality, the health-related and social costs of COVID-19 are thought to be as much as significant. The impact on mental health is expected to be especially severe as the coronavirus epidemic has shown to enhance several relevant risk factors for mental illness, spanning from the loss of community life to widespread poverty, from unemployment to disruption of critical mental health and social services. Noteworthily, the compulsory quarantine enforced for preventing the propagation of the virus led to a sharp increase in social isolation and to a significant decrease in social support, which are among the most important risk factors for any kind of suicidal behavior [21,22]. Conversely, although data on deaths by suicide during the lockdown are still scarce, the first months of the pandemic might have been characterized by a lower suicide mortality rate [23]. For instance, a decrease of suicidal behaviors was observed in France during the strict lockdown. This decrease may be explained by several factors: the so-called "pulling-together effect", observed in times of national tragedies, the work adaptation (reduced working hours and work-from-home policies), the subsidies limiting financial distress, the reduced access to illegal drugs. However, the absolute number of violent or severe suicide attempts remained relatively stable [24].

Italy was the first western country struck from the coronavirus pandemic. The first hotbed of contagion emerged at the end of February 2020 in Codogno, in the province of Lodi, about forty kilometers southeast of Milan, leading quickly to a quarantine setting enforced by law and to the rapid spread of fear. Besides the closure of schools, bars, restaurants and shops, the ED of Codogno was also temporarily closed to new admissions, and most patients were diverted to the neighboring hospitals of Pavia and Lodi. At the beginning of March, as the coronavirus reached the metropolitan area of Milan and started circulating across northern Italy, the entire Lombardy was placed on lockdown.

The main objective of the study was to describe the sociodemographic and clinical features of subjects accessing the psychiatric emergency service for suicidality during the first Sars-CoV-2 epidemic wave in three EDs in Lombardy, and to compare rates and characteristics of accesses between 8 March and 3 June 2020 to those occurring during the same period in 2019. We included accesses prompted by the whole spectrum of suicidal behaviors [4] (i.e., suicidal thoughts, suicidal self-injuring, suicide attempts, completed suicide) hereafter referred to as "suicidality" throughout the manuscript. The three EDs were chosen as differently hit by the epidemic, according to their distance from the first epicenter of the outbreak. In particular, Lodi-Codogno was the first center struck by Sars-CoV-2 epidemic in Italy and very severe restrictions were soon enforced in the attempt to prevent further spreading of the contagion. Pavia was involved in a second time in the epidemic wave, while the overflow of patients from Codogno was diverted to its hospital. Only in a later time the Sars-CoV-2 wave reached the metropolitan area of Milan, as the epidemic was already spreading across the whole of Lombardy.

2. Materials and Methods

2.1. Materials and Methods

A retrospective observational study was conducted at three EDs (Lodi-Codogno, San Matteo-Pavia, Fatebenefratelli-Milan) in Lombardy. The ED of Lodi-Codogno, where the first indigenous case of COVID-19 in Italy was confirmed, comprises two emergency rooms located in southern Lombardy, with a catchment area of about 230,000 inhabitants. The ED of San Matteo Hospital in Pavia, located 38 Km west of Lodi-Codogno and usually covering a district of about 550,000 inhabitants, during the first outbreak served to handle the overflow from the neighboring hospitals of Codogno and Lodi, which rapidly became overwhelmed. The ED of Fatebenefratelli Hospital is located in the metropolitan area of Milan (30 and 40 Km north of Lodi and Pavia respectively) serving a district of about 400,000 residents and more than one million professionals commuting daily from suburbs and surrounding areas. All three EDs offer psychiatric emergency service 24/7 and provide treatment for a range of psychiatric conditions.

2.2. Study Population and Data Collection

A retrospective chart review of medical records was carried out at the three EDs using hospitals' computer databases of emergency rooms reports. All subjects (i) older than 18 years and (ii) accessing the three EDs for suicidality between 8 March and 3 June 2020 were selected for inclusion in the analyses. In addition, subjects meeting the inclusion criteria throughout the same period of 2019 were included as a comparison group. The total number of subjects referring to the EDs and going through a psychiatric evaluation during the two periods was also annotated. The flow-chart illustrating the recruitment process is shown in Figure 1.

Data were extracted anonymously including sex, age, nationality (Italian vs. other), marital, cohabitation and occupational status, usual care provider (private/public Mental Health/Addiction Service), history of alcohol and substance use, phase of access (8 March–4 May vs. 5 May–3 June), type of suicidality (suicidal thoughts, suicide attempt, self-injuring, drug ingestion), presence of triggering conflicts, triage priority level (high vs. low), psychopharmacological treatment prescribed before/during/after ED consultation, discharge diagnosis (anxiety/mood/psychotic/personality disorder/no mental disorder-harmful substance use), and admission to the inpatient psychiatric service. The period between 8 March and 4 May 2020, when the number of COVID-19 cases rose and the lock-down measures were implemented, was designated as the peak epidemic stage (phase 1), while the period between 5 May and 3 June, as the outbreak began to subside and the measures of lock-down were removed, was defined as the late-epidemic stage (phase 2). The study was performed in accordance with the principles of the Declaration of Helsinki regarding medical research in humans and it satisfied local research ethical requirements. In particular, the privacy of research subjects and the confidentiality of their personal information were protected by anonymization of all collected data. As a retrospective, non-interventional, low-risk study, the institutional review boards at each participating site approved the study protocol and the local ethic committee was notified before study initiation.

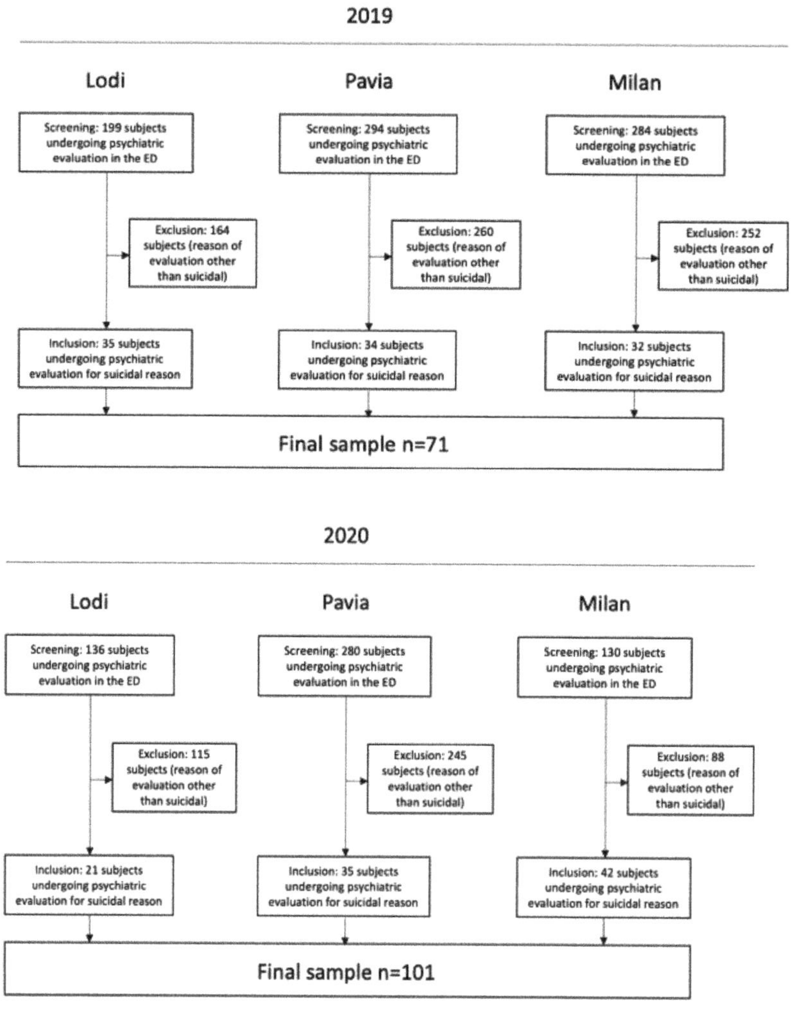

Figure 1. Recruitment Flow-chart.

2.3. Statistical Analyses

Demographic and clinical characteristics of patients accessing the EDs for suicidality in 2019 and 2020, respectively, were compared using a *t*-test for continuous variables and Chi-square test for categorical variables. The number of accesses for suicidality out of the total number of ED visits were compared between the two years using Chi-square test. Additional analyses were conducted within each year group to compare subjects based on sex, phase of the outbreak (phase 1/phase 2) and site of enrollment. Chi-square test with Odd Ratios (OR) values and 95% confidence intervals (CI) were used to find significant predictors of admission to the psychiatric inpatient unit only for the year 2020. A p value of less than 0.05 was considered statistically significant. All statistical analyses were carried out using SPSS, version 26 (IBM, Armonk, NY, USA) [25].

3. Results

3.1. Characteristics of Patients Accessing the ED for Suicidality during the First Wave of COVID-19 in 2020

Demographic characteristics of patients referred to the ED for suicidality between March 8th and June 3rd 2020 are displayed in Table 1. Overall, 94 subjects accessed the ED for suicidality (22.3% in Lodi-Codogno, 52.1% in Pavia, 25.5% Milan) with 58.5% accessing in Phase 1 and 41.5% in Phase 2. Most of them (77.7%) were Italian, with no differences in the percentage of foreigners/Italians accessing the ED during Phases 1 and 2. Across the three months, the majority of subjects were unemployed and unmarried. As shown in Table 2, half of the subjects did not usually refer to any mental health/addiction service, and the majority (52.1%) were admitted to the ED after an episode of intentional prescription drug ingestion. Overall, 12.8% accessed the ED for current suicide attempt; the distribution of suicide attempts vs. any other suicidality feature did not significantly differ between phase 1 and phase 2 in the overall sample (9.1% of suicide attempts in phase 1 vs. 17.9 in phase 2; Chi-square = 1.608, $p = 0.205$) nor considering each center separately. At the end of ED consultation, the vast majority, 87.2%, received a mental disorder diagnosis, while the remaining 12.8% were discharged with no psychiatric diagnosis/substance harmful use. Thirty subjects (31.9%) were admitted to the psychiatric inpatient unit. Among a range of possible risk factors (sex, taking antidepressants/anxiolytics/mood stabilizers/antipsychotics, suicide attempt vs. others, having/not having a psychiatric diagnosis, self-referred detrimental impact of COVID-19) only female sex (39.7% vs. 19.4%, OR = 2.7, IC 1.0–7.2) and having a psychiatric diagnosis (36.6% vs. 0%, OR = 0.81, IC 0.72–0.91) were shown to be significant risk for being admitted to the psychiatric inpatient unit. Females were also more likely to present with an episode of intentional prescription drug ingestion ($p = 0.043$), while males were more likely to show acute alcohol/drug intoxication; no differences were found in the prevalence of substance abuse. The majority of males did not usually refer to any mental health/addiction service (63.9%), while the majority of women (58.6%) did (chi = 4.502, $p = 0.034$). A significantly higher percentage of men than women were discharged with antipsychotic (22.2% vs. 6.9%, chi = 4.685, $p = 0.030$) and antidepressant (30.6% vs. 13.8%, chi = 3.870, $p = 0.49$) prescription. At the time of discharge from ED, the majority of females (65.9%) were diagnosed with a psychiatric disorder, while the majority of men (66.7%) were diagnosed with harmful substance use/no psychiatric disorder (4.685, $p = 0.030$).

Table 1. Demographic characteristics of the study sample. Values presented in parentheses are per cent, unless otherwise indicated.

	Year 2019 (n = 101)	Year 2020 (n = 94)	Chi Square	Sig.
Sex				
female	61 (60.4)	58 (61.7)	0.035	0.852
male	40 (39.6)	36 (38.3)		
Nationality				
Italian	76 (75.2)	73 (77.7)	0.157	0.692
Other	25 (24.8)	21 (22.3)		
Occupation				
employed	17 (16.8)	13 (13.8)		
unemployed	40 (39.6)	41 (43.6)		
student	12 (11.9)	6 (6.4)	3.338	0.503
retired	10 (9.9)	7 (7.4)		
other/not known	22 (21.8)	27 (28.7)		

Table 1. *Cont.*

	Year 2019 (n = 101)	Year 2020 (n = 94)	Chi Square	Sig.
Marital status				
Married	15 (14.9)	18 (19.1)		
unmarried	54 (53.5)	48 (51.1)		
separated/divorced	10 (9.9)	14 (14.9)	3.955	0.412
widowed	7 (6.9)	7 (7.4)		
other/unknown	15 (14.9)	7 (7.4)		
Cohabitation status				
partner/children	25 (24.8)	40 (42.6)		
parents/siblings	21 (20.8)	20 (21.3)		
alone	24 (23.8)	19 (20.2)	9.407	0.052
institution	18 (17.8)	9 (9.6)		
other/unknown	13 (12.9)	6 (6.4)		
Phase of access				
8 March–4 May	66 (65.3)	−58.5	0.966	0.326
5 May–3 June	35 (34.7)	−41.5		
			T	**Sig.**
Age (mean, SD)	42.5 ± 17.6	42.4 ± 15.4	0.051	0.959

Table 2. Clinical characteristics of the study sample.

	Year 2019 (n = 101)	Year 2020 (n = 94)	Chi^2	Sig.
Usual care provider				
None	49 (48.5)	48 (51.1)		
Public/private MHS+	40 (39.6)	37 (39.4)	0.305	0.859
Addiction Service	12 (11.9)	9 (9.6)		
History of alcohol substance abuse	26 (25.7)	27 (28.7)	0.219	0.64
Triage priority level				
high	51 (50.5)	47 (50)	0.005	0.945
low	50 (49.5)	47 (50)		
Conflicts triggering suicidality	47 (46.5)	38 (40.4)	0.739	0.39
Suicidality *				
Suicidal thoughts	16 (16)	19 (20.2)	0.582	0.446
Suicide attempt	1 (1)	3 (3.2)	1.174	0.279
Self-injuring	21 (21)	14 (14.9)	1.222	0.269
Drug ingestion	54 (54)	49 (52.1)	0.068	0.794
Discharge diagnosis				
Anxiety disorder	7 (6.9)	6 (6.4)	0.023	0.878
Mood disorder	38 (37.6)	31 (33)	0.459	0.498
Psychotic disorder	2 (2)	7 (7.4)	3.305	0.069
Personality disorder	49 (48.5)	38 (43.7)	1.289	0.256
No mental disorders/harmful substance use	5 (5)	12 (12.8)	3.737	0.05
Admission to psychiatric inpatient care	32 (31.7)	30 (31.9)	0.001	0.972

+ MHS: Mental Helath Service. * all the features listed relate to the aim of ending own life. 'Suicide attempt' refer to a potentially life-threatening behavior; 'self-injuring' and 'drug ingestion' refer to self-harming acts with a declared suicidal intent but lacking life-threatening potential.

3.2. *Comparisons between 2020 and 2019*

A total number of 777 subjects were referred to the ED and went through PES evaluation in the three centers between 1st March and 31st May in 2019. Of those subjects, 101 (13.0%) did so for suicidality. In the same period of 2020, 546 patients overall accessed the

ED and underwent psychiatric consultation, 94 (17.2%) for suicidality, with a statistically significant difference between the two years (Chi-Square: 4.5386; $p = 0.03$). Considering every single center, the difference was not significant for the center of Lodi (14.6% suicide in 2019 vs. 15.4% in 2020, chi: 0.046; $p = 0.83$), nor for Milan (12.8 suicide in 2019 vs. 15.8 in 2020, chi = 0.639, $p = 0.42$), but was so in Pavia (11.6% suicide in 2019 vs. 19.0% in 2020, chi = 5.934; $p = 0.02$). Comparisons of clinical characteristics of patients accessing in 2019 and 2020, respectively, are presented in Table 2. No differences were found for sex, triage priority level and history of substance abuse between the two years. No differences were found about factors triggering suicidality (conflicts with family members vs. anxiety/exacerbation of psychopathology) in the overall sample, nor considering each center separately. However, the difference was significant considering only Phase 2, with 71.8% of subjects accessing in Phase 2 doing so for anxiety/exacerbation of psychopathology, and 42.9% in the same period of the previous year (Chi = 6.345; $p = 0.012$). No differences were found in the percentage of subjects who were admitted to the psychiatric inpatient unit between 2019 and 2020 in the overall sample, nor considering each center or each period separately. No differences were found in the prevalence of each diagnostic group (psychotic disorders, mood disorders, anxiety disorders, personality disorders) as discharge diagnoses between 2019 and 2020. While dichotomizing discharge diagnoses between psychopathological or no mental disorders/harmful substance use, a difference close to significance was found between 2019 and 2020 with 5% of subjects with no mental disorders in 2019 and 12.8% in 2020 (Chi = 3.737, $p = 0.050$).

As shown in Table 3, a significant difference was found between 2019 and 2020 regarding the percentage of subjects treated with any psychotropic drug at the moment of ED consultation, with a minority of patients (26.7%) who were psychotropic drug-free in 2019 compared to 40.4% in 2020 (Chi 4.108, $p = 0.043$). No differences were found between 2019 and 2020 in the type of treatment used before/prescribed after ED consultation, except for patients accessing in 2019 having greater likelihood of being treated with anxiolytic drugs before ED consultation compared to those accessing in 2020 (33.0% vs. 50.5% Chi = 6.130, $p = 0.013$).

Table 3. Treatment characteristics of the study sample.

	Year 2019 (n = 101)	Year 2020 (n = 94)	Chi^2	Sig.
Psychotropic treatment at the moment of ED consultation				
Any psychotropic treatment	74 (73.3)	56 (59.6)	4.108	0.043
Anxiolytics	51 (50.5)	31 (33)	6.130	0.013
Antidepressants	43 (42.6)	41 (43.6)	0.022	0.883
Antipsychotics	33 (32.7)	23 (24.5)	1.601	0.206
Mood stabilizers	12 (11.9)	9 (9.6)	0.270	0.604
Psychotropic treatment administered during ED consultation				
Anxiolytics	12 (11.9)	26 (27.7)	7.725	0.005
Antidepressants	0 (0)	1 (1.1)	1.080	0.299
Antipsychotics	6 (5.9)	5 (5.3)	0.035	0.851
Mood stabilizers	0 (0)	2 (2.1)	2.171	0.141
Psychotropic treatment prescribed at discharge from PES				
Anxiolytics	17 (16.8)	15 (16)	0.027	0.869
Antidepressants	22 (21.8)	19 (20.2)	0.072	0.788
Antipsychotics	14 (13.9)	12 (12.8)	0.051	0.822
Mood stabilizers	5 (5)	3 (3.2)	0.383	0.536

4. Discussion

The main aim of the study was to compare the characteristics of patients accessing the ED for suicidality during the first wave of COVID-19 in 2020 with those accessing in the same period of 2019 in three Italian EDs differently affected by the SARS-CoV2 outbreak (Codogno, the first struck by the epidemic wave, Pavia and Milan). First, out of all the people referring to the psychiatric services of the EDs, the proportion of consultations due to suicidality was significantly higher in 2020 that in 2019. This finding is in line with previous data suggesting that massive events may trigger suicidality and contribute to the existing literature about the direct and indirect consequences of the pandemic [12–14]. Analyses separately carried out for each center further indicated that the difference in the rate of psychiatric consultations due to suicidality in the two years was actually significant in the center of Pavia but not in the centers of Lodi-Codogno and Milan. The absence of significance for the center of Lodi-Codogno may appear in contrast with early exposure to the COVID-19 of this area. Codogno was indeed the first epicenter of the outbreak in Italy and its population was subjected for an especially long time to severe restrictions, social isolation, and risk of infection. However, there is the possibility that a number of people needing psychiatric emergency consultation during the first epidemic wave was shifted to the nearby Department of Pavia, in which the number of accesses for psychiatric consultation was in fact especially high compared to the other two centers and significantly higher than in 2019. While no differences were found regarding the reasons triggering suicidality in the phase 1, a greater proportion of suicidal behaviors during the phase 2 was caused by relapsing psychopathology—instead of being triggered by interpersonal problems—compared with the same period of 2019. One hypothesis could be that the stress suffered during the epidemic phase contributed to starting the process of relapse that became fully manifested only during the post-epidemic phase [26]. On the other hand, it is also possible that feelings of uncertainty and the fear of contagion withheld people with relapsing symptoms from seeking for help in the ED during the peak epidemic phase, with some sort of rebound in patients with relapsing psychopathology as soon as the contagion started to subside in the post-epidemic phase [26]. This interpretation could also be in line with the decrease in the overall number of psychiatric emergency consultations from 2019 to 2020, confirming that the epidemic wave led to fear and avoidance of the ED to some extent. This also stands as a caveat to the increased suicidality in 2020, as the total number of accesses for suicidality remained substantially constant from 2019 to 2020, while the increase percentage of accesses for suicidality was mostly due to a drop in the amount of psychiatric emergency consultations for other reasons.

The overall severity of suicidal gestures was not more severe in 2020 than in 2019. In fact, no differences between years were found in the percentage of psychiatric emergency visits leading to inpatient treatment admission nor in the distribution of different features of suicidality. Dichotomizing discharge diagnoses between psychopathological or no psychopathological, a difference very close to significance by year was found, with a higher proportion of subjects with no mental disorders accessing for suicidality in 2020 than in 2019. Although not significant, this result suggests the need of further investigation and might indicate a large impact of COVID-19 on psychological wellbeing and suicidal behaviors, severely involving not only people with preexisting psychiatric disorders but also a broader group of people somehow vulnerable to the multifaced effect of the pandemic [27,28]. Such a hypothesis is corroborated by the finding of a greater proportion of subjects free from psychopharmacological treatments accessed in 2020 compared with 2019 and by the greater likelihood of being already treated with anxyolitics among subjects seeking consultation in 2019. Interestingly, a recent study hypothesized a mediating role of HPA activity and inflammation between social isolation and suicidality, providing a possible neurobiological framework to the increased suicidality observed in our study [29].

Some noteworthy features also emerged from cross-sex comparisons within the 2020 year. While in 2019 sex was not shown to affect the probability of being admitted to a psychiatric inpatient unit, in 2020 women were more likely than men to receive inpatient treatment as a result of psychiatric emergency consultation. Moreover, women were more likely to be already in treatment in outpatient mental health or addiction services at the time of consultation and to receive a mental disorder diagnosis at the time of discharge. On the other hand, men were mostly not referring to any community-based service and were more likely to seek for help in the ED after suicidal behavior arising from substance use unrelated to any mental disorder. Overall, females looked especially prone to enact suicidal gestures in the context of a preexisting mental disorder, while men appeared likely to show a suicidal behavior mostly independently from mental illness, highlighting the role of environmental risk factors for suicidality in the context of the COVID-19 pandemic. For example, one hypothesis could be that men are more vulnerable to react with externalizing behaviors to psychological stress and less likely to seek psychological and social support [30]. Additionally, the economic and employment strains following the pandemic could especially affect men as far as they are bound to endorse the traditional role of family breadwinners [31]. Indeed, unemployment has been shown to contribute differently to the risk of suicide among men and women [32,33].

We acknowledge some limitations of this study. First, results would be more reliable if comparisons were made not only with 2019 but with multiple years preceding the pandemic. Second, the sample is relatively small, and data were brought from few EDs in Northern Italy. Despite involving three departments differently hit by the pandemic in Lombardy, results cannot be assumed to be representative of the whole region. Third, the study has a retrospective design and data were not collected for the purpose of research. Further, no distinction about the violent/not violent nature of suicidal behaviors was provided. Lastly, as cases were recruited based on ED records, we could not include data about completed suicide, lacking information about the extreme end of suicidal spectrum both in 2019 and 2020.

5. Conclusions

Our study suggests that the proportion of subjects accessing the ED for suicidalty during the first wave of the COVID-19 epidemic was significantly higher in 2020 compared to the same period of 2019. Although this could be due to an overall drop of ED accesses during the first peak epidemic phase, we also found that a greater percentage of subjects enacting suicidal behaviors during this period was psychotropic drug-free compared to 2019, suggesting that suicidality might not be directly related to a pre-existing treated mental disorder. Our study provides some hints to be used by clinicians managing suicidality during the ongoing emergency and may be of primary ground for further studies on suicidality arising during large-scale health emergencies. Further investigations in later phases of the ongoing pandemic will help to elucidate the overall impact of such emergency on suicidal spectrum behaviors.

Author Contributions: Conceptualization, C.G., F.G., F.D., M.V., S.P., P.P., C.M. and G.C.; methodology, F.G., F.D. and P.P.; validation, P.P., C.M. and G.C.; formal analysis, C.G.; investigation, F.G. and F.D.; writing—original draft preparation, C.G. and F.G.; writing—review and editing, C.G., F.G., M.V. and S.P.; supervision, G.C. and C.M. All authors have read and agreed to the published version of the manuscript.

Funding: This research received no external funding.

Institutional Review Board Statement: The study was conducted according to the guidelines of the Declaration of Helsinki, and approved by the Ethics Committee of Milano Area 1—ASST FBF SACCO—ASST Fatebenefratelli Sacco Milano. Prot. N 0023880, date of approval 25/05/2021.

Informed Consent Statement: Not applicable. Data were collected retrospectively and anonymously from the emergency services database.

Data Availability Statement: The data presented in this study are available on request from the corresponding author. The data are not publicly available due to their collection from the hospital database. Data are not available in a publicly accessible repository.

Conflicts of Interest: The authors declare no conflict of interest.

References

1. World Health Organization. *Suicide Dates*; WHO: Geneva, Switzerland, 2014.
2. Bertolote, J.M.; Fleischmann, A. Suicide and psychiatric diagnosis: A worldwide perspective. *World Psychiatry* **2002**, *1*, 181–185.
3. Silverman, M.M.; Berman, A.L.; Sanddal, N.D. Rebuilding the Tower of Babel: A revised nomenclature for the study of suicide and suicidal behaviors. Part 1: Background, rationale, and methodology. *Suicide Life Threat Behav.* **2007**, *37*, 248–263. [CrossRef] [PubMed]
4. Hamza, C.A.; Stewart, S.L.; Willoughby, T. Examining the link between nonsuicidal self-injury and suicidal behavior: A review of the literature and an integrated model. *Clin. Psychol. Rev.* **2012**, *32*, 482–495. [CrossRef] [PubMed]
5. Klonsky, E.D.; May, A.M.; Saffer, B.Y. Suicide, Suicide Attempts, and Suicidal Ideation. *Annu. Rev. Clin. Psychol.* **2016**, *12*, 307–330. [CrossRef] [PubMed]
6. Owens, P.L.; Mutter, R.; Stocks, C. Mental Health and Substance Abuse-Related Emergency Department Visits among Adults, 2007: Statistical Brief #92. In *Healthcare Cost and Utilization Project (HCUP) Statistical Briefs*; Agency for Healthcare Research and Quality: Rockville, MD, USA, 2006. Available online: https://www.ncbi.nlm.nih.gov/books/NBK52659/ (accessed on 7 May 2021).
7. Miller, I.W.; Camargo, C.A., Jr.; Arias, S.A.; Sullivan, A.F.; Allen, M.H.; Goldstein, A.B.; Manton, A.P.; Espinola, J.A.; Jones, R.; Hasegawa, K.; et al. Suicide Prevention in an Emergency Department Population: The ED-SAFE Study. *JAMA Psychiatry* **2017**, *74*, 563–570. [CrossRef] [PubMed]
8. Claassen, C.A.; Larkin, G.L. Occult suicidality in an emergency department population. *Br. J. Psychiatry* **2005**, *186*, 352–353. [CrossRef]
9. Boudreaux, E.D.; Cagande, C.; Kilgannon, H.; Kumar, A.; Camargo, C.A. A prospective study of depression among adult patients in an urban emergency department. *Prim. Care Companion J. Clin. Psychiatry* **2006**, *8*, 66–70. [CrossRef]
10. Brenner, J.M.; Marco, C.A.; Kluesner, N.H.; Schears, R.M.; Martin, D.R. Assessing psychiatric safety in suicidal emergency department patients. *J. Am. Coll. Emerg. Physicians Open* **2020**, *1*, 30–37. [CrossRef] [PubMed]
11. Stratta, P.; Capanna, C.; Riccardi, I.; Carmassi, C.; Piccinni, A.; Dell'Osso, L.; Rossi, A. Suicidal intention and negative spiritual coping one year after the earthquake of L'Aquila (Italy). *J. Affect. Disord.* **2012**, *136*, 1227–1231. [CrossRef]
12. Kõlves, K.; Kõlves, K.E.; De Leo, D. Natural disasters and suicidal behaviours: A systematic literature review. *J. Affect. Disord.* **2013**, *146*, 1–14. [CrossRef] [PubMed]
13. Carmassi, C.; Stratta, P.; Calderani, E.; Bertelloni, C.A.; Menichini, M.; Massimetti, E.; Rossi, A.; Dell'Osso, L. Impact of Mood Spectrum Spirituality and Mysticism Symptoms on Suicidality in Earthquake Survivors with PTSD. *J. Relig. Health* **2016**, *55*, 641–649. [CrossRef] [PubMed]
14. Orui, M.; Suzuki, Y.; Maeda, M.; Yasumura, S. Suicide Rates in Evacuation Areas After the Fukushima Daiichi Nuclear Disaster. *Crisis* **2018**, *39*, 353–363. [CrossRef]
15. Wasserman, D.; Iosue, M.; Wuestefeld, A.; Carli, V. Adaptation of evidence-based suicide prevention strategies during and after the COVID-19 pandemic. *World Psychiatry* **2020**, *19*, 294–306. [CrossRef]
16. Jafari, H.; Cheraghi, M.A.; Pashaeypoor, S.; Hoseini, A.S. Human death: A concept analysis study. *J. Nurs. Midwifery Sci.* **2020**, *7*, 170–179.
17. Mamelund, S.E. Spanish Influenza Mortality of Ethnic Minorities in Norway 1918–1919. *Eur. J. Popul.* **2003**, *19*, 83–102. [CrossRef]
18. Tzeng, T.T.; Chen, P.L.; Weng, T.C.; Tsai, S.Y.; Lai, C.C.; Chou, H.I.; Chen, P.W.; Lu, C.C.; Liu, M.T.; Sung, W.C.; et al. Development of high-growth influenza H7N9 prepandemic candidate vaccine viruses in suspension MDCK cells. *J. Biomed. Sci.* **2020**, *27*, 47. [CrossRef] [PubMed]
19. Huang, C.C.; Yen, D.H.T.; Huang, H.H.; Kao, W.F.; Wang, L.M.; Huang, C.I.; Lee, C.H. Impact of severe acute respiratory syndrome (SARS) outbreaks on the use of emergency department medical resources. *J. Chin. Med. Assoc.* **2005**, *68*, 254–259. [CrossRef]
20. Breitbart, W. A COVID-19 Obituary. *Palliat. Supportive Care* **2021**, *19*, 1–2. [CrossRef] [PubMed]
21. Van Orden, K.A.; Witte, T.K.; Cukrowicz, K.C.; Braithwaite, S.R.; Selby, E.A.; Joiner, T.E., Jr. The interpersonal theory of suicide. *Psychol. Rev.* **2010**, *117*, 575–600. [CrossRef]
22. Calati, R.; Ferrari, C.; Brittner, M.; Oasi, O.; Olié, E.; Carvalho, A.F.; Courtet, P. Suicidal thoughts and behaviors and social isolation: A narrative review of the literature. *J. Affect. Disord* **2019**, *245*, 653–667. [CrossRef]
23. Qin, P.; Mehlum, L. National observation of death by suicide in the first 3 months under COVID-19 pandemic. *Acta Psychiatr. Scand.* **2021**, *143*, 92–93. [CrossRef]
24. Olié, E.; Nogue, E.; Picot, M.; Courtet, P. Hospitalizations for suicide attempt during the first COVID-19 lockdown in France. *Acta Psychiatr. Scand.* **2021**. [CrossRef]
25. International Business Machines Corporation. *IBM SPSS Statistics for Macintosh*; Version 26.0; IBM Corp: Armonk, NY, USA, 2019.
26. Butt, A.A.; Kartha, A.; Asaad, N.; Azad, A.M.; Bertollini, R.; Abou-Samra, A.B. Impact of COVID-19 upon changes in emergency room visits with chest pain of possible cardiac origin. *BMC Res. Notes* **2020**, *13*, 1–4. [CrossRef]
27. Lai, J.; Ma, S.; Wang, Y.; Cai, Z.; Hu, J.; Wei, N.; Wu, J.; Du, H.; Chen, T.; Li, R.; et al. Factors associated with mental health outcomes among health care workers exposed to coronavirus disease 2019. *JAMA Netw. Open* **2020**, *3*, e203976. [CrossRef] [PubMed]

28. Reynolds, D.L.; Garay, J.R.; Deamond, S.L.; Moran, M.K.; Gold, W.; Styra, R. Understanding compliance and psychological impact of the SARS quarantine experience. *Epidemiol. Infect.* **2008**, *136*, 997–1007. [CrossRef]
29. Conejero, I.; Nobile, B.; Olié, E.; Courtet, P. How Does COVID-19 Affect the Neurobiology of Suicide? *Curr. Psychiatry Rep.* **2021**, *23*, 16. [CrossRef] [PubMed]
30. Hicks, B.M.; Blonigen, D.M.; Kramer, M.D.; Krueger, R.F.; Patrick, C.J.; Iacono, W.G.; McGue, M. Gender differences and developmental change in externalizing disorders from late adolescence to early adulthood: A longitudinal twin study. *J. Abnorm. Psychol.* **2007**, *116*, 433–447. [CrossRef]
31. Crowley, M.S. Men's Self-Perceived Adequacy as the Family Breadwinner: Implications for Their Psychological, Marital, and Work-Family Weil-Being. *J. Fam. Econ. Issues* **1998**, *19*, 7–23. [CrossRef]
32. Lundin, A.; Lundberg, I.; Allebeck, P.; Hemmingsson, T. Unemployment and suicide in the Stockholm population: A register-based study on 771,068 men and women. *Public Health* **2012**, *126*, 371–377. [CrossRef]
33. Deady, M.; Tan, L.; Kugenthiran, N.; Collins, D.; Christensen, H.; Harvey, S.B. Unemployment, suicide and COVID-19: Using the evidence to plan for prevention. *Med. J. Aust.* **2020**, *213*, 153–154. [CrossRef] [PubMed]

Journal of
Clinical Medicine

MDPI

Article

Psychological Interventions for Children with Autism during the COVID-19 Pandemic through a Remote Behavioral Skills Training Program

Flavia Marino [1,†], Paola Chilà [1,†], Chiara Failla [1], Roberta Minutoli [1], Noemi Vetrano [1], Claudia Luraschi [1], Cristina Carrozza [1], Elisa Leonardi [1], Mario Busà [1], Sara Genovese [1], Rosa Musotto [1], Alfio Puglisi [1], Antonino Andrea Arnao [1], Giuliana Cardella [1], Francesca Isabella Famà [1], Gaspare Cusimano [1], David Vagni [1], Pio Martines [2], Giovanna Mendolia [2], Gennaro Tartarisco [1], Antonio Cerasa [1,3,4,*], Liliana Ruta [1,*] and Giovanni Pioggia [1]

1 Institute for Biomedical Research and Innovation (IRIB), National Research Council of Italy (CNR), 98164 Messina, Italy; flavia.marino@cnr.it (F.M.); paola.chila@irib.cnr.it (P.C.); chiara.failla@irib.cnr.it (C.F.); roberta.minutoli@irib.cnr.it (R.M.); noemi.vetrano@irib.cnr.it (N.V.); claudia.luraschi@irib.cnr.it (C.L.); cristina.carrozza@irib.cnr.it (C.C.); elisa.leonardi@irib.cnr.it (E.L.); mario.busa@irib.cnr.it (M.B.); sara.genovese@irib.cnr.it (S.G.); rosy.musotto@irib.cnr.it (R.M.); alfio.puglisi@irib.cnr.it (A.P.); antoninoandrea.arnao@cnr.it (A.A.A.); giuliana.cardella@irib.cnr.it (G.C.); francescaisabella.fama@irib.cnr.it (F.I.F.); gaspare.cusimano@irib.cnr.it (G.C.); david.vagni@cnr.it (D.V.); gennaro.tartarisco@cnr.it (G.T.); giovanni.pioggia@cnr.it (G.P.)
2 Azienda Sanitaria Provinciale, U.O.C. Neuropsichiatria Infantile, 91100 Trapani, Italy; pio.martines@asptrapani.it (P.M.); giovanna.mendolia@asptrapani.it (G.M.)
3 S'Anna Institute, 88900 Crotone, Italy
4 Pharmacotechnology Documentation and Transfer Unit, Preclinical and Translational Pharmacology, Department of Pharmacy, Health Science and Nutrition, University of Calabria, 87036 Arcavacata, Italy
* Correspondence: antonio.cerasa@cnr.it (A.C.); liliana.ruta@cnr.it (L.R.)
† These authors contributed equally to the study.

Citation: Marino, F.; Chilà, P.; Failla, C.; Minutoli, R.; Vetrano, N.; Luraschi, C.; Carrozza, C.; Leonardi, E.; Busà, M.; Genovese, S.; et al. Psychological Interventions for Children with Autism during the COVID-19 Pandemic through a Remote Behavioral Skills Training Program. *J. Clin. Med.* **2022**, *11*, 1194. https://doi.org/10.3390/jcm11051194

Academic Editor: Nuri B. Farber

Received: 18 December 2021
Accepted: 21 February 2022
Published: 23 February 2022

Abstract: COVID-19 has impacted negatively on the mental health of children with autism spectrum disorder (ASD), as well as on their parents. Remote health services are a sustainable approach to behavior management interventions and to giving caregivers emotional support in several clinical domains. During the COVID-19 pandemic, we investigated the feasibility of a web-based behavioral skills training (BST) program for 16 parents and their children with ASD at home. The BST parent training package was tailored to each different specific behavioral disorder that characterizes children with ASD. After training, we found a significant reduction in the frequency of all the targeted behavioral disorders, as well as an improvement in psychological distress and the perception of the severity of ASD-related symptoms in parents. Our data confirm the efficacy of remote health care systems in the management of behavioral disorders of children with ASD, as well as of their parents during the COVID-19 pandemic.

Keywords: autism; telehealth; behavioral skills training; parent training

1. Introduction

The COVID-19 pandemic has had a profound impact on the health of children with autistic spectrum disorders (ASD) and their parents. In fact, these children have been identified as part of a group at higher risk of medical complications and social distress [1] from COVID-19. Moreover, parents of children with ASD often have trouble accessing behavioral services for their children [2]. This common condition has been significantly exacerbated by the COVID-19-related containment measures, with the risk of increasing lifelong impairments and comorbidities related to this disorder. More accessible interventions are urgently needed to support the families of children with ASD by promoting new techniques that can also facilitate clinical and supportive interventions at a distance.

Some studies have discussed the possible consequences the COVID-19 pandemic could have on individuals and their parents. Research suggests that people with autism are particularly vulnerable to conditions of prolonged isolation, as they have to adapt to new routines which can negatively affect their progress [3,4], and an online survey found that people with ASD exhibited an increase in problem behavior during lockdown periods [5].

To manage the spread of COVID-19, since March 2020, an international effort has been made to adapt all healthcare services to work "remotely by default" [6]. Telehealth has therefore become of primary interest, continually evolving to encompass new approaches, new clinical demands, and digital developments.

In several clinical domains, remote digital health services foster patient–clinician relationships, ensure continuity in treatments, and support families by simultaneously reducing burdens on health systems [7]. Technology-mediated care includes live video calls, monitoring health status by medical devices, e-mail, audio, and instant messaging. This service connects clinicians virtually with patients or caregivers by removing any physical distance. Remote health services have also been used to support families of children with ASD. Hyman et al. [8] clarified the definitions of various health services by establishing the validity of this method in a similar way to traditional face-to-face clinical settings, although evidence-based protocols are lacking.

In this neuropsychiatric domain, remote health services may be more effective than in-person meetings. In fact, children with ASD have shown a positive sensitivity to the novelty of this method and the physical separation may allow clinicians to perform more naturalistic observations of the family setting [9]. Technologies related to remote health services also offer a cost-effective solution for extending the reach of behavioral interventions to families who do not live near a qualified provider, thus addressing inequalities in access to health care [10–12]. This method also has the advantage of easily training parents to be effective behavior-analytic teachers of their children [13]. Through technology-mediated care systems, it is thus possible to promote new kinds of online parent coaching by providing "anytime, anywhere" assistance to a parent who has access to the Internet during the pandemic era [14].

In this study, our aim was to demonstrate the feasibility and efficacy of a new web-based training approach aimed at reducing the frequency of targeted behavioral disorders in ASD children and improving parents' reported sense of competence related to child-related behavioral dysfunctions during the lockdown. Our online parent program was focused on behavioral skills training (BST). This is a teaching procedure that involves the use of instructions, feedback, modeling, and rehearsal [15]. This method has been used to develop new ways to support children with ASD with specific problem behaviors. The intervention typically includes modeling and prompting procedures [16] in the context of function-based treatments [17], and functional analyses [18]. The effectiveness of the BST procedure has been widely demonstrated in several clinical contexts [15–18], although its implementation in remote health service programs has been poorly investigated.

2. Materials and Methods

2.1. Enrollment

Twenty-eight parents of young children with autism were enrolled in the study. Parents were recruited and tested at the clinical facilities of the Institute for Biomedical Research and Innovation of the National Research Council of Italy (IRIB-CNR) in Messina and at the Centre for Autism Spectrum Disorders, Child Neuropsychiatry Unit, Provincial Health Agency of Trapani, Italy.

Inclusion criteria for the parents were: (1) being a native Italian speaker; (2) being biological parents; (3) having a home internet connection; and (4) being able to use web-based and telehealth tools. The inclusion criteria for ASD children were as follows: (1) being over 3 years of age; (2) clinical diagnosis of ASD based on DSM-5 criteria by a licensed neuropsychiatrist with the support of the Autism Diagnostic Observation Schedule, second edition (ADOS-2, Module 3); (3) a verbal development and performance quotient greater than 45;

(4) no hearing, visual or physical disability preventing participation; and (5) not being on psychopharmacological treatment. All participants had had a previous diagnosis which was further confirmed through the evaluation and consent of experienced professionals from the research group (i.e., a child neuropsychiatrist and a clinical psychologist). Data were collected from October 2020 to May 2021 during the second and third waves of the pandemic in Italy.

2.2. Ethics

All subjects provided informed consent for inclusion prior to their participation in the study. The study was conducted according to the guidelines of the Declaration of Helsinki and approved by the Committee of the Research Ethics and Bioethics Committee (http://www.cnr.it/ethics, accessed on 17 December 2021) of the National Research Council of Italy (CNR) (Prot. No. CNR-AMMCEN 54444/2018 01/08/2018) and by the Ethics Committee Palermo 1 (http://www.policlinico.pa.it/, accessed on 17 December 2021) of Azienda Ospedaliera Universitaria Policlinico Paolo Giaccone Palermo (report No. 10/2020–25/11/2020).

2.3. Study Design

The objective of the study was to assess the effectiveness of tele-assisted BST for parents in reducing the frequency of specific problem behaviors in children with ASD. To this end, given the wide behavioral variability and the absence of a control group a between-group design was not feasible and a multiple single subject design was also not feasible due to the wide range of techniques used and difficulty in assessing protocol adherence, fidelity and gathering data on a daily basis. Therefore, we applied a repeated measures design with four-time steps, using the frequency of undesired behavior as the outcome variable.

2.4. Treatment

The protocol was conducted through a web platform [G-Suite; Google LLC; Mountain view, CA, USA)] that gave access to video-conferencing tools. The Teleconsultation Center at IRIB-CNR in Messina had one teleconferencing workstation, with a basic webcam and headset, while parents at home were equipped with a tablet which was used to receive parent training and to record sessions for subsequent data coding and analysis (see Sections 2.5 and 2.7).

Parents and therapists briefly met via videoconferencing or telephone before and after each training session as needed in order to review the procedures, prepare the room and materials, discuss the results obtained, and to plan for the subsequent week's session.

While both parents were expected to participate in the training, video-recording of the target behaviour and behavioural data gathering was only mandatory for one parent.

2.5. Protocol Phases and Parent Training Procedures

The experimental protocol consisted of a total of eight phases (see Table 1) divided into 13 sessions/meetings lasting 45 min each, in accordance with the ABA procedure, with the participation of both parents and children. The first four sessions were of pure training, eight central sessions were for active treatment, and the last session was for feedback. The final target was to match the treatment to the identified functions of problem behavior.

During Phase 0, an online meeting was arranged with families, and the therapists informed the parents of the study's aims and procedures. Parent-report questionnaires were given to parents and gathered at the beginning of phase 1.

In Phase 1, the first operative meeting was scheduled. The therapist collected information on the individual child's behaviors and discussed them with the parents. At the end of the meeting, the therapist provided them with an individualized frequency checklist in order to have an operationalized definition of the problem behaviors reported by the parents. Identified behaviour must have been observable, measurable, and repeatable.

In the following week, the parents observed and monitored their child's problem behaviors whilst completing the behavior frequency checklist.

Table 1. Protocol structure.

Phases	Therapist's Tasks	Parent's Tasks
Phase 1	Protocol explanation, Data collection	Behaviours frequency checklist
Phase 2	First baseline, selection of target behaviour, instruction for video recording	Selection of target behaviour, starts video recording
Phase 3	Insert examples in the ABC worksheet from gathered observations. Gives Instruction on ABC worksheet and functional analysis	ABC worksheet recording
Phase 4	Analysis of the type of problem behavior, instruction on functional analysis trough ABC worksheet and videos	Receives instruction, starts the protocol and gather the objective baseline (T0)
Phase 5	Gather T0. Start BST parent training program, teaches procedures for behavioural change	Receive BST
Phase 6	Debrief and fidelity	Receive feedback
Phase 7	Data analysis; external review of fidelity	-
Phase 8	Debrief	Gives feedback

In Phase 2, the second operative meeting was scheduled. The therapist and the parents discussed the results reported in the checklist and selected the target behaviour. During the online meeting, the therapist established a first baseline related to the problem behavior. The behavior selected for treatment was the more frequently observed behavior that reduced learning opportunities or social inclusion or was either physically or emotionally harmful for the child or their family. At the end of the meeting, the parents were instructed to record videos of the target behavior during the following week.

In Phase 3, the therapist, during the third meeting, compiled the Antecedent-Behavior-Consequence (ABC) worksheet using information collected through the recorded videos. Parents received live coaching on functional analysis procedures in order to understand and identify the antecedents [events that precede] and consequences [events that follow] of the problem behavior using the recorded videos as examples. The therapist provided instructions on filling out the Antecedent-Behavior-Consequence (ABC) worksheet. At the end of the meeting, the use of short videos helped parents to interpret the problem behavior and to complete the ABC worksheet with the assistance of the therapist. The therapist then asked the parents to record the data on the ABC worksheet during the following week while continuing to record the videos.

In Phase 4 (fourth meeting), the therapist focused on analyzing the ABC worksheet compiled by the parents in order to identify the function of the monitored behavior through the recorded videos. Through a careful analysis of the antecedents and the consequences of the problem behavior over time, the therapist explained to parents why and how to follow the correct behavioral procedures that would favor a positive change. At the end of the meeting, parents were instructed to continue monitoring the behavior, recording video data, and filling out the ABC worksheet. Parents were now instructed to record videos with the same duration (45 min), in the same home location, and in the same context (i.e., presence/absence of parents) in order to gather the baseline (T0) for the BST.

In Phase 5, the fifth online meeting was held. The BST approach was integrated into the meeting sessions. This training utilizes instructions, modeling, rehearsal, and feedback in order to teach a new skill. The therapist first explains the skill to the parent, then models his/her behavior, who in turn models that of their child. The rehearsal phase is associated with role-playing used to train parents and model their behaviour during online meetings. At the end of each instance of the BST, the operator provided feedback on the performance. Feedback is positive when parents perform in accordance with the

BST procedure, or corrective when the parents have difficulty in following the instructions correctly. In our study, we used both types of feedback to aid parents in following the BST instructions. Online coaching was complemented by homework with written instructions on the procedure, which was sent to parents at the end of meetings.

In Phase 6, a debriefing session was held between the therapist and the parents regarding the tasks that had been previously assigned. The procedural fidelity was evaluated in order to assess the adherence to the treatment and to maintain it if the behavioral change was moving towards the expected goal. In the case of lapses in the procedures, phase 5 was briefly resumed and the fidelity reestablished.

During the 6th to 12th online meetings, parents and therapists moved between phases 5 and 6 according to the training needs and continued to record videos.

Parents were instructed to continue to apply the procedures explained during BST and record a new session with the same duration (45 min), in the same home location, and in the same context (i.e., presence/absence of parents) every day. The idea was to reproduce the same procedures presented by the therapist during the sessions, leading to comparable outcome measurements over time. These sessions at home without a consultant's input were recorded digitally using video-conferencing software for data collection. Specific reminders (by email or phone calls) were delivered to the parents in order to ensure that the videos were recorded during T1, T2 and T3.

Phase 7 was dedicated to monitoring fidelity and analyzing the progress of tasks. The results were analysed through a visual inspection of recorded materials during T0, T1, T2 and T3. Two additional experienced behavioral consultants, blind to any other result, evaluated the frequency of the problem behavior and the fidelity of the parental behavioral procedure. During the video analysis, the behavioral consultant marked the presence/absence (using "+" or "−" signs on a datasheet) of the problem behavior, obtaining a trend of the behavior over time, and marked the correct/incorrect procedure performed by the parents according to the schedule given by the therapist. Fidelity was dichotomized using "p" or "n" letters for each instance (pass or no-pass).

In the final phase (Phase 8), the feedback from the participants and parent-reported questionnaires was gathered. A timetable of the protocol, treatment and phases is reported in Table 2.

2.6. Training Experience

The therapists who delivered the interventions were all chartered psychologists, or psychotherapists, with behavioral analyst training and at least 5 years' experience in working with children on the autism spectrum.

2.7. Outcome Measurements

Outcome measurements were divided into: (a) objective measurement of problem behavior in children occurring on the day immediately after each session; and (b) psychological assessment of parents recorded before and after treatment.

For children with ASD, the main outcome was the frequency of the problem behavior which was recorded for statistical purposes at four different timepoints: Baseline (T0), and 20 days (T1), 40 days (T2), and 60 days (T3) after training (phase 5).

In terms of the parents, we collected outcome measurements on parenting stress together with a scale for assessing the parent's perception of the child's behavioral manifestations. This evaluation was carried out twice, at the baseline and at the end of treatment. The main outcome measures were the Parenting Stress Index (PSI) to assess the level of stress before and after treatment and the Home Situation Questionnaire (HSQ-ASD), which provides objective measures of the perception and influence of children's behavior on the parents' lives.

Table 2. Timetable of the protocol and data acquisition.

Protocol (days)	Treatment (days)	Week	Phase	Meetings	Data Gathering
-	-	-	0	0	Psychological Assessment T0
0	-	1	1	1	
7	-	2	2	2	
14	-	3	3	3	
21	-	4	4	4	
22	0	-	-	-	Behavioral T0
28	6	5	5	5	
35	13	6	5–6	6	
42	20	7	5–6	7	Behavioral T1
49	27	8	5–6	8	
56	34	9	5–6	9	
62	40	-	-	-	Behavioral T2
63	41	10	5–6	10	
70	48	11	5–6	11	
77	55	12	5–6	12	
82	60	-	-	-	Behavioral T3
83–90	-	13	7	-	
91	-	13	8	13	Psychological Assessment T1

2.7.1. Parenting Stress Index/Short Form (PSI-SF)

The PSI-SF is a self-assessment questionnaire [19]. It takes about 10–15 min to complete the questionnaire. Parenting stress levels are assessed by analyzing three different factors: 1. characteristics of the children, 2. characteristics of the parent, and 3. aspects related to the parental situation. The short module is made up of 36 items, divided into three subscales. (1) Parenting Distress (PD), referring to the feelings of the parents; (2) dysfunctional parent–child interaction (P—CDI), which focuses on the child's perception as unresponsive to parental expectations; and (3) Difficult Child (DC), which focuses on some of the characteristics of the child that make him/her easy or difficult to manage.

2.7.2. Home Situation Questionnaire (HSQ-ASD)

The HSQ-ASD [20] is a caregiver-rated scale designed to assess the severity of disruptive and non-compliant behaviors in children. The scores obtained with this scale refer to the parent's perception of their child's behavioral manifestations. Within the scale, data are collected on the inflexibility (HSQ-I) and avoidance (HSQ-A) manifested by the child. This modified and revised version for ASD consists of 27 elements. Parents were asked to indicate whether their children had problems with compliance in these situations and, if so, to rate the severity on a Likert scale of 0 to 9, with higher scores indicating greater non-compliance.

2.8. Statistical Analysis

Statistical analyses were performed using SPSS v. 23.0 (IBM, Armonk, NY, USA). The Kolmogorov–Smirnov test was carried out which confirmed the assumptions of normality only for psychological outcome measures.

Families who dropped out and families who continued with treatment were compared using a t-test for continuous variables and chi-square test for categorical variables.

For children, although the sample size was small, based on our experience in treating behavioral disorders in young children with ASD, we expected large effects. Therefore, we applied repeated measures ANOVA, reporting the post hoc power observed. The Greenhouse–Geisser correction was used if conditions of sphericity were not met.

The initial frequency of behavior can differ considerably for different children and different behaviors. For each participant, we therefore used the ratio of frequencies measured at different time steps with the initial frequency.

Inter-rater agreement was computed using Cohen's kappa (k).

For the parents' measures (PSI-SF; HSQ-ASD), we expected a smaller effect size, and therefore used non-parametric (Wilcoxon signed-rank test) and parametric statistics (paired t-test) aimed at analyzing the effects of the treatment on parents' outcome measures. We adjusted the alpha level using a Šidák correction for hierarchical multiple comparisons, with alpha = 0.025 for the primary measures (SI/SF and HSQ-ASD scores).

3. Results

The attrition rate was 42%. Indeed, six families dropped out before the beginning of phase 1, due to difficulties in managing weekly online connections, work commitments and/or family management of other children. Eight children with ASD and their relative parents (n°16), completed the treatment and were finally analyzed. Table 3 shows the demographic and psychological characteristics of children with ASD and their parents. The between-groups comparison showed no significant differences on any descriptive and psychological characteristic ($p > 0.05$).

Table 4 shows each individual behavioral symptom which was intended to be eliminated or reduced and its function. In Table 5, the behavioral treatment for each case is presented through the web-based training protocol with a brief explanation. The different procedures were performed as reported by Cooper and colleagues [18]. As expected, children with ASD showed heterogeneous behavioral spectrum disorders. Treatments were tailored to each specific behavioral symptom with the aim of reducing its frequency.

3.1. Fidelity

No parent reported with videos every day. On average, 2.93 (0.73) [2.10–4.32] videos were reported per week. There were no weeks with less than one video for each participant. No video was missing at T0, T1, T2 and T3. For all the families, behavioural data were gathered only by the main caregiver (in all families, it was the mother).

Procedural fidelity of the parent was 0.81 (0.13) [0.75–1.00] at T1, 0.97 (0.07) [0.80–1.00] at T1, 1.00 (0.00) [1.00–1.00] at T3. It should be noted that the number of instances on which fidelity was based decreased with the increase in time-steps.

3.2. Inter-Rater Agreement

Inter-rater agreement was excellent. Raters agreed in 94% of 224 instances for behavioral frequency, $k = 0.883$, and 92% of 119 instances for parents' procedural fidelity, $k = 0.849$. No disagreement was present in instances at T3. For the other time-steps, a final agreement was reached in all cases through discussion between the raters.

3.3. Behavioural Results

During active treatment, there was an immediate trend towards a better clinical outcome (Table 6), which at the end of the treatment was significantly improved (Figure 1).

Table 3. Demographic and psychological characteristics of children with ASD and their parents.

Measure	Completed	Dropped
Number of children/parents	8/16	6/12
Gender (M/F)	6/2	6/0
Age (months)	72.0 ± 30.4 68 (40–138)	57 ± 14.1 51 (48–84)
Total DQ Griffiths	67.0 ± 19.3 67.5 (45.5–95.5)	63.9 ± 14.2 69.4 (39.0–75.0)
Age of Mother (years)	41.0 ± 5.8 39 (33–52)	37.7 ± 2.3 38 (35–40)
Age of Father (years)	48.4 ± 5.0 49 (41–57)	43.0 ± 4.8 49 (41–57)
Education of Mother (years)	16.1 ± 2.6 18 (13–18)	13.8 ± 2.0 13 (13–18)
Education of Father (years)	16.8 ± 2.3 18 (8–21)	14.7 ± 2.6 18 (8–21)
Working Mother/Father (ratio)	0.50/1.00	0.83/1.00
Number of siblings	0.25 ± 0.46 0 (0–1)	1.33 ± 1.37 1 (0–3)

Data are given as mean values (SD), and median (range). ASD: autism spectrum disorders; DQ: Developmental Quotient. Data are expressed as mean ± SD or median (range) values if assumptions of normality are proved or otherwise.

Table 4. Problem behaviors and relative function in the ASD children enrolled.

	Problem Behavior	Behavioral Function	Context
ASD S1	Difficulties in accepting Stop Signal ("no")	Access to the tangible	At home when routine activities in the presence of both parents are changed or interrupted
ASD S2	Repetitive requests	Access to the tangible	At home during routine activities in the presence of both parents
ASD S3	Unshared laughter	Seeking attention	At home when the child carries out independent activities requested by the parents
ASD S4	Shouting when faced with a task proposed by the mother	Task avoidance/escape	At home when following the mother's request to perform tasks
ASD S5	Climbing on furniture, shouting, taking dangerous objects	Attention-seeking	At home in the presence of both parents engaged in other activities
ASD S6	Echolalia	Automatic reinforcement	At home when engaged in independent play activities
ASD S7	Throwing objects	Automatic reinforcement	At home while carrying out independent activities, with the mother engaged in other activities
ASD S8	Expressing denial and rejection as a for of idiosyncratic behavior	Task avoidance	At home when following requests by both parents

Table 5. Problem procedures and relative explanation in the ASD children enrolled [21].

	Behavioral Procedure	Explanation
ASD S1	Extinction	Parents physically remove themselves from the child when the target behaviour occurs (consequence intervention).
ASD S2	Desensitization	Gradual reduction of the number of requests the child can make and to which the parents can respond (antecedent intervention) according to the established criterion.
ASD S3	Differential reinforcement/Extinction	Extinction: Parents ignore the child when he/she emits the target behavior (consequence intervention) DRO (Differential Reinforcement of Other Behavior): parents were instructed to provide a reinforcement, agreed during the session, whenever the child did not exhibit the problem behavior in a given period of time.
ASD S4	High-p/fading of the prompt	Rapid presentation of a high-probability prompt followed by a low-probability prompt (antecedent intervention). Fading of the prompt: gradual reduction of the help provided by the parents on the task with low probability of the issue (intervention on the antecedent)
ASD S5	Differential reinforcement/Extinction	Extinction: Parents ignore the child when they display the target behavior (consequence intervention) DRO: parents were instructed to provide reinforcement, agreed during the session, whenever the child did not exhibit the problem behavior in a given period of time.
ASD S6	Expanding interests/Direction of Attention	Associating disliked objects/activities with liked, albeit restricted, objects/activities (antecedent intervention)
ASD S7	Expanding interests	Presenting functional auditory stimuli through songs or videos
ASD S8	Token economy	Child had the opportunity to earn tokens during the day (tangible tokens). After reaching an agreed number of tokens, they had the opportunity to exchange them for a reward they liked. The token economy was built on a billboard on which the child could attach points, thus favoring the visual channel for collecting points, and did not use a response cost.

Mauchly's test of sphericity was not significant, Mauchly's W = 0.440, $X^2 = 4.70$, $df = 5$, $p = 0.460$.

The multivariate test was significant, F (3, 5) = 247, $p < 0.001$, $n^2 = 0.993$ with an observed power (OP) of 1.00. The within-subject effect was also significant F (3, 21) = 92.3, $p < 0.001$, $n^2 = 0.930$, OP = 1.00. However, the between-subject effects were also significant, F (1, 7) = 398, $p < 0.001$, $n^2 = 0.983$, OP = 1.00.

In order to better understand the structure of change, we tried different polynomial models of frequency-change in time, and the best fit was for a linear model with F (1, 7) = 770, $p < 0.001$, $n^2 = 0.991$, OP = 1.00.

A decrease in behavioral frequency was present in all children in all the time steps, and a pairwise comparison showed that differences were significant between T1 and T0 (M = 38% [17%; 58%], $p = 0.002$), T2 and T1 (M = 26% [5%; 47%], $p = 0.016$), and T3 and T2 (M = 26% [2%; 50%], $p = 0.032$).

Table 6. Frequency of behavioral symptoms during active treatment.

	Main Behavioral Symptoms	Frequency * T0	Frequency T1 (20 days)	Frequency T2 (40 days)	Frequency T3 (60 days)
ASD S1	Difficulties in accepting Stop Signal ("no")	6	5	2	0
ASD S2	Repetitive requests	20	16	10	5
ASD S3	unshared' laughter	10	5	5	1
ASD S4	Shouting when faced with a task proposed by the mother	10	5	2	1
ASD S5	Climbing on furniture, shouting, and taking dangerous objects	12	8	3	2
ASD S6	Echolalia	26	18	16	2
ASD S7	Throwing objects	8	3	1	1
ASD S8	Expressing denial and rejection as a for of idiosyn-cratic behavior	8	5	3	0

* Frequency is expressed as the number of events during the session.

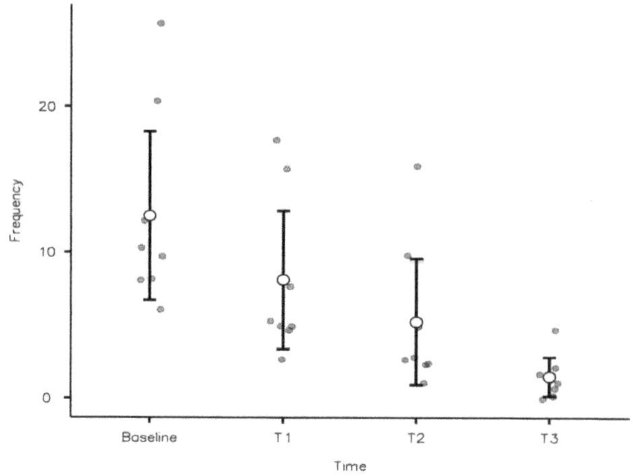

Figure 1. Significant reduction in the frequency of behavioral symptoms during web-based treatment with the BST approach.

3.4. Parental Wellbeing

We also evaluated the effects of our web-based training on the psychological wellbeing and perception of severity in parents of ASD children, measured before and after the treatment (Table 7). As concerns the PSI-SF scale, we found a significant reduction in total psychological stress and PD and P-CDI subscales after treatment. A similar beneficial effect was also detected in the HSQ-ASD scale, where parents showed a significant reduction in the perception of the severity of inflexibility (HSQ-I) and avoidance behaviors manifested by their children after treatment (HSQ-A).

Table 7. Psychological effects on parents before and after BST treatment.

	Before Treatment	After Treatment	W/p-Level	Paired t-Test/p-Level
		PSI-SF Scale		
Total Value	105.7 ± 7.3 105 (90–114)	95.4 ± 8.1 98 (84–107)	105/0.001	6.2/<0.001
PD	35.6 ± 7.9 36 (21–47)	29.3 ± 8.1 30 (16–43)	67/0.03	2.7/0.02
P-CDI	36.2 ± 8.7 33 (26–52)	29 ± 5.4 29.5 (19–38)	73.5/0.008	3.6/0.003
DC	32.9 ± 12.4 30 (19–53)	36.9 ± 7.1 37 (21–50)	n.s	n.s
		HSQ-ASD Scale		
Total Value	4.8 ± 1.8 4.6 (1.9–7.4)	3.5 ± 1.6 3 (1–7)	66/0.003	6.3/<0.001
Inflexibility	5.3 ± 1.6 5.4 (2–8.2)	3.4 ± 1.2 3.3 (2–5)	78/0.002	4.3/0.001
Avoidance	4.8 ± 2.1 4.4 (1.8–7.8)	3.2 ± 2 2.8 (1–6)	91/0.001	7.9/<0.001

Data are given as mean values (SD), and median (range). PSI-SF: Parenting Stress Index/Short Form; HSQ-ASD: Home Situation Questionnaire; PD: Parenting Distress; P-CDI: Dysfunctional parent–child interaction; DC: Difficult Child.

4. Discussion

In this study, we demonstrated that a well-known behavioral approach, that is, BST, could be efficiently offered to children with ASD and their parents using a low-cost and commercial web-based training approach. We found a significant reduction in the frequency of behavioral disorders detected in children with ASD after treatment, as well as a general reduction in psychological distress and the perception of the severity of ASD-related symptoms in parents.

This study demonstrated the feasibility of live coaching on BST procedures as a valid approach to managing behavioral disorders in children with ASD and for helping their parents deal with such disorders during COVID-19 pandemic. Distance behavioral training programs should be encouraged, and public awareness should be raised among parents and clinicians aimed at regarding telehealth as an alternative and valid means of providing treatment [22,23]. In the future, such programs could help tackle the lack of therapists available to support the growing demand for their services and the role of primary caregivers as a critical component in the success of treatments [24,25].

In our study, all the children showed a marked progressive reduction in the frequency of their targeted behavioral symptoms during the follow-up period. In fact, after 20 days (T1), the lowest reduction was 17% and the median was 35%; after 40 days, the lowest was 38% and the median 65%; and finally, at the end of the protocol (60 days), the lowest was 75% (ASD S2) with a median reduction of 90%, with two out of eight children no longer showing the target inappropriate behavior.

We also found a reduction in parent-reported stress, a decrease in child inflexibility and avoidance, and a more functional parent–child interaction. The only scale that showed no significant reduction (and showed a slight increase) was PSI-DC. This scale is designed to assess the parent's perception of child-related disorders. To explain this finding we propose that, although our remote BST parent training might induce a better understanding of the difficulties they are facing, the adaptation to stressful events associated with caring for an autistic depends on several factors (family demands; family adaptive resources, the family's definition of the stressful situation and family adaptive coping mechanisms) [23].

There are several studies demonstrating the effectiveness of parental training on the behavioral patterns of children with ASD [26,27]. In fact, parent training can effectively help in improving parent–child interactions and social communication [28]. A study by Tonge et al. [29] demonstrated that both parental education and training in behavioral procedures for children with autism can be beneficial for parental mental health. In Tonge's study [29], parents received a manual-based education and behavior management skills training package. Sessions were skills-based and action-oriented through the provision of workbooks, modeling, videos, rehearsal, homework tasks, and feedback. At a 6-month follow-up evaluation, the combination of parent education and behavioral teaching led to a significant reduction in anxiety, insomnia, and somatic symptoms. Hassan et al. [30] demonstrated the effectiveness of BST in developing parental skills and treatment strategies to support specific social behaviors in their children. In Hassan's study, free-play sessions with parents and their children were structured. These authors demonstrated that treatment carried out according to the BST procedure improved functional skills and communication by decreasing the manifestation of destructive behaviors.

A recent systematic review provided evidence of the utility of telehealth as a service delivery model for providing analytic-based services and for training caregivers to implement behavioral assessments and procedures [31]. Despite this evidence, there are a few studies which evaluated the feasibility of telehealth for families with ASD. Boutain et al. [32] evaluated the success of a remote web-based BST training package to teach parents to implement new treatments with their children for the independent completion of three self-care skills (washing hands, washing faces, and applying lotions). Another study on online coaching in daily living skills, with four children ranging in age from 5 to 9 years, showed that parents faithfully implemented treatment which led to increases in independent daily living skills for all the participants [33]. In line with all this evidence, we demonstrated that a remote BST service is useful in managing behavioral disorders and improving parent awareness by reducing the frequency of various behavioral disorders in children, as well as lowering psychological distress in parents.

Limitations

The first limitation of this study was the high attrition rate (42%). Nevertheless, it should be noted that all the drop-outs happened at the beginning of the study and none dropped after the initial assessment. Even if we found no significant difference between drop-outs and families who continued till the end of the protocol, it could be noted that the families who dropped out tended to have working mothers with more children and lower educational levels. This agrees with the concerns expressed during the interviews about the difficulties in reconciling BST with family and work schedules. This is further reinforced by the fact that in all families that continued with the protocol, even if both parents participated in the training, only the mothers actively reported behavioral data. As a consequence, we cannot account for the effect of the involvement and support of the fathers in the therapeutic outcome. Furthermore, we did not record other undesired behaviors, and we therefore do not know whether parents independently applied the learned procedures to other behaviours and if that could partly explain the decrease observed in parental psychological measures. Future studies should improve the feasibility of this procedure and study its contextual needs and accommodations to remotely intercept different populations and family organizations.

Another limitation of the current study was the limited number of participants. A larger sample could provide a more accurate analysis of the effects of treatment. One internal limitation was the lack of a control group which prevented a direct comparison with another type of intervention. Furthermore, the analysis was performed on a group of heterogeneous behavioral disorders and procedures. This limitation is evident due to the large between-subject effect size of the study. Nevertheless, this limitation is also a strength, given the lack of online behavioral studies on the topic. In fact, we believe we have shown the feasibility of the training for a wide set of procedures and hope that this will foster a larger variety of new studies that no longer focus exclusively on a single procedure.

Finally, we gathered only the frequency of undesired behaviours to avoid overwhelming the parents with too many tasks. Therefore, we did not know of the occurrence of alternative behaviours or the emergence of new undesired behaviours. We recommend that future studies include a larger number of participants and a parallel control group receiving a traditional behavioral treatment. In addition, future research could include an analysis of treatments with homogeneous behaviors. Another important topic would be to assist practicing clinicians in determining an appropriate protocol for the delivery of a 1:1 telehealth service. Some proposals are already in place, but still lack experimental support [31].

5. Conclusions

The COVID-19 pandemic has created an enormous amount of suffering for all levels of society, but especially for more vulnerable people. At the same time, it has also led researchers to search for new solutions and to challenge long-held assumptions regarding therapy. Remote health services can provide a sustainable model for both conducting assessments and training healthcare professionals and staff in order to implement several behavioral strategies, as proposed by Ferguson et al. [34]. In this study, we confirm that parental coaching can also be carried out through an easily accessible remote service aimed at making the parents of children with ASD increasingly competent in the daily management of their children and being more empowering in their role. Such remote services can provide support through skills and behavior management treatments not only during global health crises, but also as a sustainable and standard model for the future.

Author Contributions: Conceptualization, F.M., P.C., A.C. and G.P.; methodology, F.M., P.C., C.F., R.M. (Roberta Minutoli), N.V., D.V. and A.C.; software, M.B., A.P., G.T. and D.V.; validation, F.M., P.C., R.M. (Roberta Minutoli), N.V. and L.R.; formal analysis, A.A.A., A.P., R.M. (Rosa Musotto), G.T., D.V., A.C. and G.P.; investigation, F.M., C.F., N.V., C.L., C.C., E.L., G.C. (Giuliana Cardella), F.I.F. and G.C. (Gaspare Cusimano); resources, F.M., C.F., R.M. (Rosa Musotto), S.G., P.M., G.M., D.V., L.R. and G.P.; data curation, F.M., C.F., N.V., C.L., C.C., E.L., S.G., G.C. (Giuliana Cardella), F.I.F., G.C. (Gaspare Cusimano), A.A.A., G.T. and D.V.; writing—original draft prepa-ration, F.M., C.F., D.V., A.C. and G.P.; writing—review and editing, F.M., D.V., A.C. and G.P.; vis-ualization, F.M., D.V. and G.P.; supervision, F.M., D.V., A.C., L.R. and G.P.; project administration, G.P.; funding acquisition, P.M., G.M., G.C. (Gaspare Cusimano) and G.P. All authors have read and agreed to the published version of the manuscript.

Funding: This research was funded by the Assessorato Regionale delle Attività Produttive, Sicily, grant number n. 08SR2620000204, entitled LAB@HOME—Una Casa Intelligente per l'Autismo, P.O. F.E.S.R. Sicilia 2014/2020, Azione 1.1.5, and funded by the Azienda Sanitaria Provinciale—ASP-di Trapani: Grant number n. 08SR2620000204 Assessorato Regionale delle Attività Produttive Sicilia and Deliberation n. 20190003196-10/12/2019 ASP Trapani.

Institutional Review Board Statement: The study was conducted according to the guidelines of the Declaration of Helsinki and approved by the Ethics Committee of the Research Ethics and Bioethics Committee (http://www.cnr.it/ethics, accessed on 17 December 2021) of the National Research Council of Italy (CNR) (Prot. N. CNR-AMMCEN 54444/2018 01/08/2018) and by the Ethics Committee Palermo 1 (http://www.policlinico.pa.it/, accessed on 17 December 2021) of Azienda Ospedaliera Universitaria Policlinico Paolo Giaccone Palermo (report n. 10/2020–25/11/2020).

Informed Consent Statement: Informed consent was obtained from all subjects involved in the study.

Data Availability Statement: The datasets generated during the current study are available from the corresponding author on reasonable request.

Conflicts of Interest: The authors declare no conflict of interest.

References

1. Eshraghi, A.A.; Li, C.; Alessandri, M.; Messinger, D.S.; Eshraghi, R.S.; Mittal, R.; Armstrong, F.D. COVID-19: Overcoming the challenges faced by individuals with autism and their families. *Lancet Psychiatry* **2020**, *7*, 481–483. [CrossRef]
2. Kogan, M.D.; Strickland, B.B.; Blumberg, S.J.; Singh, G.K.; Perrin, J.M.; van Dyck, P.C. A National Profile of the Health Care Experiences and Family Impact of Autism Spectrum Disorder Among Children in the United States, 2005–2006. *Pediatrics* **2008**, *122*, e1149–e1158. [CrossRef] [PubMed]
3. Colizzi, M.; Sironi, E.; Antonini, F.; Ciceri, M.L.; Bovo, C.; Zoccante, L. Psychosocial and Behavioral Impact of COVID-19 in Autism Spectrum Disorder: An Online Parent Survey. *Brain Sci.* **2020**, *10*, 341. [CrossRef] [PubMed]
4. Narzisi, A. Handle the autism spectrum condition dur- ing coronavirus (COVID-19) stay at home period: Ten tips for helping parents and caregivers of young children. *Brain Sci.* **2020**, *10*, 207. [CrossRef] [PubMed]
5. Amaral, D.G.; de Vries, P.J. COVID-19 and autism research: Perspectives from around the globe. *Autism Res.* **2020**, *13*, 844–869. [CrossRef]
6. Greenhalgh, T.; Rosen, R.; Shaw, S.E.; Byng, R.; Faulkner, S.; Finlay, T.; Grundy, E.; Husain, L.; Hughes, G.; Leone, C.; et al. Planning and Evaluating Remote Consultation Services: A New Conceptual Framework Incorporating Complexity and Practical Ethics. *Front. Digit. Health* **2021**, *3*, 726095. [CrossRef]
7. Jordan, C.; Leslie, K.; Roder-DeWan, H.H.; Adeyi, O.S.; Barker, P.; Daelmans, B.; Doubova, S.V.; English, M.; Elorrio, E.G.; Guanais, F.; et al. High-quality health systems in the Sustainable Development Goals era: Time for a revolution. *Lancet Glob. Health* **2018**, *6*, e1196–e1252.
8. Hyman, S.L.; Levy, S.E.; Myers, S.M. Council on Children with Disabilities, Section on Developmental and Behavioral Pediatrics. Identification, Evaluation, and Management of Children with Autism Spectrum Disorder. *Pediatrics* **2020**, *145*, e20193447. [CrossRef]
9. Pakyurek, M.; Yellowlees, P.; Hilty, D. The child and adolescent telepsychiatry consultation: Can it be a more effective clinical process for certain patients than conventional practice? *Telemed J. E Health* **2010**, *16*, 289–292. [CrossRef]
10. Boisvert, M.; Lang, R.; Andrianopoulos, M.; Boscardin, M.L. Telepractice in the assessment and treatment of individuals with autism spectrum disorders: A systematic review. *Dev. Neurorehabilit.* **2010**, *13*, 423–432. [CrossRef]
11. Lindgren, S.; Wacker, D.P.; Suess, A.; Schieltz, K.; Pelzel, K.; Kopelman, T.; Lee, J.; Romani, P.; Waldron, D. Telehealth and Autism: Treating Challenging Behavior at Lower Cost. *Pediatrics* **2015**, *137*, 167–175. [CrossRef]
12. Ingersoll, B.; Gergans, S. The effect of a parent-implemented imitation intervention on spontaneous imitation skills in young children with autism. *Res. Dev. Disabil.* **2007**, *28*, 163–175. [CrossRef]
13. Vismara, L.A.; McCormick, C.; Young, G.S.; Nadhan, A.; Monlux, K. Preliminary findings of a telehealth approach to parent training in autism. *J. Autism Dev. Disord.* **2013**, *43*, 2953–2969. [CrossRef]
14. Dittman, C.K.; Farruggia, S.P.; Palmer, M.L.; Sanders, M.R.; Keown, L.J. Predicting success in an online parenting intervention: The role of child, parent, and family factors. *J. Fam. Psychol.* **2014**, *28*, 236–243. [CrossRef]
15. Miltenberger, R.G. Behavior skills training procedures. In *Behavior Modification Principles and Procedures*; Miltenberger, R.G., Ed.; Thompson Wadsworth: Belmont, CA, USA, 2004; pp. 237–249.
16. Koegel, R.L.; Glahn, T.J.; Nieminen, G.S. Generalization of parent-training results1. *J. Appl. Behav. Anal.* **1978**, *11*, 95–109. [CrossRef]
17. Robertson, R.E.; Wehby, J.H.; King, S.M. Increased parent reinforcement of spontaneous requests in children with autism spectrum disorder: Effects on problem behavior. *Res. Dev. Disabil.* **2013**, *34*, 1069–1082. [CrossRef]
18. Stokes, J.V.; Luiselli, J.K. In-home parent training of functional analysis skills. *Int. J. Behav. Consult. Ther.* **2008**, *4*, 259–263. [CrossRef]
19. Haskett, M.E.; Ahern, L.S.; Ward, C.S.; Allaire, J.C. Factor Structure and Validity of the Parenting Stress Index-Short Form. *J. Clin. Child Adolesc. Psychol.* **2006**, *35*, 302–312. [CrossRef]
20. Chowdhury, M.; Aman, M.G.; Lecavalier, L.; Smith, T.; Johnson, C.; Swiezy, N.; McCracken, J.T.; King, B.; McDougle, C.J.; Bearss, K.; et al. Factor structure and psychometric properties of the revised Home Situations Questionnaire for autism spectrum disorder: The Home Situations Questionnaire-Autism Spectrum Disorder. *Autism* **2015**, *20*, 528–537. [CrossRef]
21. Cooper, J.O.; Heron, T.E.; Heward, W.L. *Applied Behavior Analysis*; Merrill: New York, NY, USA, 2007.
22. Schieltz, K.M.; Wacker, D.P. Functional assessment and function-based treatment delivered via telehealth: A brief summary. *J. Appl. Behav. Anal.* **2020**, *53*, 1242–1258. [CrossRef]
23. McStay, R.L.; Trembath, D.; Dissanayake, C. Stress and Family Quality of Life in Parents of Children with Autism Spectrum Disorder: Parent Gender and the Double ABCX Model. *J. Autism Dev. Disord.* **2014**, *44*, 3101–3118. [CrossRef]
24. Heitzman-Powell, L.S.; Buzhardt, J.; Rusinko, L.C.; Miller, T.M. Formative Evaluation of an ABA Outreach Training Program for Parents of Children with Autism in Remote Areas. *Focus Autism Other Dev. Disabil.* **2014**, *29*, 23–38. [CrossRef]
25. Friesen, K.A.; Weiss, J.A.; Howe, S.J.; Kerns, C.M.; McMorris, C.A. Mental Health and Resilient Coping in Caregivers of Autistic Individuals during the COVID-19 Pandemic: Findings from the Families Facing COVID Study. *J. Autism Dev. Disord.* **2021**, 1–11. [CrossRef]
26. Powell, D.; Dunlap, G.; Fox, L. Prevention and Intervention for the Challenging Behaviors of Toddlers and Preschoolers. *Infants Young-Child.* **2006**, *19*, 25–35. [CrossRef]

27. Brookman-Frazee, L.; Stahmer, A.; Baker-Ericzén, M.J.; Tsai, K. Parenting Interventions for Children with Autism Spectrum and Disruptive Behavior Disorders: Opportunities for Cross-Fertilization. *Clin. Child Fam. Psychol. Rev.* **2006**, *9*, 181–200. [CrossRef]
28. Patterson, S.Y.; Smith, V.; Mirenda, P. A systematic review of training programs for parents of children with autism spectrum disorders: Single subject contributions. *Autism* **2012**, *16*, 498–522. [CrossRef]
29. Tonge, B.; Brereton, A.; Kiomall, M.; Mackinnon, A.; King, N.; Rinehart, N. Effects on Parental Mental Health of an Education and Skills Training Program for Parents of Young Children With Autism: A Randomized Controlled Trial. *J. Am. Acad. Child Adolesc. Psychiatry* **2006**, *45*, 561–569. [CrossRef]
30. Hassan, M.; Simpson, A.; Danaher, K.; Haesen, J.; Makela, T.; Thomson, K. An Evaluation of Behavioral Skills Training for Teaching Caregivers How to Support Social Skill Development in Their Child with Autism Spectrum Disorder. *J. Autism Dev. Disord.* **2018**, *48*, 1957–1970. [CrossRef]
31. Unholz-Bowden, E.; McComas, J.J.; McMaster, K.L.; Girtler, S.; Kolb, R.L.; Shipchandler, A. Caregiver Training Via Telehealth on Behavioral Procedures: A Systematic Review. *J. Behav. Educ.* **2020**, *29*, 246–281. [CrossRef]
32. Boutain, A.R.; Sheldon, J.B.; Sherman, J.A. Evaluation of a telehealth parent training program in teaching self-care skills to children with autism. *J. Appl. Behav. Anal.* **2020**, *53*, 1259–1275. [CrossRef]
33. Gerow, S.; Radhakrishnan, S.; Akers, J.S.; McGinnis, K.; Swensson, R. Telehealth parent coaching to improve daily living skills for children with ASD. *J. Appl. Behav. Anal.* **2021**, *54*, 566–581. [CrossRef] [PubMed]
34. Ferguson, J.; Craig, E.A.; Dounavi, K. Telehealth as a Model for Providing Behaviour Analytic Interventions to Individuals with Autism Spectrum Disorder: A Systematic Review. *J. Autism Dev. Disord.* **2019**, *49*, 582–616. [CrossRef] [PubMed]

Journal of
Clinical Medicine

MDPI

Article

PTSD Symptoms and Coping with COVID-19 Pandemic among Treatment-Seeking Veterans: Prospective Cohort Study

Marina Letica-Crepulja [1,2,*], Aleksandra Stevanović [1,2,3], Diana Palaić [2], Iva Vidović [1] and Tanja Frančišković [1,2,3]

1 Department of Psychiatry and Psychological Medicine, Faculty of Medicine, University of Rijeka, 51000 Rijeka, Croatia; aleksandras@medri.uniri.hr (A.S.); vidoviiva@gmail.com (I.V.); tanja.franciskovic@medri.uniri.hr (T.F.)

2 Department of Psychiatry, Clinical Hospital Center Rijeka, Referral Center of the Ministry of Health of the Republic of Croatia, 51000 Rijeka, Croatia; diana.palaic@gmail.com

3 Department of Basic Medical Sciences, Faculty of Health Studies, University of Rijeka, 51000 Rijeka, Croatia

* Correspondence: marinalc@medri.uniri.hr; Tel.: +385-51658321

Abstract: Background: The aim of this study was to examine post-traumatic stress disorder (PTSD) symptom levels and coping strategies during the COVID-19 pandemic among treatment-seeking veterans with pre-existing PTSD. Method: A cohort of 176 male treatment-seeking veterans with pre-existing PTSD during the first COVID-19 pandemic lockdown (T1) and 132 participants from the same cohort one year after the onset of the pandemic (T2) participated in a longitudinal study. All participants responded to a COVID-19-related questionnaire and the following measures: the Life Events Checklist for DSM-5 (LEC-5), PTSD Checklist for DSM-5 (PCL-5) and the Brief COPE. Results: The intensity of overall PTSD symptoms, avoidance symptoms and negative alterations in cognitions and mood was lower at T2. PTSD symptoms were not significantly correlated with SARS-CoV-2 potentially traumatic events (PTE) at T2. Veterans scored higher on emotion-focused and problem-focused coping than on dysfunctional coping. Conclusions: Veterans with pre-existing PTSD who were receiving long-term treatment coped with COVID-19 stressors without the effects of retraumatization and a consequent worsening of PTSD symptoms.

Keywords: COVID-19; PTSD; war-related stress; pandemic-related stress; treatment-seeking

Citation: Letica-Crepulja, M.; Stevanović, A.; Palaić, D.; Vidović, I.; Frančišković, T. PTSD Symptoms and Coping with COVID-19 Pandemic among Treatment-Seeking Veterans: Prospective Cohort Study. *J. Clin. Med.* **2022**, *11*, 2715. https://doi.org/10.3390/jcm11102715

Academic Editors: Alfonso Troisi and Ursula Werneke

Received: 20 February 2022
Accepted: 9 May 2022
Published: 11 May 2022

Publisher's Note: MDPI stays neutral with regard to jurisdictional claims in published maps and institutional affiliations.

1. Introduction

The coronavirus disease-19 (COVID-19) pandemic has caused multiple health, social, and economic stressors and presents a progressively emerging and potentially long-lasting life threat [1]. Pandemic stressors have a broad spectrum of impacts including mental health risk for individuals around the world. Extensive research has documented the negative psychiatric consequences of the COVID-19 pandemic [2–4]. A study that examined the global impacts of the pandemic on major depressive and anxiety disorders showed that prevalence of major depressive disorder and anxiety disorders had increased by more than 25 percent worldwide [3].

Patients with pre-existing mental disorders appeared to be at higher risk for wide-ranging mental health effects [5–7]. Regarding the veteran population, the results from recent studies revealed resilience to mental health problems and lower rates of suicidal ideation among US military veterans nearly 10 months into the pandemic [8,9]. However, these studies also showed that the prevalence of generalized anxiety disorder increased and the prevalence of major depressive disorder and post-traumatic stress disorder (PTSD) remained stable during the pandemic [10]. A recent longitudinal study, conducted during the period between two lockdowns among treatment-seeking veterans with pre-existing mental health difficulties in the UK, did not find any significant changes in symptoms of PTSD, common mental health disorders, anger, or alcohol use between the lockdowns [11].

A study that compared prepandemic and peripandemic levels of PTSD symptoms among Croatian treatment-seeking veterans with pre-existing PTSD demonstrated a reduction in PTSD symptom levels during the onset of the COVID-19 pandemic [12]. As the COVID-19 pandemic is often referred to as a "marathon, not a sprint," and is spread around the world, there remains a need for further longitudinal studies to examine long-term changes in mental health of veterans with pre-existing difficulties in different settings.

Coping reflects a form of adaptation elicited by stressful circumstances. The previous research has repeatedly shown that combat veterans with PTSD use a non-adaptive and avoidance coping style [13–15]. The coping strategies veterans use when facing the pandemic stressors are important, because they can either alleviate or cause additional stress. There is a lack of systematic research on coping with pandemic stressors among veterans with pre-existing mental health difficulties including PTSD.

Almost thirty years after the Homeland War in Croatia (1991–1995), veterans still suffer from numerous health problems. In 2020, there were 33,089 treatment-seeking veterans with PTSD, which is 7.76% of the overall veteran population in Croatia [16]. A recent study revealed high rates of overall symptoms and greater severity of post-traumatic symptoms (i.e., complex PTSD) among treatment-seeking veterans years after the war ended [17]. The aim of this study was to follow the trajectories of PTSD symptom levels and examine coping strategies during the onset and one year after the onset of the COVID-19 pandemic among treatment-seeking veterans with pre-existing PTSD.

2. Materials and Methods

2.1. Participants and Procedure

All participants were male veterans from the Homeland War in Croatia (1991–1995) and had been in treatment for war-related PTSD for an average of 18.8 years (range 3 to 30 years at the second measurement) at the Referral Center of the Ministry of Health of the Republic of Croatia (RCPTSD) at the Clinical Hospital Center (CHC) Rijeka. Of 250 treatment-seeking veterans whom we approached, 176 (70.4%) participated at the first measurement (T1), which took place from April 15 to the end of May 2020 (i.e., during the onset of the COVID-19 pandemic). Sixty-four veterans could not be reached, five refused to participate, and five were excluded from further analysis due to incomplete data. They were recontacted during April and May 2021 (T2) when the third wave of the COVID-19 pandemic reached its peak. One hundred thirty-two (132) responded and consented to participate in the second measurement. Of the 44 who did not take part in the second measurement, five refused to participate, one had died, and the remaining 39 could not be reached even after three phone calls. Since their first referral, and before T1, participants had been involved in one or more outpatient treatment options: intensive PTSD program for day-care hospital (78.2%), long-term psychotherapy (26.3%), low-level treatment groups such as PTSD Club (11.3%), and regular outpatient psychiatric appointments (89.5%). Every other participant had received inpatient care (49.6%) at some point during their treatment. At T1 and T2, and in between, participants had been treated in regular outpatient psychiatric appointments with no changes in the administration of regular medication.

Due to the ongoing COVID-19 restrictions, the assessments were conducted by telephone or face-to-face with participants who attended the check-up. After the participants had been given detailed information about the study, all participants provided their written informed consent. In cases when the assessments were made by telephone, the written informed consent was provided at the next regular onsite appointment. The two parts of the evaluation consisted of a structured clinical interview and self-report questionnaires. Besides sociodemographic items, the structured interview at T2 included additional questions on difficulties with specific aspects of the COVID-19 pandemic. The study was approved by the Ethical Committee of CHC Rijeka, ethical approval code 003-05/20-1/85.

2.2. Measures

The measures used in the study were the Life Events Checklist for DSM-5 (LEC-5), PTSD Checklist for DSM-5 (PCL-5) and the Brief COPE. At the second assessment, the participants were asked whether they had experienced any traumatic life event in the past twelve months since the lifetime traumatization was assessed at T1.

The Life Events Checklist for DSM-5 (LEC-5) was used to assess possible traumatic events experienced by participants in the past twelve months [18]. The self-report measure lists 16 traumatic events and an additional item indicating any other stressful event. For the study, the total score of lifetime trauma, calculated as the sum of traumatic events, ranged from 0 to 17. The checklist was reported to have good psychometric properties [18,19].

The PTSD Checklist for DSM-5 (PCL-5) with Criterion A is a self-report measure revised to match the adapted DSM-5 criteria for PTSD [20]. A provisional PTSD diagnosis can be made considering items rated 2 = moderately or higher according to the DSM-5 diagnostic rule (at least one B, one C, two D, and two E symptoms present). Symptom severity was calculated as the sum of all items (0–80) or as the sum within a specific cluster of symptoms. Authors reported the score of 33 or above to be indicative of probable PTSD diagnosis and was thus used as the cut-off score in this study. Validation studies showed excellent psychometric properties for evaluating PTSD [20–23]. PCL-5 showed good internal consistency in our study, with Cronbach alphas ranging from 0.72 to 0.85 for clusters and 0.90 for total PCL-5.

The Brief COPE is a 28-item multidimensional measure of coping strategies used for regulating cognitions and behaviors in response to stressors [24]. Fourteen two-item scales are rated on the four-point rating scales (1 = I have not been doing this at all to 4 = I have been doing this a lot). The score of each scale is the sum of two items, with the possible range of 0–8. Each scale can be viewed independently or as part of emotion-focused, problem-focused, or dysfunctional coping strategies [24,25]. The Brief COPE is reported to have good psychometric properties [24]. Good psychometric properties were also reported for the Croatian version of Brief COPE in the study with a large adult online sample [26]. The Cronbach alpha in our study was 0.81.

The COVID-19-related questionnaire was created for specifically this study, and consisted of three parts. The first part was related to severe acute respiratory syndrome coronavirus 2 (SARS-CoV-2) infection of the participants and their close relatives, severity of the COVID-19 symptoms, the need for hospitalization, the level of recovery and death of a close family member. The second part was related to the level of compliance to the government COVID-19 measures. The third part was related to COVID-related stressors: pandemic duration, pandemic uncertainty, media coverage/exposure, restricted family gatherings, restricted access to medical services, fear of COVID-19, physical distancing, financial burden, self-isolation, restricted access to domestic supplies, and other.

2.3. Data Analysis

The existing dataset from T1 and the data collected at T2 were used for the analysis. Descriptive statistics were used to present frequencies/percentages or means and standard deviations for parametric measures. Pearson's chi-square test was used to test for differences between groups on categorical variables. In cases where the cells' frequency was below five, the Yates correction was applied. Group differences on continuous variables were tested with *t*-tests or Mann–Whitney U tests when number of cases was <20. Differences between measurements on continuous variables were tested with t-tests for repeated measurement. Spearman's correlation coefficient was applied to test for significant correlations. Statistical significance was set as $p < 0.05$. Statistical analysis was performed with Statistica software, version 12 (Dell Inc., Tulsa, OK, USA).

3. Results

3.1. Demographics and War-Related Characteristics

Of 176 male participants in the first measurement, 132 (75%) war veterans participated in the second measurement. The sociodemographic characteristics are presented in Table 1. The missing 44 participants and those who participated at T2 did not differ significantly on any of the sociodemographic characteristics or war-related measures. Therefore, the functional equivalence and representativeness of the sample allowed for further analysis.

Table 1. Sociodemographic characteristics of study participants at the first assessment (T1). Data are presented as count (percentage) unless otherwise indicated.

	The 1st Measurement Participants n = 176		Statistics	
	Participants Assessed at T1 and T2 **n = 132**	**Participants Missing at T2** **n = 44**		
	X (SD)	X (SD)		
Age	53.38 (6.39)	54.16 (5.97)	t = −0.201	p = 0.113
	n (%)	n (%)		
Educational level				
Elementary school	11 (8.3)	4 (9.1)		
High school	108 (81.8)	36 (81.8)	χ^2 = 0.042	p = 0.979
Higher education	13 (9.9)	4 (9.1)		
Work status				
Employed	34 (25.8)	6 (13.6)		
Unemployed	16 (12.1)	10 (22.7)	χ^2 = 4.658	p = 0.097
Retired	82 (62.1)	28 (63.6)		
Marital status				
Married/cohabitating	93 (70.5)	36 (81.8)		
Single	20 (15.2)	5 (11.4)	χ^2 = 2.767	p = 0.429
Divorced	16 (12.1)	2 (4.5)		
Other	3 (2.3)	1 (2.3)		
Economic status (self-reported)				
High	2 (1.5)	0 (0)		
Medium	83 (62.9)	27 (61.4)	χ^2 = 0.762	p = 0.683
Low	47 (35.6)	17 (38.6)		
	X(SD)	X(SD)		
Treatment duration (in years)	17.8 (8.61)	15.71 (8.55)	t = 1.370	p = 0.173
Deployment duration (in months)	31.5 (19.43)	30.86 (22.73)	t = 0.164	p = 0.870
Life events (LEC-5)	10.04 (4.6)	9.44 (4.34)	t = 0.748	p = 0.455

Since the previous assessment, none of the participants changed their educational level, four (3%) relocated, and six (4.5%) had their marital status changed. In the last year, 16 (12.1%) participants had their employment status changed as 4 participants found employment, 1 lost his job, and 11 retired. Eighteen participants (13.6%) reported a change in their economic status with 16 (12.1%) reporting lower economic status and 2 (1.5%) better economic status. The majority of participants (n = 101, 76.5%) did not experience a potentially traumatic event (PTE) over the past twelve months, 28 (21.2%) reported one PTE, and 3 (2.3%) participants reported from two to six PTE in the last year (assessed by LEC).

3.2. COVID-19 Related Characteristics

Since the first assessment when only one participant had been infected, 14 (10.6%) participants were infected with SARS-CoV-2 between T1 and T2. Five participants had mild, four had moderate and four had severe COVID-19 symptoms. One participant with severe COVID-19 symptoms had been treated in the intensive care unit. Eight had wholly recovered, and six reported they had partially recovered from COVID-19. Compared to the previous year when only 2 participants had a close family member who tested positive, at the second measurement, 46 (34.8%) reported a family member or a close person with COVID-19, and 5 participants had lost a close relative due to the illness.

The majority of the participants said that they had entirely followed (n = 71, 53.8%) or mostly followed (n = 41, 31.1%) the precautionary measures introduced by the government during the past year.

The participants were asked to assess if they were affected by COVID-19-related non-PTE stressors. The most challenging COVID-19-related non-PTE stressful aspect was pandemic duration, since 99 (75%) of participants reported to be affected by it. Other stressors were pandemic uncertainty (69.7%), media coverage/exposure to pandemic (67.4%) and restriction of family gatherings (65.9%). The least frequent COVID-19-related non-PTE stressor was self-isolation (35.6%) (Figure 1). The increase in number of experienced COVID-19-related non-PTE stressors was not significantly related to the overall PTSD symptom intensity at T2 (r = 0.15, p = 0.08).

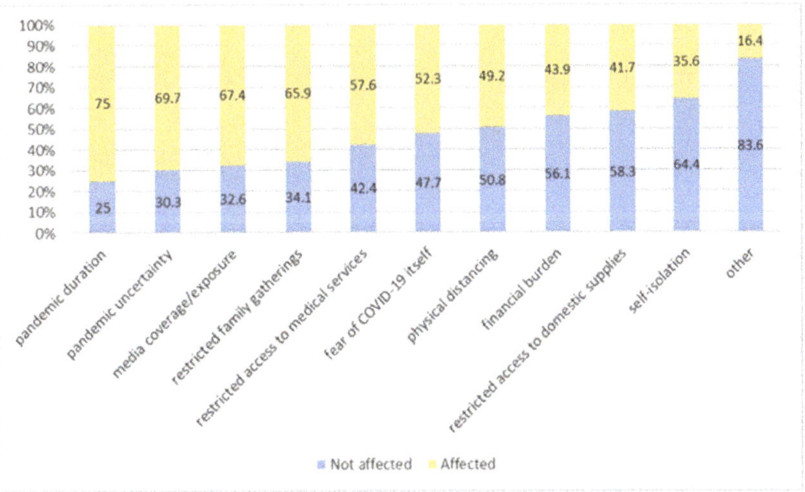

Figure 1. The proportion of the participants affected by COVID-19-related non-PTE stressors.

3.3. PTSD Symptom Severity

Most of the participants scored 33 or higher on total symptom severity, indicative of probable PTSD diagnosis (T1 83.8%, T2 80.6%). The intensity of the overall PTSD symptoms, avoidance symptoms and negative alterations in cognitions and mood was significantly lower at T2. The change in intrusion symptoms and alterations in arousal and reactivity was not statistically significant (Table 2).

The PTSD symptoms were neither significantly correlated with SARS-CoV-2 (personally or a close one's) infection nor the intensity of the COVID-19 symptoms (personally or of a close one) at T2. Of 37 participants with at least one PTE in the last year assessed by LEC, 9 experienced COVID-19-related PTE. A comparison between participants with COVID-19-related PTE (severe personal COVID-19 illness and death of a close one due to COVID-19) and participants with at least one other PTE in the last 12 months was made. The participants with COVID-19-related PTE (n = 9) did not differ in the intensity of overall PTSD symptoms at T2 compared to participants with other PTE ($n = 28$) in the last 12 months ($U = 101.5$, $p = 0.39$). In the overall sample, the number of experienced PTEs in the last year was not significantly related to overall PTSD symptom intensity ($r = 0.12$, $p = 0.19$).

Table 2. Overall PTSD symptom severity and PTSD symptom clusters severity on two measurements during the COVID-19 pandemic *.

	T1		T2			
	Range	**Mean (SD)**	**Range**	**Mean (SD)**	**t**	***p***
Cluster B symptoms (intrusion symptoms)	2–20	13.31 (4.05)	0–20	12.83 (4.60)	1.081	0.282
Cluster C symptoms (avoidance symptoms)	2–8	5.84 (1.78)	0–8	5.29 (2.24)	2.380	0.019
Cluster D symptoms (negative alterations in cognitions and mood)	1–29	16.83 (6.49)	0–32	15.45 (6.3)	1.998	0.048
Cluster E symptoms (alterations in arousal and reactivity)	2–24	13.18 (4.84)	2–24	12.41 (5.02)	1.440	0.152
PCL-5 total score	16–75	47.24 (12.87)	7–76	44.1 (14.09)	2.234	0.027

* Abbreviations: PTSD—post-traumatic stress disorder; SD—standard deviation; PCL-5—PTSD Checklist for DSM-5 (PCL-5) with Criterion A.

The overall PTSD symptoms and cluster D symptoms were significantly correlated with perceived difficulties in dealing with media coverage (overall symptoms: $r = 0.19$, $p < 0.05$; cluster D symptoms: $r = 0.23$, $p < 0.05$) and with restricted access to domestic supplies (overall symptoms: $r = 0.22$, $p < 0.05$; cluster D symptoms: $r = 0.24$, $p < 0.05$). The increase in number of experienced COVID-19-related non-PTE was not significantly related to the overall PTSD symptom intensity at T2 ($r = 0.15$, $p = 0.08$).

3.4. Coping with COVID-19-Related Issues

In general, the average scores of individual coping strategies had diminished over a year. The average means for individual coping strategies in two measurements are presented in Figure 2. Acceptance and self-distraction continued to be the most frequently used coping strategies one year into the pandemic. The participants reported a significant decrease in self-distraction ($t = 6.402$, $p < 0.001$), active coping ($t = 3.788$, $p < 0.001$), denial ($t = 2.825$, $p = 0.005$), emotional support ($t = 5.368$, $p < 0.001$), venting ($t = 3.489$, $p = 0.001$), positive reframing ($t = 3.821$, $p < 0.001$), planning ($t = 2.815$, $p = 0.006$), and religion ($t = 2.55$, $p = 0.012$).

In an alternative way of grouping coping strategies, in the second measurement, veterans scored higher on emotion-focused coping (Mean = 4.07, SD = 1.01) and problem-focused coping (Mean = 3.71, SD = 1.57) than on dysfunctional coping (Mean = 3.13, SD = 0.96). Compared to the first measurement, there was a significant decrease in all three types of coping (emotion-focused coping: $t = 4.72$, $p < 0.001$; problem-focused $t = 3.589$, $p < 0.001$; dysfunctional coping: $t = 3.45$, $p < 0.001$) (Table 3).

Table 3. Average scores for alternative grouping of the coping strategies on two measurements during the COVID-19 pandemic.

	T1	T2		
	Mean (SD)	**Mean (SD)**	**t**	***p***
Emotion focused	4.64 (1.06)	4.07 (1.01)	4.718	<0.001
Problem focused	4.31 (1.40)	3.71 (1.57)	3.589	<0.001
Dysfunctional	3.51 (0.87)	3.13 (0.96)	3.447	<0.001

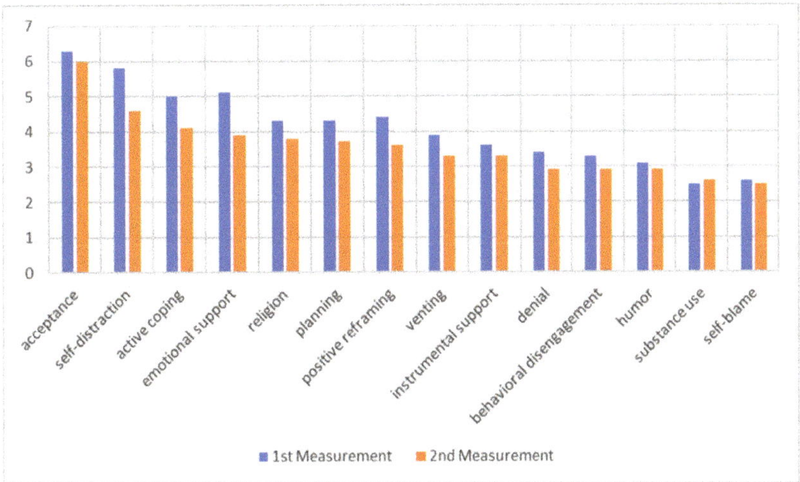

Figure 2. The average scores on individual coping strategies (the Brief COPE) in overall sample (range of 0–8).

4. Discussion

The aim of this study was to compare PTSD symptom levels and examine coping strategies at the onset and one year after the onset of the COVID-19 pandemic among treatment-seeking male veterans with pre-existing PTSD. The main finding was that the intensity of the overall PTSD symptoms (T1= 47.28, SD = 12.81; T2= 43.82, SD = 14.46; $p = 0.016$), avoidance symptoms and negative alterations in cognitions and mood decreased despite the greater exposure to COVID-19-related PTEs and the twelve-month longer exposure to COVID-19-related non-PTE stressors. The findings suggested that veterans with PTSD receiving a long-term treatment experienced COVID-19 stressors without the effects of retraumatization and a consequent worsening of PTSD symptoms. Stressful experiences to which the participants were exposed during the lockdown differ from the initial traumatic war-related stressors. Therefore, they had a lower potential for retraumatization (i.e., PTSD exacerbation after experiencing a new traumatic event). War-related stressors are central in the personal life experience of the participants and are the most substantial factors associated with PTSD [27–29]. The stressful experiences related to the COVID-19 pandemic appeared to be far from the central negative event to the participants' life and identity. The findings of this study are consistent with emerging results regarding the mental health of veteran populations during the pandemic. In a nationally representative sample of US military veterans, the prevalence of major depressive disorder and PTSD positive screens remained stable while the prevalence of generalized anxiety disorder positive screens increased [10] and the rate of suicidal ideation decreased nearly 10 months into the pandemic [9]. Regarding the mental health among treatment-seeking veterans with pre-existing mental health difficulties, the UK study revealed no significant changes in symptoms of PTSD during the pandemic [11] and a study conducted in Croatia revealed a decrease in PTSD symptoms during the onset of the pandemic as compared to the measurement a year before [12]. PTSD symptoms and particularly avoidance symptoms may have reduced because of the restrictive measures that prevented greater extent of exposure to reminders of trauma in everyday life. Adherence to treatment, regularity of appointments, and stability of treatment as all participants continued to be treated as usual (TAU) may also be viewed as a functional coping strategy that prevented considerable risk of worsening PTSD symptoms [12]. The results emphasize the importance of treatment engagement of veterans who meet criteria for mental disorder, since approximately 60% of them do not seek help because of concerns about stigma, with many expecting to face prejudice and discrimination [30]. Appropriate treatment options during the COVID-19 pandemic to prevent, treat, and mitigate the effects of COVID-19 are likely to promote mental health and prevent its deterioration [5].

PTSD symptoms were neither significantly correlated with exposure to the COVID-19-related PTEs nor were they significantly correlated with the number of experienced PTEs between the two pandemic timepoints. Regarding COVID-19-related non-PTEs in general, the higher number of experienced stressors was not significantly related to the overall PTSD symptom intensity at the second measurement ($r = 0.15$, $p = 0.08$). Recent research on the correlation between pandemic-related stressors and mental health problems in the general population revealed higher levels of symptoms of adjustment disorder in those with a variety of COVID-19-related stressors [31]. Among veterans with an increased level of mental health suffering, different COVID-related stressors appeared to be the strongest risk factors for increased suicidality [9], increased distress [10], common mental disorders, and hazardous drinking [32]. In treatment-seeking veterans, those who reported more COVID-related stressors and lower levels of social support may have been particularly vulnerable to an increasing severity of a range of mental health difficulties [11,33]. The results of this study indicating no correlation of PTSD symptom level with COVID-related PTE and non-PTE can be explained by a lower potential of COVID-related stressful experiences worsening PTSD symptoms because they differ from the central negative traumatic events (war-related criterion A) [12,29]. As the veteran cohort in this study was aged 54 (SD = 5.97), the results could be explained in light of the recent findings indicating that older adults may be more resilient and less affected by the mental health effects of the pandemic than younger age groups [3].

The veterans used coping strategies to a lesser extent one year after than during the onset of the pandemic, which points to a certain level of adjustment to "the new normal" circumstances. Moreover, they used emotion-focused and problem-focused strategies, which prevented worsening of their PTSD symptoms and enabled better adjustment to the pandemic circumstances. Current literature suggests that certain coping strategies, such as avoidance coping, are associated with a greater PTSD severity [34,35] and others, such as problem- or emotion-focused coping strategies without the aid of social support, are protective and associated with lower levels of PTSD [36]. These findings are in line with recent reports from Canada, where veterans reported predominantly adaptive coping strategies in dealing with COVID-related stressors and dysfunctional strategies such as increased alcohol intake the least [37]. US veterans reported greater appreciation of life, closer interpersonal relationships, and an increased sense of personal strength due to coping with COVID-related stressors [8]. Most of the participants ($n = 111$, 84.8%) followed the protective measures introduced by the government during the pandemic. Compliance with the measures may be viewed as an adaptive coping strategy of acceptance. A possible explanation for compliance with the measures may be returning to "combat mode" and military subordination [12].

Despite the decreased intensity between the two measurements, the PTSD symptoms and symptoms of negative alterations in cognitions and mood were significantly correlated with perceived difficulties in dealing with media coverage (overall symptoms: $r = 0.19$, $p < 0.05$; negative alterations in cognitions and mood: $r = 0.19$, $p < 0.05$) and with restricted access to domestic supplies (overall symptoms: $r = 0.22$, $p < 0.05$; negative alterations in cognitions and mood $r = 0.22$, $p < 0.05$). It has been repeatedly emphasized after the exploration of the psychological, social, and neuroscientific effects of COVID-19 that one of the immediate mental health priorities is to establish longer-term strategies for mental health since intensive media consumption may amplify distress and anxiety, and optimal patterns of consumption may enhance wellbeing [38,39]. In research carried out on the general population, both participants who had been directly exposed to COVID-19 and participants who had been indirectly exposed to COVID-19 (e.g., via media) experienced PTSD-like symptoms [40], which points to a recommendation of minimizing COVID-related media consumption.

The current findings should be considered within the context of several limitations. The sample size was relatively small, which increases the risk of type II errors. The present findings may not be generalized to the wider population of treatment-seeking veterans with PTSD as the context of traumatization and the context of the pandemic were related to Croatia. Therefore, further research is needed to evaluate the generalizability of the current findings to female, younger or more diverse veteran samples.

Author Contributions: Conceptualization, M.L.-C.; methodology, M.L.-C., A.S., D.P., I.V. and T.F.; software, A.S.; validation, M.L.-C. and A.S.; formal analysis, A.S.; investigation, M.L.-C., A.S., I.V. and D.P.; resources, M.L.-C.; data curation, M.L.-C., A.S., I.V. and D.P.; writing—original draft preparation, M.L.-C. and A.S.; writing—review and editing, M.L.-C., A.S., D.P. and T.F.; visualization, M.L.-C. and A.S.; project administration, M.L.-C. and A.S. All authors have read and agreed to the published version of the manuscript.

Funding: This research was funded in part by the University of Rijeka, grant number uniri-pr-biomed-19-3.

Institutional Review Board Statement: The study was conducted in accordance with the Declaration of Helsinki, and approved by the Ethics Committee of Clinical Hospital Center Rijeka (003-05/20-1/85; 12 June 2020).

Informed Consent Statement: Informed consent was obtained from all subjects involved in the study.

Data Availability Statement: The data that support the findings of this study are available on doi: 10.5281/zenodo.5801404.

Acknowledgments: The authors would like to thank the participants of the study, without whom this research could not have been undertaken. The authors would also like to thank their colleagues Marica Čargonja, Karlo Damiš, Vlatka Fanjkutić, Irena Jedriško, Paola Jovanović, Ingrid Modrčin, Ivana Popović, and Ornela Šebelić for their cooperation and support.

Conflicts of Interest: The authors declare no conflict of interest.

References

1. Gersons, B.P.R.; Smid, G.E.; Smit, A.S.; Kazlauskas, E.; McFarlane, A. Can a 'second disaster' during and after the COVID-19 pandemic be mitigated? *Eur. J. Psychotraumatol.* **2020**, *11*, 1815283. [CrossRef] [PubMed]
2. Krishnamoorthy, Y.; Nagarajan, R.; Saya, G.K.; Menon, V. Prevalence of psychological morbidities among general population, healthcare workers and COVID-19 patients amidst the COVID-19 pandemic: A systematic review and meta-analysis. *Psychiatry Res.* **2020**, *293*, 113382. [CrossRef] [PubMed]
3. COVID-19 Mental Disorders Collaborators. Global prevalence and burden of depressive and anxiety disorders in 204 countries and territories in 2020 due to the COVID-19 pandemic. *Lancet* **2021**, *398*, 1700–1712. [CrossRef]
4. Emodi-Perlman, A.; Eli, I.; Uziel, N.; Smardz, J.; Khehra, A.; Gilon, E.; Wieckiewicz, G.; Levin, L.; Wieckiewicz, M. Public Concerns during the COVID-19 Lockdown: A Multicultural Cross-Sectional Study among Internet Survey Respondents in Three Countries. *J. Clin. Med.* **2021**, *10*, 1577. [CrossRef]
5. Campion, J.; Javed, A.; Sartorius, N.; Marmot, M. Addressing the public mental health challenge of COVID-19. *Lancet* **2020**, *7*, 657–659. [CrossRef]
6. Holman, E.A.; Thompson, R.R.; Garfin, D.R.; Silver, R.C. The unfolding COVID-19 pandemic: A probability-based, nationally representative study of mental health in the United States. *Sci. Adv.* **2020**, *6*, eabd5390. [CrossRef]
7. Daly, M.; Robinson, E. Psychological distress and adaptation to the COVID-19 crisis in the United States. *J. Psychiatr. Res.* **2021**, *136*, 603–609. [CrossRef]
8. Pietrzak, R.H.; Tsai, J.; Southwick, S.M. Association of symptoms of posttraumatic stress disorder with posttraumatic psychological growth among US veterans during the COVID-19 pandemic. *JAMA* **2021**, *4*, e214972. [CrossRef]
9. Nichter, B.; Hill, M.L.; Na, P.J.; Kline, A.C.; Norman, S.B.; Krystal, J.H.; Southwick, S.M.; Pietrzak, R.H. Prevalence and trends in suicidal behavior among US Military veterans during the COVID-19 pandemic. *JAMA* **2021**, *78*, 1218–1227. [CrossRef]
10. Hill, M.L.; Nichter, B.; Na, P.J.; Norman, S.B.; Morland, L.A.; Krystal, J.H.; Pietrzak, R.H. Mental health impact of the COVID-19 pandemic in U.S. military veterans: A population-based, prospective cohort study. *Psychol. Med.* **2021**, 1–12. [CrossRef]
11. Hendrikx, L.J.; Williamson, C.; Baumann, J.; Murphy, D. The impact of the COVID-19 pandemic on treatment-seeking veterans in the United Kingdom with preexisting mental health difficulties: A longitudinal study. *J. Trauma. Stress* **2022**, *35*, 330–337. [CrossRef] [PubMed]

12. Letica-Crepulja, M.; Stevanović, A.; Grković, J.; Rončević-Gržeta, I.; Jovanović, N.; Frančišković, T. Posttraumatic stress disorder symptoms and coping with the lockdown among help-seeking veterans before and during the COVID-19 pandemic. *Croat. Med. J.* **2021**, *62*, 241–249. [CrossRef] [PubMed]
13. Nemeroff, C.B.; Bremner, J.D.; Foa, E.B.; Mayberg, H.S.; North, C.S.; Stein, M.B. Posttraumatic stress disorder: A state-of-the-science review. *J. Psychiatr. Res.* **2006**, *40*, 1–21. [CrossRef] [PubMed]
14. Badour, C.L.; Blonigen, D.M.; Boden, M.T.; Feldner, M.T.; Bonn-Miller, M.O. A longitudinal test of the bi-directional relations between avoidance coping and PTSD severity during and after PTSD treatment. *Behav. Res. Ther.* **2012**, *50*, 610–616. [CrossRef] [PubMed]
15. Rice, V.J.; Boykin, G.; Jeter, A.; Villarreal, J. How do I handle my life now? Coping and the post traumatic stress disorder checklist—Military version. *Proc. Hum. Factors Ergon. Soc. Annu. Meet.* **2014**, *58*, 1252–1256. [CrossRef]
16. Croatian Institute of Public Health. Indicators of Health Status and Use of Health Care of Croatian Veterans of the Homeland War—The State of 2020 [Translated Title]. Croatian Institute of Public Health. 2021. Available online: https://www.hzjz.hr/wp-content/uploads/2021/09/Branitelji_2020.pdf (accessed on 4 April 2021).
17. Letica-Crepulja, M.; Stevanović, A.; Protuđer, M.; Grahovac Juretić, T.; Rebić, J.; Frančišković, T. Complex PTSD among treatment-seeking veterans with PTSD. *Eur. J. Psychotraumatol.* **2020**, *11*, 1716593. [CrossRef]
18. Weathers, F.W.; Litz, B.T.; Keane, T.M.; Palmieri, P.A.; Marx, B.P.; Schnurr, P.P. The PTSD Checklist for DSM-5 (PCL-5). National Center for PTSD. Available online: www.ptsd.va.gov (accessed on 15 March 2020).
19. Gray, M.J.; Litz, B.T.; Hsu, J.L.; Lombardo, T.W. Psychometric properties of the life events checklist. *Assessment* **2004**, *11*, 330–341. [CrossRef]
20. Blevins, C.A.; Weathers, F.W.; Davis, M.T.; Witte, T.K.; Domino, J.L. The Posttraumatic Stress Disorder Checklist for DSM-5 (PCL-5): Development and initial psychometric evaluation. *J. Trauma. Stress* **2015**, *28*, 489–498. [CrossRef]
21. Bovin, M.J.; Marx, B.P.; Weathers, F.W.; Gallagher, M.W.; Rodriguez, P.; Schnurr, P.P.; Keane, T.M. Psychometric properties of the PTSD Checklist for Diagnostic and Statistical Manual of Mental Disorders-Fifth Edition (PCL-5) in veterans. *Psychol. Assess.* **2016**, *28*, 1379–1391. [CrossRef]
22. Sveen, J.; Bondjers, K.; Willebrand, M. Psychometric properties of the PTSD checklist for DSM-5: A pilot study. *Eur. J. Psychotraumatol.* **2016**, *7*, 30165. [CrossRef]
23. Wortmann, J.H.; Jordan, A.H.; Weathers, F.W.; Resick, P.A.; Dondanville, K.A.; Hall-Clark, B.; Foa, E.B.; Young-McCaughan, S.; Yarvis, J.S.; Hembree, E.A.; et al. Psychometric analysis of the PTSD Checklist-5 (PCL-5) among treatment-seeking military service members. *Psychol. Assess.* **2016**, *28*, 1392–1403. [CrossRef]
24. Carver, C.S. You want to measure coping but your protocol's too long: Consider the brief COPE. *Int. J. Behav. Med.* **1997**, *4*, 92–100. [CrossRef] [PubMed]
25. Carver, C.S.; Scheier, M.F.; Weintraub, J.K. Assessing coping strategies: A theoretically based approach. *J. Appl. Soc. Psychol.* **1989**, *56*, 267–283. [CrossRef]
26. Margetić, B.; Peraica, T.; Stojanović, K.; Ivanec, D. Predictors of emotional distress during the COVID-19 pandemic; a Croatian study. *Pers. Individ. Differ.* **2021**, *175*, 10691. [CrossRef]
27. Schock, K.; Böttche, M.; Rosner, R.; Wenk-Ansohn, M.; Knaevelsrud, C. Impact of new traumatic or stressful life events on pre-existing PTSD in traumatized refugees: Results of a longitudinal study. *Eur. J. Psychotraumatol.* **2016**, *9*, 32106. [CrossRef] [PubMed]
28. Rubin, D.C.; Boals, A.; Hoyle, R.H. Narrative centrality and negative affectivity: Independent and interactive contributors to stress reactions. *J. Exp. Psychol. Gen.* **2014**, *143*, 1159–1170. [CrossRef] [PubMed]
29. Boals, A.; Ruggero, C. Event centrality prospectively predicts PTSD symptoms. *Anxiety Stress Coping* **2016**, *29*, 533–541. [CrossRef]
30. Amsalem, D.; Lazarov, A.; Markowitz, J.C.; Gorman, D.; Dixon, L.B.; Neria, Y. Increasing treatment-seeking intentions of US veterans in the COVID-19 era: A randomized controlled trial. *Depress. Anxiety* **2021**, *38*, 639–647. [CrossRef]
31. Lotzin, A.; Krause, L.; Acquarini, E.; Ajdukovic, D.; Ardino, V.; Arnberg, F.; Böttche, M.; Bragesjö, M.; Dragan, M.; Figueiredo-Braga, M.; et al. Risk and protective factors, stressors, and symptoms of adjustment disorder during the COVID-19 pandemic: First results of the ESTSS COVID-19 pan-European ADJUST study. *Eur. J. Psychotraumatol.* **2021**, *12*, 1964197. [CrossRef]
32. Sharp, M.L.; Serfioti, D.; Jones, M.; Burdett, H.; Pernet, D.; Hull, L.; Murphy, D.; Wessely, S.; Fear, N.T. UK veterans' mental health and well-being before and during the COVID-19 pandemic: A longitudinal cohort study. *Brit. Med. J.* **2021**, *11*, e049815. [CrossRef]
33. Murphy, D.; Williamson, C.; Baumann, J.; Busuttil, W.; Fear, N.T. Exploring the impact of COVID-19 and restrictions to daily living as a result of social distancing within veterans with pre-existing mental health difficulties. *Brit. Med. J. Mil. Health* **2020**, *168*, 29–33. [CrossRef] [PubMed]
34. Clohessy, S.; Ehlers, A. PTSD symptoms, response to intrusive memories and coping in ambulance service workers. *Br. J. Clin. Psychol.* **1999**, *8*, 251–265. [CrossRef] [PubMed]
35. Hooberman, J.; Rosenfeld, B.; Rasmussen, A.; Keller, A. Resilience in trauma exposed refugees: The moderating effect of coping style on resilience variables. *Am. J. Orthopsychiatry* **2010**, *80*, 557–563. [CrossRef] [PubMed]
36. Linley, P.A.; Joseph, S. Positive change following trauma and adversity: A review. *J. Trauma. Stress* **2004**, *17*, 11–21. [CrossRef] [PubMed]

37. Mahar, A.; Reppas-Rindlisbacher, C.; Edgelow, M.; Siddhpuria, S.; Hallet, J.; Rochon, P.A.; Cramm, H. Concerns and coping strategies of older adult veterans in Canada at the outset of the COVID-19 pandemic. *J. Mil. Veteran Fam. Health* **2021**, *7*, e20210712. [CrossRef]
38. Holmes, E.A.; O'Connor, R.C.; Perry, V.H.; Tracey, I.; Wessely, S.; Arseneault, L.; Ballard, C.; Christensen, H.; Cohen Silver, R.; Everall, I.; et al. Multidisciplinary research priorities for the COVID-19 pandemic: A call for action for mental health science. *Lancet Psychiatry* **2020**, *7*, 547–560. [CrossRef]
39. Khubchandani, J.; Wiblishauser, M.J.; Price, J.H.; Webb, F.J. COVID-19 related information and psychological distress: Too much or too bad? *Brain Behav. Immun.* **2021**, *12*, 100213. [CrossRef]
40. Bridgland, V.M.E.; Moeck, E.K.; Green, D.M.; Swain, T.L.; Nayda, D.M.; Matson, L.A.; Hutchison, N.P.; Takarangi, M. Why the COVID-19 pandemic is a traumatic stressor. *PLoS ONE* **2021**, *16*, e0240146. [CrossRef]

Journal of
Clinical Medicine

Article

Adverse Mental Health Sequelae of COVID-19 Pandemic in the Pregnant Population and Useful Implications for Clinical Practice

Dariusz Wojciech Mazurkiewicz [1,*], Jolanta Strzelecka [2] and Dorota Izabela Piechocka [3]

1 St. Mark's Place Institute for Mental Health, 57 St. Mark's Place, New York, NY 10003, USA
2 Department of Neurology and Pediatrics, Medical University of Warsaw, Żwirki and Wigury 61 Street, 02-091 Warsaw, Poland; jolanta.strzelecka@wum.edu.pl
3 Department of Gynecology and Practical Obstetrics, Medical University of Bialystok, Szpitalna 37 Street, 15-295 Bialystok, Poland; dorota.piechocka@umb.edu.pl
* Correspondence: dwmazurkiewicz@aol.com

Abstract: The COVID-19 pandemic has increased risk of disturbances in the functioning of everyday life, directly or indirectly has influenced the risk of mental disorders in the most vulnerable populations, including pregnant women. The aim of this study was to analyze adverse mental health effects in the pregnant population during the COVID-19 pandemic, investigate risk factors for adverse mental health outcomes, identify protective factors, and create practical implications for clinical practice, bearing in mind the need to improve perinatal mental healthcare during such pandemics. Qualitative research was conducted in the electronic databases PubMed and Web of Sciences for the keywords COVID-19, pregnancy, depression, anxiety, and telemedicine for relevant critical articles (n = 3280) published from 2020 until October 2021, outlining the outcomes of control studies, meta-analysis, cross-sectional studies, face-to-face evaluation survey studies, remotely administered survey studies, and observational studies regarding the main topic; all were evaluated. Mental health problems among pregnant women linked to the COVID-19 pandemic, in most cases, show symptoms of depression, anxiety, insomnia, and PTSD and may cause adverse outcomes in pregnancy and fetus and newborn development, even at later stages of life. Therefore, useful implications for clinical practice for improving the adverse mental health outcomes of pregnant women associated with the COVID-19 pandemic are highly desirable. Our research findings support and advocate the need to modify the scope of healthcare provider practice in the event of a disaster, including the COVID-19 pandemic, and may be implemented and adopted by healthcare providers as useful implications for clinical practice.

Keywords: COVID-19; psychological distress; anxiety; depression; pregnancy; disaster; telemedicine; theory–practice gap; stress; trauma

Citation: Mazurkiewicz, D.W.; Strzelecka, J.; Piechocka, D.I. Adverse Mental Health Sequelae of COVID-19 Pandemic in the Pregnant Population and Useful Implications for Clinical Practice. *J. Clin. Med.* **2022**, *11*, 2072. https://doi.org/10.3390/jcm11082072

Academic Editor: Alfonso Troisi

Received: 9 February 2022
Accepted: 3 April 2022
Published: 7 April 2022

1. Introduction

The COVID-19 pandemic, as a public health emergency of international concern, constitutes a challenge to psychological resilience [1], heavily impacting global mental health [2] by causing acute respiratory coronavirus 2 (SARS-CoV-2) [3], with a rapid increase in the number of cases and deaths since its first identification in Wuhan, China, in December 2019 [4]. The vulnerable population of women who became mothers during the COVID-19 emergency appear to be at high risk for developing mental health problems [5]. Respiratory fluid droplets containing the SARS-CoV-2 virus may spread from person to person—in some cases, through contact with an infected surface when the person touches their eyes, nose, or mouth—and the average SARS-CoV-2 incubation period is 3–7 days [6]. The symptoms of COVID-19 thus may or may not be observed, and this disease can be confirmed by laboratory test results. Pregnant women may suffer from asymptomatic

COVID-19 and an increased leukocyte count, raised lymphopenia, and higher C-reactive protein (CRP) levels, requiring extracorporeal membranous oxygenation (ECMO) and invasive ventilation more than nonpregnant women do [7]. The risk factors of severe COVID-19 in pregnancy are directly linked to preexisting diabetes, chronic hypertension, pre-eclampsia, and high body mass index (BMI); in the long term, outcomes such as higher risk of preterm birth (PTB) and/or pre-eclampsia may occur in pregnant women who have suffered from COVID-19 [8]. The risk of vertical SARS-CoV-2 infection in pregnancy, and its related fetal growth restriction, miscarriage, and preterm births are still quite unclear and under deliberation [9], and neonates born to mothers infected with SARS-CoV-2 have an overall favorable prognosis [6]. However, there is a clear link between poor mental health in pregnant women and pregnancy complications [10]. Mental health problems have been observed and reported to increase in the pregnant population in general, including an increase in the incidence of depression, antenatal, postpartum depression, and anxiety, all associated with adverse effects on intrauterine growth, birth weight, prematurity, behavioral, and/or mood in offspring, increasing the risk of depression during adolescence and adulthood, and linked to perinatal suicides and maternal mortality in the first 12 months after delivery [11–13]. The COVID-19 pandemic changed people's health behavior and sparked a psychological response reaction in society [14], especially in the pregnant population, currently suffering from an overall increased severity of anxiety [15] and an increased incidence of anxiety and depression [16]. There has been a noted sensitivity to social risks, an increase in negative emotions linked to anxiety and depression, indignation, and a decrease in positive emotions and life satisfaction after the declaration of COVID-19 in China related to the general human population [17].

The aim of this study was to analyze adverse mental health effects in the pregnant population during the COVID-19 pandemic, investigate risk factors for adverse mental health outcomes, identify protective factors, and create practical implications of mental health prophylaxis for clinical practice, bearing in mind the need to increase efforts in perinatal mental healthcare during such a pandemic.

2. Materials and Methods

A systematic scoping review [18] was conducted in electronic databases PubMed and Web of Sciences for keywords COVID-19, pregnancy, depression, anxiety, telemedicine for relevant critical articles (n = 3280) published from 2020 until October 2021 outlining the outcomes of control studies, meta-analysis, cross-sectional studies, face-to-face evaluation survey studies, remotely administered survey studies, and observational studies regarding the main topic, which were then evaluated. The equator checklist document used in this systematic scoping review was PRISMA Extension for Scoping Reviews [19] to analyze the presence of adverse mental health symptoms in pregnant women linked to the COVID-19 pandemic in domains as follows: social and medical consequences of COVID-19, psychological factors responsible for adverse COVID-19 mental health outcomes in pregnant women, the determination of COVID-19 mental health problems, including symptoms and diagnosis among pregnant women in different countries of the world, the influence of COVID-19 on psychological and medical factors related to adverse pregnancy and offspring development outcomes, and dilemmas and hopes in ways to improve the provision of services to pregnant women during disasters, including the COVID-19 pandemic.

2.1. Literature Search and Study Selection

A search was conducted on the PubMed and Web of Science databases. The search strategy included keywords linked to coronavirus, psychological symptoms, depression, and pregnancy. MESH terms (e.g., "pregnancy" (Mesh) AND "coronavirus" (Mesh) AND ("depression" (Mesh) OR "depressive disorder" (Mesh) OR "anxiety" (Mesh) OR "telemedicine" (Mesh) and text word search terms ("pregnancy" AND "coronavirus" AND ("mental health" OR "depression" OR "anxiety" OR "telemedicine") were used.

2.2. Inclusion and Exclusion Criteria

The inclusion criteria were as follows: (1) any study including outcomes of control studies, meta-analysis, cross-sectional studies, face-to-face evaluation survey studies, remotely administered survey studies, and observational studies that recruited pregnant women with adverse mental health outcomes that resulted from the pregnant women's experience with, exposure to, or infection with COVID-19; (2) studies written in English; (3) articles published from 2020 until October 2021; and (4) any original paper appearing in a peer-reviewed journal.

2.3. Data Collection

Two researchers used a multistep approach to select eligible studies. In total, 3280 publications were retrieved in our study; duplicates, publications, upon title and abstract review, not meeting the research criteria, publications not linked to the research topic, or those not meeting the inclusion criteria after full-text evaluation were removed. In the case of disagreement among researchers, it was resolved during a consensus session with a third researcher. After a full-text review, 16 articles met the inclusion criteria. Figure 1 represents the PRISMA flow diagram summarizing the screening process.

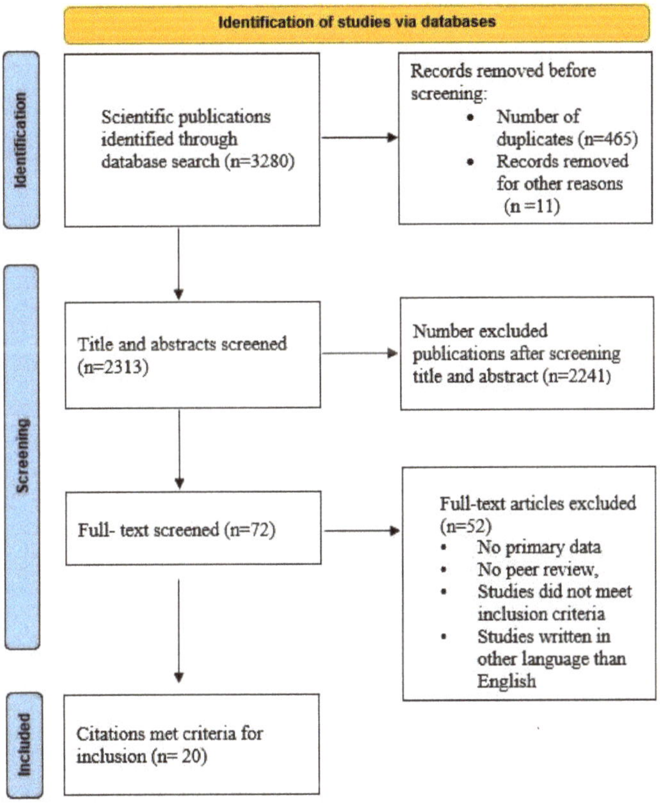

Figure 1. PRISMA flow diagram of the screening process.

2.4. Data Extraction and Investigated Variables

Two researchers independently extracted the following data: the aim of the study, country of the study, sample size, study design and assessment tool, and summary of study benefits and limitations. The publications strictly focused on the adverse mental health outcomes of the COVID-19 pandemic in pregnant women population, and research topic publications that met the criteria for inclusion were linked. Data were processed independently by two researchers and are summarized in Table 1.

Table 1. Qualitative synthesis findings.

Aim of Study	Country	Sample Size	Study Design and Assessment Tool	Study Summary Benefits	Limitations	Study Quality
Prevalence of psychiatric symptoms of pregnant and non-pregnant women during the COVID-19 epidemic (Zhou et al., 2020) [20]	China	N = 544 pregnant; *n* = 315 nonpregnant.	Cross-sectional study: used social media application; online patient health questionnaire (PHQ-9); generalized anxiety disorder scale (GAD-7); somatization subscale of the symptom checklist 90 (SCL-90); insomnia severity index (ISI); post-traumatic stress disorder checklist-5 (PCL-5).	Pregnant women have an advantage of facing mental problems caused by COVID-19, showing fewer depression, anxiety, insomnia, and PTSD symptoms than nonpregnant women do.	Lacks longitudinal follow-up, limiting the generalization of findings to other regions; No data on psychological interventions for pregnant women.	8/10
Vulnerability and resilience to pandemic-related stress among U.S. woman pregnant at the start of the COVID-19 pandemic (Preis et al., 2020.a.) [21]	U.S.	N = 4451	Cross-sectional study: secure online software survey Questionnaire. The Pandemic-Related Pregnancy Stress Scale (PREPS).	Two major pandemic-related stress domains for pregnant women in Poland, the U.S., Germany, Israel: fears of perinatal COVID-19 infection, and being unprepared for birth.	Excluded women without access to the Internet and social media.	7/10
Risk factors for anxiety and depression among pregnant women during the COVID-19 pandemic: web-based cross-sectional survey (Kajdy et al., 2020) [22]	Poland	N = 500	Web-based cross-sectional survey: GAD-7; PHQ-9. Available in 15 languages.	Pregnant women are worried about the COVID-19 pandemic and have difficulty in accessing professional medical help; feel insecure about exposure risk to the coronavirus when accessing medical facilities; infection of the infant in the peripartum period; financial problems lead to conflict in the family; a single mother may be more prone to anxiety isolation, fear of being trapped and rumors spreading on social media, growing anxiety and social panic; fear of blame, guilt and stigmatization related to being infected with COVID-19.	Survey may reach more women of a higher socioeconomic status and from larger agglomerations.	9/10
Pandemic-related pregnancy stress and anxiety among women pregnant during the coronavirus disease 2019 pandemic. (Preis et al., 2020.b.) [23]	U.S.	N = 788	Cross-sectional study: social media to complete online questionnaire GAD-7; PREPS.	COVID-19 pandemic-related stress predicts heightened anxiety in women pregnant during this crisis: preparation for birth; worries about COVID-19 infection to self and baby.	Inclusion criteria: pregnant at the time of questionnaire completion and older than 18 years; exclusion was inability to read or write English.	8/10

Table 1. *Cont.*

Aim of Study	Country	Sample Size	Study Design and Assessment Tool	Study Summary Benefits	Limitations	Study Quality
Effects of the COVID-19 pandemic on anxiety and depressive symptoms in pregnant women: preliminary study. (Durankuş and Aksu, 2020) [24]	Turkey	N = 260 out of 318	Cross-sectional study: online questionnaire survey study EPDS-Edinburgh Postpartum Depression Scale.	Urgent need to provide psychosocial support to this population during the crisis. Adverse events may otherwise occur during pregnancy, and thus affect both mother and fetus.	Survey was administered online, thus preventing a face-to-face evaluation of participants; authors used their own created questionnaire on the pandemic, and its psychological effects were subjective.	6/10
Anxiety and depression symptoms in the same pregnant women before and during the COVID-19 pandemic (Ayaz et al., 2020) [25]	Turkey	N = 63	Cross-sectional study: Beck Anxiety Inventory (BAI) questionnaire; Depression and Anxiety Symptoms II (IDAS II) questionnaire.	Depressive and anxiety symptoms were significantly increased during the SARS-CoV-2 pandemic compared with pre-pandemic surveys. Effective screening strategies for depression and anxiety symptoms during the pandemic should be prioritized to allow for timely treatment.	Sample size, but power analysis indicated that the effect of this limitation was reduced.	3/10
Elevated depression and anxiety symptoms among pregnant individuals during the COVID-19 pandemic (Lebel et al., 2020) [26]	Canada	N = 1987 <35 weeks gestation	Cross-sectional study: Online survey of standardized measures of depression, anxiety, pregnancy-related anxiety, and social support. EPDS; PROMIS Anxiety Adult 7-item short form; social support effectiveness questionnaire (SSEQ); interpersonal support evaluation list (ISEL); Godin-Shephard Leisure-Time Exercise Questionnaire.	Elevated anxiety and depression symptoms that may have a long-term impact on offspring related to COVID-19 worries about threats to their own lives, their baby's health, not getting enough prenatal care, and social isolation.	Inclusion criteria: living in Canada, able to read and write English, and having a confirmed pregnancy <35 weeks gestation.	9/10
Psychological impact of coronavirus disease 2019 in pregnant women (Saccone et al., 2020) [27]	Italy	N = 100	Cross-sectional study: Event Scale-Revised (IES-R) questionnaire; Spielberger State-Trait Anxiety Inventory (STAI); visual analog scale (VAS).	Psychological impact and anxiety of the COVID-19 epidemic found be more severe in women who are in the first trimester of pregnancy during the outbreak; high anxiety regarding the vertical transmission of the disease was reported by almost half of the respondents.	Findings from the study were limited by the single-center study design and small sample size.	5/10
Depression, stress, anxiety, and their predictors in Iranian pregnant women during the outbreak of COVID-19 (Effati-Daryani et al., 2020) [28]	Iran	N = 205	Online descriptive–analytical cross-sectional study; Depression, Anxiety and Stress Scale 21 (DASS-21).	Promoting marital life satisfaction and socioeconomic status can play an effective role in controlling anxiety, and reducing stress and depression in pregnant women.	Those who had a mobile phone with Internet connection could participate in this study.	7/10

Table 1. *Cont.*

Aim of Study	Country	Sample Size	Study Design and Assessment Tool	Study Summary Benefits	Limitations	Study Quality
Attitudes and collateral psychological effects of COVID-19 in pregnant women in Colombia (Parra-Saavedra et al., 2020) [29]	Colombia	N = 946 out of 1021	Cross-sectional web survey.	Rate of psychological consequences of the pandemic was much larger than the number of patients clinically affected by the virus, with symptoms of anxiety, insomnia, and depression.	Excluded women without access to the Internet and social media.	8/10
Distress and anxiety associated with COVID-19 among Jewish and Arab pregnant women in Israel. (Taubman-Ben-Ari et al., 2020) [30]	Israel	N = 336 comprising 225 Jewish and 111 Arab pregnant women	Cross-sectional study: social media to complete online questionnaire. Mental Health Inventory-Short Form based on the original MHI.	COVID-19-related anxieties were quite high, especially in Arab women, with concern over the health of the fetus, public transportation and place, being infected themselves, and the delivery of the baby.	Cannot be considered representative of population of pregnant women in Israel, questionnaire only in Hebrew.	6/10
The effect of COVID-19 pandemic and social restrictions on depression rates and maternal attachment in immediate postpartum women: a preliminary study. (Oskovi-Kaplan et al. 2020) [31]	Turkey	N = 223	Cross-sectional study: EPDS and Maternal Attachment Inventory (MAI).	Positive impact on the depressive symptoms of new mothers may have providing appropriate isolation in hospitals; psychological status of pregnant and postpartum women may help in the improvement of psychosocial support.	Lack of a control group that was evaluated before the onset of pandemic and due to ongoing cases with a high incidence; a lack of any validated questionnaire for COVID-19 infection on psychological status.	7/10
Unprecedented reduction in births of very low birthweight (VLBW) and extremely low birthweight (ELBW) infants during the COVID-19 lockdown in Ireland: a 'natural experiment' allowing analysis of data from the prior two decades. (Philip et al., 2020) [32]	Ireland	N = 473,000	Descriptive cohort study: VON international benchmarking; labor ward weekly statistics for live and stillbirths; early pregnancy assessment unit (EPAU) statistics for early pregnancy loss/miscarriage information; inpatient ward statistics for early or late fetal loss during hospital admission.	100% reduction in ELBW infants was noted in one designated health region of Ireland from January to April 2020 compared with the preceding 20 years.	Retrospective nature of birth cohort data from one health region of Ireland; completion of the study prior to the official finish of lockdown; 3. ELBW cohort analyzed with the small number of births.	8/10
Danish premature birth rates during the COVID-19 lockdown. (Hedermann et al., 2020) [33]	Denmark	N = 31,180 live singleton infants	Cross-sectional study; Nationwide prevalence proportion study with premature births as cases, term pregnancies as controls, and birth during lockdown from 12 March to 14 April 2015–2020.	Lockdowns (e.g., reduced infection load and reduced physical activity) are possibly beneficial for reducing extreme prematurity and potentially reducing infant mortality; a nonsignificant but slightly increased number of very premature births.	Study summary benefits data need to be confirmed in other countries.	8/10

Table 1. *Cont.*

Aim of Study	Country	Sample Size	Study Design and Assessment Tool	Study Summary Benefits	Limitations	Study Quality
SARS-CoV-2 vertical transmission with adverse effects on the newborn revealed through integrated immunohistochemical, electron microscopy and molecular analyses of Placenta. (Facchetti et al., 2020) [34]	Italy	N = 101	Cross-sectional study; Research: comprehensive immunohistochemical and immune-fluorescence analysis: RNA-in situ hybridization and RT-PCR for S transcripts, and by electron microscopy.	First evidence for maternal–fetal transmission of SARS-CoV-2, likely propagated by circulating virus-infected fetal mononuclear cells.	No limitation reported.	9/10
Pandemic stress and its correlates among pregnant women during the second wave of COVID-19 in Poland (Ilska et al., 2021) [35]	Poland	N = 1119	Cross-sectional study design, online survey; PREPS.	38.5% of participants reported high preparedness stress; 26% reported high perinatal infection stress, pregnant women are most vulnerable to pandemic-related stress.	Excluded women who had no access to the Internet or social media.	8/10

2.5. Quality Assessment Tool

The qualitative Newcastle–Ottawa Quality Assessment Scale (NOQAS) [36] and the adapted version for cross-sectional studies to score each study (Supplementary Materials) were used. This tool on the basis of the criteria included 3 categories ("selection", "comparability", and "outcome"), with a maximal score of 9 and 10 points for cohort and cross-sectional studies, respectively. The "selection" category, which accounted for a maximum of 4 points (5 points for cross-sectional studies), the "comparability" category, which accounted for a maximum of 2 points, and "outcome," which accounted for a maximum of 3 points. The quality of each study is shown in Table 1.

3. Results

3.1. Characteristics of Included Studies

Qualitative synthesis findings were concluded on the basis of 16 articles out of 3280 researched publications. A total of sixteen studies included in the final analysis: one study was conducted in China, Canada, Iran, Colombia, Ireland, Denmark, and Israel; two studies were done in the U.S., Poland, and Italy; three studies were conducted in Turkey. These publications described research into adverse mental health outcomes that resulted from a total number of 515,803 pregnant women's experience with, exposure to, infection with COVID-19 in the following studies (Figure 2): China (N = 544) [20]; Poland, the U.S., Germany, and Israel (N = 4451) [21]; the U.S. (N = 788) [23]; Israel (N = 336) [30]; Turkey (N = 260) [24], (N = 63) [25], and (N = 223) [31]; Canada (N = 1987) [26]; Italy (N = 100) [27] and (N = 101) [34]; Iran (N = 205) [28]; Colombia (N = 946) [29]; Ireland (N = 473,000) [32]; Denmark (N = 31,180) [33]; Poland (N = 500) [22] and (N = 1119) [35].

3.2. Quality of Included Studies

A qualitative analysis was conducted with necessary reciprocal translations for interpreting the evaluation score of 16 articles out of 3280 published studies, outlining the outcomes of control studies, meta-analysis, cross-sectional studies, face-to-face evaluation survey studies, remotely administered survey studies, and observational studies regarding the main topic, which were then evaluated. Overall, 75% (12/16) of the studies evaluated using the Newcastle–Ottawa scale had an overall low risk of bias. The risk of bias for medium in three of the 16 studies (18.75%), and high in one (6.25%). Our study analyzes the presence of adverse mental health symptoms in pregnant women linked to the COVID-19 pandemic, and allows for us to divide and describe findings in five domains as follows.

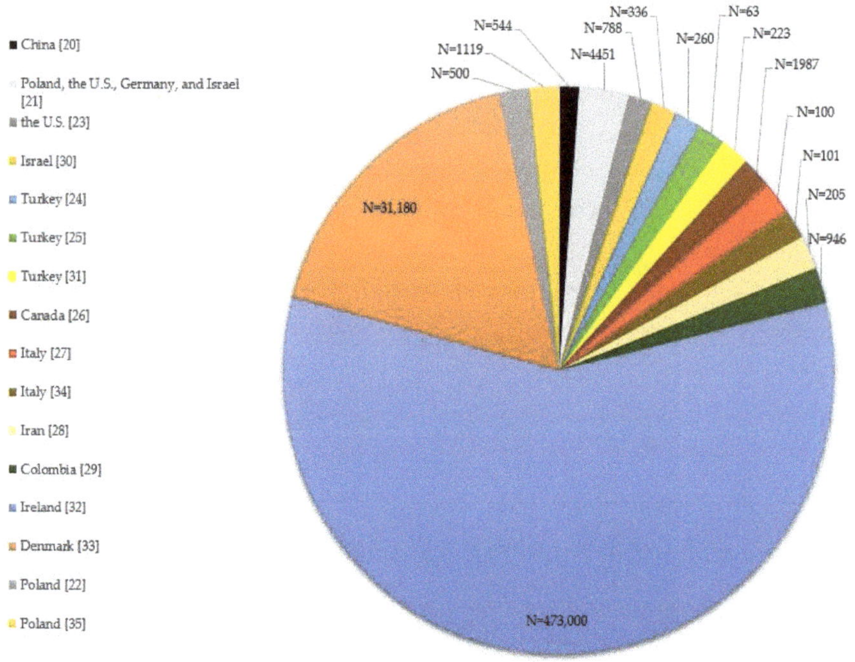

Figure 2. A total number of 515, 803 pregnant participants by the included sixteen studies.

3.3. Domain 1: Social and Medical Consequences of COVID-19 in Pregnant Women Population

Pregnant women are worried about the COVID-19 pandemic and have difficulty in accessing professional medical help; feel insecure about exposure risk to the coronavirus when accessing medical facilities; infection of the infant in the peripartum period; financial problems lead to conflict in the family; a single mother may be more prone to anxiety isolation, fear of being trapped and rumors spreading on social media, growing anxiety and social panic; and fear of blame, guilt and stigmatization related to being infected with COVID-19 [22]. A fear of infection, anger, and confusion related to financial status, ennui, inadequate information and supplies, and quarantine duration increased post-traumatic stress disorder (PTSD) symptoms and feelings of vulnerability [26,37–41], and all undeniably badly affect the emotional and mental statuses of pregnant women. Pregnant women are more likely to develop mental health problems than nonpregnant women of childbearing age are, and this was confirmed on the basis of a cross-sectional study of pregnant (n = 544) and nonpregnant (n = 315) women in Beijing, China [20]. The findings about the suppression of immune system function in pregnant women allow for us to classify the population of pregnant women into a group at high risk of SARS-CoV-2 infection [42]; on other hand, this population does not appear to be at increased risk of contracting SARS-CoV-2, since there is scientific confirmation that their rates of infection seem to parallel the rates of infection in their surrounding communities [43]. Women are more vulnerable and arguably less resistant to viral infection during the SARS-CoV-2 pandemic, as women and younger convalescent COVID-19 plasma donors are more likely to lack measurable neutralizing antibodies, while higher antibody levels were observed in men, older donors, and those who had been hospitalized [44]. Maternal risk factors associated with severe COVID-19 and admission to an intensive care unit are increasing age, high body mass, any preexisting maternal comorbidity, chronic hypertension, pre-eclampsia, preexisting diabetes, and both non-White ethnicity and high body mass index, are maternal risk factors for death and the need for invasive ventilation [8]. Unfortunately, evidence now exists for the maternal–fetal transmission of SARS-CoV-2, and N proteins were strongly expressed in the placenta of a COVID-19-positive pregnant woman whose newborn tested positive for viral RNA and developed COVID-19 pneumonia soon after birth [34]. The intrauterine transmission of SARS-CoV-2 appears to be rare, and this is possibly related to low levels of SARS-CoV-2 viremia and a decreased co-expression of ACE2 and TMPRSS2 needed for SARS-CoV-2 entry into the cells in the placenta [45]. The mode and timing of delivery should be individualized based on the severity of disease, existing comorbidities, and obstetric indications [46]. However, early cord clamping may minimize the risk of viral transmission by avoiding longer, close contact with the infected mother [46], and in turn, it may increase the mother's good feelings about the safety of the newborn.

3.4. Domain 2: Main Psychological Factors Responsible for Adverse COVID-19 Mental Health Outcomes in Pregnant Women

Scientific publications reported that it is unclear whether and how SARS-CoV-2 can be transmitted from the mother to the fetus [47] and whether vertical transmission or placental pathology might occur following maternal infection during pregnancy remains unknown [48]. Women experience elevated levels of stress related to being worried about perinatal infection [35]. Fears of perinatal COVID-19 infection (29.1% of 4451 pregnant women in the U.S.) and feeling unprepared for birth due to the COVID-19 pandemic (nearly 30% of 4451 pregnant women in the U.S.) are noted as two major pandemic-related stressor domains for pregnant women in Poland, the U.S., Germany, and Israel [13]. We are faced with a paradox, because quarantine in the COVID-19 pandemic exacerbates the stress of isolation in pregnant women when a social connection helps us to cope with stress and maintain resilience [49].

3.5. Domain 3: Determination of COVID-19 Mental Health Problems Including Symptoms and Diagnosis among Pregnant Women in Different Countries

Even though 3–5% of the general population is affected by anxiety symptoms, a severe stressor such as the COVID-19 pandemic can increase such a rate in the general population of pregnant women if the prevalence of gestational anxiety is between 15% and 23%, as confirmed by scientific data [22]. COVID-19 pandemic-related stress predicts heightened anxiety in pregnant women during this crisis [23]. A preliminary study in Turkey on the effects of the COVID-19 pandemic on anxiety and depressive symptoms in pregnant women confirmed such a fact in 35.4% of the population; the obtained scores were higher than 13 on the Edinburgh Postpartum Depression Scale (EPDS) among respondents ($n = 260$) [24]; a score of more than 10 on the EPDS suggests that minor or major depression may be present [50]. The level of anxiety and depressive symptoms in pregnant women during COVID-19 infection significantly increased before such an event, and the pandemic outbreak leads to adverse birth outcomes [25]. However, a Canadian study indicated that pregnant women did not have higher levels of depression, stress, and anxiety prior the COVID-19 outbreak when compared with the time after the outbreak outcomes [51]. A study on elevated depressive and anxiety symptoms among pregnant individuals during the COVID-19 pandemic in Canada were surveyed, and its results provided information about substantially elevated anxiety and depressive symptoms compared to those in similar pre-pandemic pregnancy cohorts, with 37% reporting clinically relevant symptoms of depression and 57% reporting clinically relevant symptoms of anxiety; it also indicated stressor concerns about not receiving the necessary prenatal care, having relationship strain and social isolation due to the COVID-19 pandemic; more physical activity was associated with lower psychological symptoms [26]. A study conducted in Naples, Italy highlighted that participants who had never had depression or anxiety in previous pregnancy rated the psychological impact of the COVID-19 outbreak as severe (over 50%), especially in the first trimester of pregnancy during the outbreak, reported higher than normal anxiety in general (66%), and high anxiety regarding the vertical transmission of the disease was reported by almost half of the respondents [27].

An online descriptive–analytical cross-sectional study during the outbreak of COVID-19 with the DASS-21 tool (Depression, Anxiety and Stress Scale 21, which includes 21 questions and three subscales of stress, depression, and anxiety, and contains seven questions for each subscale, scored from not at all (0) to very high (3) for each question with 205 pregnant women in Iran, produced mean (SD) scores of depression, stress, and anxiety of 3.91 (3.9), 6.22 (4.25), and 3.79 (3.39); where depression, stress, and anxiety symptoms were observed in 32.7%, 32.7%, and 43.9% of the participants, from a mild to very severe degree [28]. In 2020, the clinical impact, psychological effects, and knowledge of pregnant women during the COVID-19 outbreak in seven cities in Colombia were evaluated, where 49.1% of women reported suffering from insomnia [29]. In comparison with the Turkish study [24], findings show that a lower rate of depressive symptoms (25%) was reported in Colombian work [29], while the same Colombian study confirmed a similar anxiety symptom rate (50.4%) with findings by Italian scientists [27], and higher than that in Iran's study results [28]. A study on distress and anxiety among Jewish and Arab pregnant women in Israel in three domains on levels of all COVID-19-related anxieties were quite high, especially in Arab women, with concern over the health of the fetus, public transportation and place, being infected themselves, and the delivery of the baby [30]. In face-to-face evaluation surveys, EPDS and the Maternal Attachment Inventory were adopted in a study (conducted in COVID-19 pandemic referral hospital in Ankara, Turkey) and applied within 48 h after birth of the patients regarding the effect of the COVID-19 pandemic and social restrictions on depression rates and maternal attachment in immediate postpartum women; the study result highlighted that the rate of depression was twice lower in comparison with the reported findings of a preliminary study on depression and anxiety symptoms in pregnant Turkish women (35.4% rate of women had EPDS scores higher than 13) by Durankus and Aksu [24]; depressive symptoms of new mothers may have been positively impacted by appropriate isolation in hospitals for pregnant women, so the feeling of being safe and isolated may be the cause of better EPDS scores [31].

3.6. Domain 4: Influence of COVID-19 on Psychological and Medical Factors Related to Adverse Pregnancy and Offspring Development Outcomes

Influence of COVID-19 on medical factors may be linked to adverse pregnancy and offspring development outcomes. Hyperinflammation as a symptom of SARS-CoV-2 reported in pregnant women suffering from SARS-CoV-2 infection, and cytokine storms could hypothetically adversely increase the risk for neurodevelopmental disorders in the neonates [3]. In cases of acute respiratory syndrome coronavirus (SARS-CoV) and MERS-CoV, high incidences of spontaneous miscarriage, preterm birth, and neonatal death have been reported [52,53]. However, a study was performed in China on the effects of SARS-CoV-2 infection during pregnancy (n = 35) versus nonpregnant patients, and its findings on the clinical symptoms of COVID-19 in pregnant women were misleading and atypical (compared with those in 31 nonpregnant patients), with a significantly lower proportion of fever (54.8% vs. 87.5%, $p = 0.006$), a shorter average interval from onset to hospitalization, and a higher proportion of severe or critical COVID-19 (32.3% vs. 11.4%, $p = 0.039$) [54].

The influence of COVID-19 on psychological factors may be related to adverse pregnancy and offspring development outcomes, too. There is a clear link between poor mental health in pregnant women and pregnancy complications [10]. The exposure of pregnant women to psychological distress, even linked with depression and stress in general or anxiety, is a risk factor of schizophrenia spectrum disorders, autism spectrum disorder (ASD), antisocial behavior, and attention deficit hyperactivity disorder (ADHD) [55,56]; thus, the psychological stress of the COVID-19 pandemic during pregnancy can increase the risk of neurodevelopmental disorders in offspring [57], and the risk preterm delivery, low birth weight, and postnatal complications [58]. The COVID-19 lockdown may have adverse birth weight outcomes. An unprecedented reduction in births of very low birth weights (VLBW) and extremely low birth weights (ELBW) infants was reported in the general population during the COVID-19 lockdown in Ireland [32] and Denmark [33].

3.7. Domain 5: Dilemmas and Hopes in Ways to Improve the Provision of Services to Pregnant Women during Disasters, Including the COVID-19 Pandemic

Providing support and care in psychopsychiatric services for pregnant women is a priority. It may be difficult during the COVID-19 pandemic if a mental health provider system is lacking and healthcare professionals are not trained in the field of mental health, as was confirmed in the case of Kashmir, India [59]. In survey research conducted in Belgium, only 38.2% of women received, and 61.8% of respondents did not receive, medical help from their obstetrician because of the COVID-19 pandemic [60]. The scope of psychological and psychiatric services for pregnant women is also changing in favor of telemedicine [23] to have remote access to a psychiatrist and provide psychological therapy for pregnant women and even continue such service after the delivery of a baby. This option is recommended, especially during the COVID-19 pandemic, by the American College of Obstetricians and Gynecologists (ACOG) and the Society for Maternal and Fetal Medicine (SMFM) [61,62]. Research conducted in Poland demonstrated that 47.41% of women had at least one telehealth appointment during their pregnancy, which is a much higher percentage rate than 31.8% of telehealth appointments in New York during the COVID-19 pandemic [63]. The same study concluded that it is preferable to recommend a hybrid healthcare model over a traditional in-person care model, and patient testing and screening should be performed in person, while follow-up visits can be carried out via telehealth, and the recommended model allows for providers to lower the risk of COVID-19 infection while maintaining a high standard of prenatal care [63]. The education of midwives is a high priority to address the effects of a life-threatening mass disaster event, the health of a pregnant woman and her fetus, the course of her pregnancy and delivery, the methods of prevention and treatment, and extending professional authorizations under the midwife license in the face of terrorism and/or mass disaster [64].

4. Discussion

The COVID-19 pandemic formed a serious multi-etiological global mental health challenge influencing every aspect of life and disrupting the social fabric [65]. The COVID-19 pandemic has caused general anxiety worldwide [66] and created numerous stressful conditions, especially for vulnerable populations such as pregnant women [35]; in some cases, the increased the risk of psychological imbalance associated with changes in everyday life [67] and increased the risk of the most common mental disorders among pregnant women during this a worldwide disaster [68], including anxiety, depression, insomnia, and PTSD [20,22–24,29]. The aim of this study was to analyze adverse mental health effects in the pregnant population during the COVID-19 pandemic, investigate risk factors for adverse mental health outcomes, identify protective factors, and create practical implications for clinical practice, bearing in mind the need to improve perinatal mental healthcare during such pandemics. Qualitative research was conducted in the electronic databases PubMed and Web of Sciences for the keywords COVID-19, pregnancy, depression, anxiety, and telemedicine for relevant critical articles (n = 3280) published from 2020 until October 2021, outlining the outcomes of control studies, meta-analysis, cross-sectional studies, face-to-face evaluation survey studies, remotely administered survey studies, and observational studies regarding the main topic; all were evaluated. The qualitative synthesis findings were concluded on the basis of 16 articles out of 3280 researched publications. Our findings on a total number of 515,803 pregnant participants are linked to adverse mental health sequelae of the COVID-19 pandemic in the pregnant population. Our study analyzes the presence of adverse mental health symptoms in pregnant women associated with the COVID-19 pandemic and allows us to divide and describe findings in five domains: Domain 1: Social and medical consequences of COVID-19 in the pregnant women population. Domain 2: Main psychological factors responsible for adverse COVID-19 mental health outcomes in pregnant women. Domain 3: Determination of COVID-19 mental health problems, including symptoms and diagnosis among pregnant women in different countries. Domain 4: Influence of COVID-19 on the psychological and medical factors related to adverse pregnancy and offspring development outcomes. Domain 5: Dilemmas and hopes in ways to improve the provision of services to pregnant women during disasters, including the COVID-19 pandemic. Pregnant women are more likely to develop mental health problems than nonpregnant women of childbearing age are, and this was confirmed on the basis of a cross-sectional study of pregnant (n = 544) and nonpregnant (n = 315) women in Beijing, China [20]. Elevated anxiety and depression symptoms that may have a long-term impact on offspring related to COVID-19 worries about threats to their own lives and their baby's health [23], not getting enough prenatal care, and social isolation were the most frequently reported factors in the population of 1987 women <35 weeks gestation [26]. Evidence from 38.5% of participants reported high preparedness stress; 26% reported high perinatal infection stress, and pregnant women are most vulnerable to pandemic-related stress [35]. Pregnant women have an advantage of facing mental problems related to COVID-19, showing fewer depression, anxiety, insomnia, and PTSD symptoms than non-pregnant women do [20]. However, the effects of the COVID-19 pandemic on mental health are still not fully understood; thus, research in this area is still being conducted in many countries—among others, in Turkey, Colombia, and Italy. In comparison with the Turkish study [24], findings show that a lower rate of depressive symptoms (25%) was reported in Colombia [29], while the same Colombian study confirmed similar anxiety symptom rate (50.4%) with findings pointed out by Italian scientists [27] and higher than that in Iran's study results [28]. We noticed two major pandemic-related stress domains for pregnant women: fear of perinatal COVID-19 infection and being unprepared for birth were reported in four countries [21]. Pregnant women are worried about the COVID-19 pandemic and have difficulty in accessing professional medical help, feel insecure about the exposure risk to the coronavirus when accessing medical facilities, fear infection of the infant in the peripartum period, and have financial problems that lead to conflict in the family; additionally, a single mother may be more prone to anxiety isolation; fear of being trapped and rumors spreading on social media; growing anxiety and social panic; and fear of blame, guilt, and stigmatization related to being infected with COVID-19 [22]. Psychological impact and anxiety of the COVID-19 epidemic were found be more severe in women who were in the first trimester of pregnancy during the outbreak; high anxiety regarding the vertical transmission of the disease was reported by almost half of the respondents [27]. Notable, the rate of psychological consequences of the pandemic was much larger than the number of patients clinically affected by the virus, with symptoms of anxiety, insomnia, and depression [29]. Depressive and anxiety symptoms were significantly increased during the SARS-CoV-2 pandemic compared with pre-pandemic surveys, and effective screening strategies for depression and anxiety symptoms during the pandemic should be prioritized to allow for timely treatment [25]. Lockdowns (e.g., reduced infection load and reduced physical activity) are possibly beneficial for reducing extreme prematurity and potentially reducing infant mortality, a nonsignificant but slightly increased number of very premature births [33]. Evidence from pregnant women in China found that low levels of physical activity were associated with increased symptoms of depression during COVID-19, and in Canada, pregnant women who engaged in higher levels of physical activity tended to show lower symptoms of depression and anxiety [69]. The pregnant woman population is struggling with the COVID-19 pandemic, experiencing stressful factors such as adverse fetal outcomes and the increase in ruptured ectopic pregnancies, causing maternal deaths and stillbirths, concerns about the spread or infection of SARS-CoV-2, financial instability, limited scientific knowledge about the effects of COVID-19 on fetal wellbeing, and interruptions of prenatal care [35]. Urgent need to provide psychosocial support to the pregnant women population during the COVID-19 crisis was highlighted. Adverse events may otherwise occur during pregnancy and thus affect both mother and fetus [24].

Our study produced five overarching domains by analysis and synthesis of the current knowledge on the main topic related to adverse consequences of the COVID-19 on the mental health of pregnant women and the possibility of improving these outcomes in a medical provider practice in a way to reach the preparation of useful implications for clinical practice during the COVID-19 pandemic.

4.1. Useful Implications for Clinical Practice

Research findings support and advocate the need to modify the scope of healthcare provider practice in the COVID-19 pandemic disaster and could be implemented and adopted by healthcare providers, as useful implications for clinical practice on the following discoveries:

- psychopsychiatric consequences of the negative influence of COVID-19 globally affect women regardless of race of origin [10,20,21,23–33,35,51–54,57,59,70];
- fears of perinatal COVID-19 infection and feeling unprepared for birth due to the COVID-19 pandemic can be a major psychological problem for pregnant women [21,27];
- quarantine may involve destructive feelings of loss of freedom among pregnant women [49], and social distancing and isolation/quarantine procedures implemented during the COVID-19 pandemic increased risk of psychological problems among pregnant women and new mothers [71];
- pregnant women should be informed of the increase in severity of COVID-19, including admission to intensive care units, need for ECMO and invasive ventilation compared with non-pregnant women, and encouraged to undertake safety measures to reduce the risk of infection, and pregnant women with preexisting comorbidities will need to be considered as a high-risk group for COVID-19 [8];
- the possibility of a mother infecting her own unborn child with the SARS-CoV-2 virus is an extreme psychological burden for the mother and a serious factor that may impair the child's development [27,35];
- early cord clamping may minimize the risk of viral transmission by avoiding longer, close contact with the infected mother [46], and in turn, it may increase the mother's good feelings about the safety of the newborn;
- mental health problems among pregnant women linked to the COVID-19 pandemic in most cases establish symptoms of depression, anxiety, insomnia, and PTSD [20,22–24,29];
- the status of not receiving the necessary prenatal care, having relationship strain, and being in social isolation may become initiating factors of mental health disorders [35,59];
- a positive impact on the depressive symptoms of new mothers may be achieved by providing appropriate isolation in hospitals for pregnant women [31], including. but not limited to. quarantine;
- the psychological stress of the COVID-19 pandemic during pregnancy can increase the risk of preterm delivery, low birth weight, postnatal complications, and neurodevelopmental disorders in offspring [10,25,57,58]; in some cases, a 100% reduction in ELBW infants was noted during the COVID-19 pandemic [32,33];
- telemedicine may be used to effectively improve access to medical services for women during the pandemic, especially in quarantined areas, reducing feelings of fear, threat, and loneliness [23,61,72], and may improve access and utilization of prenatal care across the board [63,70];
- reducing feelings of fear, panic, anxiety, threat, and loneliness is a priority, especially during a disaster [23,61,72,73];
- a midwife should have the right and duty to order, prescribe, and administer pharmacological agents that, on a daily basis, are prescribed at the discretion of an OB/GYN specialist and must be prepared for sudden maternal cardiac arrest in a pregnant woman and to address the moral dilemma of delivering a fetus from a deceased mother's womb [64];
- critically important are methods of supportive parenting and using techniques to downregulate arousal in time of occurred stress, and physical activity was associated with lower psychological symptoms [26];
- effective screening strategies for depressive and anxiety symptoms during the pandemic should be prioritized to allow for timely treatment [25];

- mental health specialists and other medical providers, midwives, and nurses can prevent adverse outcomes by identifying problems early (paying special attention to the group of women with adverse mental health and psychiatric symptoms, including assessing sleep patterns, sources of fear, anxiety, swinging moods, irritability, depression, worries, and suicidal ideation or its attempt), and establishing comprehensive treatment plans for pregnant women in conditions such as emergencies and the COVID-19 natural disasters [25];
- routine assessment of trauma history and psychopathology during prenatal visits is warranted to identify women at risk; abnormalities of the early bonding of mother–offspring always must be taken into consideration, if mental health impairment symptoms occur [74], and in the case of necessity, a perinatal psychiatrist should be consulted [75];
- promoting marital and relationship wellbeing may play a valuable role in anxiety control, lowering stress, and reducing depression in pregnant women [28];
- physical exercise is often correlated with decreased depressive and anxiety symptoms in pregnant women and therefore should be recommended [69,76];
- patient testing and screening should be conducted in person, while follow-up visits can be carried out via telehealth, and the recommended model allows for providers to lower the risk COVID-19 infection while maintaining a high standard of prenatal care [63];
- women who became mothers during the COVID-19 emergency appear to be at high risk for developing mental health problems [5];
- implementing community-based strategies to support resilience and psychologically vulnerable individuals during the COVID-19 crisis is fundamental for any community [77], including pregnant women;
- copying with psychological distress of the COVID-19 pandemic during pregnancy should be more recommended to prevent adverse effects on the fetal growth and neurodevelopment disorders in offspring, because maternal psychological distress (e.g., stress, anxiety, and depression) has been found as a risk factor of child or adult neurodevelopment disorders, including, but not limited to, ADHD, ASD, schizophrenia spectrum disorder, antisocial behavior, and depressive symptoms [3,55–57];
- observation highlights the need for increased screening and treatment for perinatal mood and anxiety disorders in the postpartum period as the COVID-19 pandemic continues [75];
- providing psychological support to pregnant and lactating women may reduce the long-term negative effects of COVID-19 pandemic [76].

4.2. Strengths and Limitations

The strength of this study is that it was conducted with the use of and following up the PRISMA extension for scoping review guidelines. The limitations of this study may have resulted from the inclusion criterion of researching articles only written in English language, which could have excluded valuable scientific publications in other languages.

5. Conclusions

Our study analyzed the presence of adverse mental health symptoms in a total number of 515,803 pregnant women's experience with exposure to or infection with COVID-19. The psychological impact and anxiety of the COVID-19 crisis were found be more severe in women who were in the first trimester of pregnancy during the disaster. Depression symptoms worries about threats to their own lives, their baby's health, not getting enough prenatal care, and social isolation are some of the most important factors in group of <35 weeks gestation age; 26% pregnant women reported perinatal COVID-19 infection stress and being unprepared for birth. Depressive and anxiety symptoms were significantly increased during the SARS-CoV-2 pandemic compared with pre-pandemic surveys.

Urgent need to provide psychosocial support to this population during the crisis was highlighted and allowed us to produce the useful implications for clinical practice bearing in mind adverse mental health effects in the pregnant population during the COVID-19 pandemic and following our efforts to investigate risk factors for adverse mental health outcomes, identify protective factors and the need to improve perinatal mental healthcare during such pandemics. The useful implications for clinical practice to improve the adverse mental health outcomes of pregnant women associated with the COVID-19 pandemic are highly desirable. This is necessary to not only eliminate the long-term consequences of different forms of severe stressors' outcomes but also to reduce the economic costs of medically treating adverse severe mental problems. Improving the effectiveness of midwifery and nursing practice for such disaster responses is pivotal. To address adverse mental health issues during the pandemic, it is necessary to adopt several psychosocial interventions to reduce anxiety and other destructive mental health outcomes among the population of pregnant women with methods for controlling outbreaks like COVID-19. It is urgent to conduct cohort studies of the impact of the COVID-19 pandemic on the mental state of pregnant women, fetuses, and child development outside the mother's womb.

Supplementary Materials: The following supporting information can be downloaded at https://www.mdpi.com/article/10.3390/jcm11082072/s1: NEWCASTLE—OTTAWA QUALITY ASSESSMENT SCALE.

Author Contributions: Conceptualization, D.W.M.; methodology, D.W.M. and J.S.; formal analysis, D.W.M. and D.I.P.; resources, D.W.M., J.S. and D.I.P.; writing—original draft preparation, D.W.M. and J.S.; writing—review and editing, D.W.M. and D.I.P.; visualization, D.W.M., J.S. and D.I.P.; and supervision, D.W.M. All authors have read and agreed to the published version of the manuscript.

Funding: This research received no external funding.

Institutional Review Board Statement: Not applicable.

Informed Consent Statement: Not applicable.

Conflicts of Interest: The authors declare no conflict of interest.

References

1. Wang, C.; Pan, R.; Wan, X.; Tan, Y.; Xu, L.; Ho, C.S.; Ho, R.C. Immediate Psychological Responses and Associated Factors during the Initial Stage of the 2019 Coronavirus Disease (COVID-19) Epidemic among the General Population in China. *Int. J. Environ. Res. Public Health* **2020**, *17*, 1729. [CrossRef] [PubMed]
2. Torales, J.; O'Higgins, M.; Castaldelli-Maia, J.M.; Ventriglio, A. The Outbreak of COVID-19 Coronavirus and its Impact on Global Mental Health. *Int. J. Soc. Psychiatry* **2020**, *66*, 317–320. [CrossRef]
3. Martins-Filho, P.R.; Tavares, C.; Santos, V.S. Factors Associated with Mortality in Patients with COVID-19. A Quantitative Evidence Synthesis of Clinical and Laboratory Data. *Eur. J. Intern. Med.* **2020**, *76*, 97–99. [CrossRef] [PubMed]
4. Rasmussen, S.A.; Smulian, J.C.; Lednicky, J.A.; Wen, T.S.; Jamieson, D.J. Coronavirus Disease 2019 (COVID-19) and Pregnancy: What Obstetricians Need to Know. *Am. J. Obstet. Gynecol.* **2020**, *222*, 415–426. [CrossRef]
5. Grumi, S.; Provenzi, L.; Accorsi, P.; Biasucci, G.; Cavallini, A.; Decembrino, L.; Falcone, R.; Fazzi, E.M.; Gardella, B.; Giacchero, R.; et al. Depression and Anxiety in Mothers Who Were Pregnant During the COVID-19 Outbreak in Northern Italy: The Role of Pandemic-Related Emotional Stress and Perceived Social Support. *Front. Psychiatry* **2021**, *12*, 716488. [CrossRef] [PubMed]
6. Wróblewska-Seniuk, K.; Basiukajc, A.; Wojciechowska, D.; Telge, M.; Miechowicz, I.; Mazela, J. Clinical Characteristics of Newborns Born to Mothers with COVID-19. *J. Clin. Med.* **2021**, *10*, 4383. [CrossRef] [PubMed]
7. Celewicz, A.; Celewicz, M.; Michalczyk, M.; Wozniakowska-Gondek, P.; Krejczy, K.; Misiek, M.; Rzepka, R. Pregnancy as a Risk Factor of Severe COVID-19. *J. Clin. Med.* **2021**, *10*, 5458. [CrossRef] [PubMed]
8. Allotey, J.; Stallings, E.; Bonet, M.; Yap, M.; Chatterjee, S.; Kew, T.; Debenham, L.; Llavall, A.C.; Dixit, A.; Zhou, D.; et al. Clinical Manifestations, Risk Factors, and Maternal and Perinatal Outcomes of Coronavirus Disease 2019 in Pregnancy: Living Systematic Review and Meta-Analysis. *BMJ* **2020**, *370*, 1641–1647. [CrossRef]
9. Trad, A.T.A.; Ibirogba, E.R.; Elrefaei, A.; Narang, K.; Tonni, G.; Picone, O.; Suy, A.; Moratonas, E.C.; Kilby, M.; Ruano, R. Complications and Outcomes of SARS-CoV-2 in Pregnancy: Where and What Is the Evidence? *Hypertens. Pregnancy* **2020**, *39*, 361–369. [CrossRef] [PubMed]
10. Brooks, S.K.; Weston, D.; Greenberg, N. Psychological Impact of Infectious Disease Outbreaks on Pregnant Women: Rapid Evidence Review. *Public Health* **2020**, *189*, 26–36. [CrossRef] [PubMed]

11. Buekens, P.; Alger, J.; Bréart, G.; Cafferata, M.L.; Harville, E.; Tomasso, G. A Call for Action for COVID-19 Surveillance and Research during Pregnancy. *Lancet Glob. Health* **2020**, *8*, 877–878. [CrossRef]
12. Orsolini, L.; Valchera, A.; Vecchiotti, R.; Tomasetti, C.; Iasevoli, F.; Fornaro, M.; De Berardis, D.; Perna, G.; Pompili, M.; Bellantuono, C. Suicide during Perinatal Period: Epidemiology, Risk Factors, and Clinical Correlates. *Front. Psychiatry* **2016**, *7*, 138. [CrossRef] [PubMed]
13. Field, T.; Diego, M.; Hernandez-Reif, M.; Figueiredo, B.; Deeds, O.; Ascencio, A.; Schanberg, S.; Kuhn, C. Comorbid Depression and Anxiety Effects on Pregnancy and Neonatal Outcome. *Infant Behav. Dev.* **2010**, *33*, 23–29. [CrossRef] [PubMed]
14. Liu, B.; Han, B.; Zheng, H.; Liu, H.; Zhao, T.; Wan, Y.; Cui, F. Who Is the Most Vulnerable to Anxiety at the Beginning of the COVID-19 Outbreak in China? A Cross-Sectional Nationwide Survey. *Healthcare* **2021**, *9*, 970. [CrossRef] [PubMed]
15. Hessami, K.; Romanelli, C.; Chiurazzi, M.; Cozzolino, M. COVID-19 Pandemic and Maternal Mental Health: A Systematic Review and Meta-Analysis. *J. Matern. Fetal Neonatal Med.* **2020**, 1–8. [CrossRef] [PubMed]
16. Tomfohr-Madsen, L.M.; Racine, N.; Giesbrecht, G.F.; Lebel, C.; Madigan, S. Depression and Anxiety in Pregnancy during COVID-19: A Rapid Review and Meta-Analysis. *Psychiatry Res.* **2021**, *300*, 113912. [CrossRef] [PubMed]
17. Li, S.; Wang, Y.; Xue, J.; Zhao, N.; Zhu, T. The Impact of COVID-19 Epidemic Declaration on Psychological Consequences: A Study on Active Weibo Users. *Int. J. Environ. Res. Public Health* **2020**, *17*, 2032. [CrossRef]
18. Munn, Z.; Peters, M.D.J.; Stern, C.; Tufanaru, C.; McArthur, A.; Aromataris, E. Systematic Review or Scoping Review? Guidance for Authors When Choosing between a Systematic or Scoping Review Approach. *BMC Med. Res. Methodol.* **2018**, *18*, 143. [CrossRef]
19. Tricco, A.C.; Lillie, E.; Zarin, W.; O'Brien, K.K.; Colquhoun, H.; Levac, D.; Moher, D.; Peters, M.D.J.; Horsley, T.; Weeks, L.; et al. PRISMA Extension for Scoping Reviews (PRISMA-ScR): Checklist and Explanation. *Ann. Intern. Med.* **2018**, *169*, 467–473. [CrossRef] [PubMed]
20. Zhou, Y.; Shi, H.; Liu, Z.; Peng, S.; Wang, R.; Qi, L.; Li, Z.; Yang, J.; Ren, Y.; Song, X.; et al. The Prevalence of Psychiatric Symptoms of Pregnant and Non-pregnant Women during the COVID-19 Epidemic. *Transl. Psychiatry* **2020**, *10*, 319. [CrossRef] [PubMed]
21. Preis, H.; Mahaffey, B.; Heiselman, C.; Lobel, M. Vulnerability and Resilience to Pandemic-Related Stress among U.S. Women Pregnant at the Start of the COVID-19 Pandemic. *Soc. Sci. Med.* **2020**, *266*, 113348. [CrossRef] [PubMed]
22. Kajdy, A.; Feduniw, S.; Ajdacka, U.; Modzelewski, J.; Baranowska, B.; Sys, D.; Pokropek, A.; Pawlicka, P.; Kaźmierczak, M.; Rabijewski, M.; et al. Risk Factors for Anxiety and Depression among Pregnant Women during the COVID-19 Pandemic: A Web-Based Cross-Sectional Survey. *Medicine* **2020**, *99*, e21279. [CrossRef] [PubMed]
23. Preis, H.; Mahaffey, B.; Heiselman, C.; Lobel, M. Pandemic-Related Pregnancy Stress and Anxiety among Women Pregnant during the Coronavirus Disease 2019 Pandemic. *Am. J. Obstet. Gynecol. MFM* **2020**, *2*, 100155. [CrossRef]
24. Durankuş, F.; Aksu, E. Effects of the COVID-19 Pandemic on Anxiety and Depressive Symptoms in Pregnant Women: A Preliminary Study. *J. Matern. Fetal Neonatal Med.* **2020**, *35*, 1–7. [CrossRef] [PubMed]
25. Ayaz, R.; Hocaoğlu, M.; Günay, T.; Yardımcı, O.D.; Turgut, A.; Karateke, A. Anxiety and Depression Symptoms in the Same Pregnant Women before and during the COVID-19 Pandemic. *J. Perinat. Med.* **2020**, *48*, 965–970. [CrossRef] [PubMed]
26. Lebel, C.; MacKinnon, A.; Bagshawe, M.; Tomfohr-Madsen, L.; Giesbrecht, G. Elevated Depression and Anxiety Symptoms among Pregnant Individuals during the COVID-19 Pandemic. *J. Affect. Disord.* **2020**, *277*, 5–13. [CrossRef]
27. Saccone, G.; Florio, A.; Aiello, F.; Venturella, R.; De Angelis, M.C.; Locci, M.; Bifulco, G.; Zullo, F.; Di Spiezio Sardo, A. Psychological Impact of Coronavirus Disease 2019 in Pregnant Women. *Am. J. Obstet. Gynecol.* **2020**, *223*, 293–295. [CrossRef] [PubMed]
28. Effati-Daryani, F.; Zare, S.; Mohammadi, A.; Hemmati, E.; Ghasemi; Yngyknd, S.; Mirghafourvand, M. Depression, Stress, Anxiety and Their Predictors in Iranian Pregnant Women during the Outbreak of COVID-19. *BMC Psychol.* **2020**, *8*, 99. [CrossRef] [PubMed]
29. Parra-Saavedra, M.; Villa-Villa, I.; Pérez-Olivo, J.; Guzman-Polania, L.; Galvis-Centurion, P.; Cumplido-Romero, Á.; Santacruz-Vargas, D.; Rivera-Moreno, E.; Molina-Giraldo, S.; Guillen-Burgos, H.; et al. Attitudes and Collateral Psychological Effects of COVID-19 in Pregnant Women in Colombia. *Int. J. Gynaecol. Obstet.* **2020**, *151*, 203–208. [CrossRef]
30. Taubman-Ben-Ari, O.; Chasson, M.; Abu Sharkia, S.; Weiss, E. Distress and Anxiety Associated with COVID-19 among Jewish and Arab Pregnant Women in Israel. *J. Reprod. Infant Psychol.* **2020**, *38*, 340–348. [CrossRef] [PubMed]
31. Oskovi-Kaplan, Z.A.; Buyuk, G.N.; Ozgu-Erdinc, A.S.; Keskin, H.L.; Ozbas, A.; Moraloglu Tekin, O. The Effect of COVID-19 Pandemic and Social Restrictions on Depression Rates and Maternal Attachment in Immediate Postpartum Women: A Preliminary Study. *Psychiatr. Q.* **2020**, *92*, 675–682. [CrossRef] [PubMed]
32. Philip, R.K.; Purtill, H.; Reidy, E.; Daly, M.; Imcha, M.; McGrath, D.; O'Connell, N.H.; Dunne, C.P. Unprecedented Reduction in Births of Very Low Birthweight (VLBW) And Extremely Low Birthweight (ELBW) Infants during the COVID-19 Lockdown in Ire-Land: A 'Natural Experiment' Allowing Analysis of Data from the Prior Two Decades. *BMJ Global Health* **2020**, *5*, e003075. [CrossRef] [PubMed]
33. Hedermann, G.; Hedley, P.L.; Bækvad-Hansen, M.; Hjalgrim, H.; Rostgaard, K.; Poorisrisak, P.; Breindahl, M.; Melbye, M.; Hougaard, D.M.; Christiansen, M.; et al. Danish Premature Birth Rates during the COVID-19 Lockdown. *Arch. Dis. Childhood. Fetal Neonatal Ed.* **2020**, *106*, 93–95. [CrossRef]

34. Facchetti, F.; Bugatti, M.; Drera, E.; Tripodo, C.; Sartori, E.; Cancila, V.; Papaccio, M.; Castellani, R.; Casola, S.; Boniotti, M.B.; et al. SARS-CoV2 Vertical Transmission with Adverse Effects on the Newborn Revealed through Integrated Immunohistochemical, Electron Microscopy and Molecular Analyses of Placenta. *EBioMedicine* **2020**, *59*, 102951. [CrossRef] [PubMed]
35. Ilska, M.; Kołodziej-Zaleska, A.; Brandt-Salmeri, A.; Preis, H.; Lobel, M. Pandemic Stress and Its Correlates among Pregnant Women during the Second Wave of COVID-19 in Poland. *Int. J. Environ. Res. Public Health* **2021**, *18*, 11140. [CrossRef] [PubMed]
36. Wells, G.A.; Shea, B.; O'Connell, D.; Peterson, J.; Welch, V.; Losos, M.; Tugwell, P.; Ga, S.W.; Zello, G.A.; Petersen, J.A. The Newcastle-Ottawa Scale (NOS) for Assessing the Quality of Nonrandomised Studies in Meta-Analyses. 2014. Available online: http://www.ohri.ca/programs/clinical_epidemiology/oxford.asp (accessed on 30 November 2021).
37. Zanardo, V.; Manghina, V.; Giliberti, L.; Vettore, M.; Severino, L.; Straface, G. Psychological Impact of COVID-19 Quarantine Measures in Northeastern Italy on Mothers in the Immediate Postpartum Period. *Int. J. Gynaecol. Obstet.* **2020**, *150*, 184–188. [CrossRef]
38. Esterwood, E.; Saeed, S.A. Past Epidemics, Natural Disasters, COVID19, and Mental Health: Learning from History as we Deal with the Present and Prepare for the Future. *Psychiatr. Q.* **2020**, *91*, 1121–1133. [CrossRef]
39. Thapa, S.B.; Mainali, A.; Schwank, S.E.; Acharya, G. Maternal Mental Health in the Time of the COVID-19 Pandemic. *Acta Obstet. Et Gynecol. Scand.* **2020**, *99*, 817–818. [CrossRef] [PubMed]
40. Caparros-Gonzalez, R.A.; Alderdice, F. The COVID-19 Pandemic and Perinatal Mental Health. *J. Reprod. Infant Psychol.* **2020**, *38*, 223–225. [CrossRef] [PubMed]
41. Yassa, M.; Birol, P.; Yirmibes, C.; Usta, C.; Haydar, A.; Yassa, A.; Sandal, K.; Tekin, A.B.; Tug, N. Near-Term Pregnant Women's Attitude Toward, Concern about and Knowledge of the COVID-19 Pandemic. *J. Matern. Fetal Neonatal Med.* **2020**, *33*, 3827–3834. [CrossRef] [PubMed]
42. Okuyama, M.; Mezawa, H.; Kawai, T.; Urashima, M. Elevated Soluble PD-L1 in Pregnant Women's Serum Suppresses the Immune Reaction. *Front. Immunol.* **2019**, *10*, 86. [CrossRef]
43. Easterlin, M.C.; Crimmins, E.M.; Finch, C.E. Will Prenatal Exposure to SARS-CoV-2 Define a Birth Cohort with Accelerated Aging in the Century Ahead? *J. Dev. Orig. Health Dis.* **2020**, *12*, 1–5. [CrossRef] [PubMed]
44. Mehew, J.; Johnson, R.; Roberts, D.; Harvala, H. Convalescent Plasma for COVID-19: Male Gender, Older Age and Hospitalization Associated with High Neutralizing Antibody Levels, England, 22 April to 12 May 2020. *Eurosurveillance* **2020**, *25*, 2001754. [CrossRef] [PubMed]
45. Jamieson, D.J.; Rasmussen, S.A. An Update on COVID-19 and Pregnancy. *Am. J. Obstet. Gynecol.* **2022**, *226*, 177–186. [CrossRef] [PubMed]
46. Wang, C.L.; Liu, Y.Y.; Wu, C.H.; Wang, C.Y.; Wang, C.H.; Long, C.Y. Impact of COVID-19 on Pregnancy. *Int. J. Med. Sci.* **2021**, *18*, 763–767. [CrossRef]
47. Vivanti, A.J.; Vauloup-Fellous, C.; Prevot, S.; Zupan, V.; Suffee, C.; Do Cao, J.; Benachi, A.; De Luca, D. Transplacental Transmission of SARS-CoV-2 Infection. *Nat. Commun.* **2020**, *11*, 3572. [CrossRef]
48. Sharps, M.C.; Hayes, D.; Lee, S.; Zou, Z.; Brady, C.A.; Almoghrabi, Y.; Kerby, A.; Tamber, K.K.; Jones, C.J.; Adams Waldorf, K.M.; et al. A Structured Review of Placental Morphology and Histopathological Lesions Associated with SARS-CoV-2 Infection. *Placenta* **2020**, *101*, 13–29. [CrossRef]
49. Van Bavel, J.J.; Baicker, K.; Boggio, P.S.; Capraro, V.; Cichocka, A.; Cikara, M.; Crockett, M.J.; Crum, A.J.; Douglas, K.M.; Druckman, J.N.; et al. Using Social and Behavioural Science to Support COVID-19 Pandemic Response. *Nat. Hum. Behav.* **2020**, *4*, 460–471. [CrossRef] [PubMed]
50. Van der Zee-van den Berg, A.I.; Boere-Boonekamp, M.M.; Groothuis-Oudshoorn, C.; Reijneveld, S.A. The Edinburgh Postpartum Depression Scale: Stable Structure but Subscale of Limited Value to Detect Anxiety. *PLoS ONE* **2019**, *14*, e0221894. [CrossRef]
51. Berthelot, N.; Lemieux, R.; Garon-Bissonnette, J.; Drouin-Maziade, C.; Martel, É.; Maziade, M. Uptrend in Distress and Psychiatric Symptomatology in Pregnant Women during the Coronavirus Disease 2019 Pandemic. *Acta Obstet. Et Gynecol. Scand.* **2020**, *99*, 848–855. [CrossRef]
52. Wong, S.F.; Chow, K.M.; Leung, T.N.; Ng, W.F.; Ng, T.K.; Shek, C.C.; Ng, P.C.; Lam, P.W.; Ho, L.C.; To, W.W.; et al. Pregnancy and Perinatal Outcomes of Women with Severe Acute Respiratory Syndrome. *Am. J. Obstet. Gynecol.* **2004**, *191*, 292–297. [CrossRef] [PubMed]
53. Alfaraj, S.H.; Al-Tawfiq, J.A.; Memish, Z.A. Middle East Respiratory Syndrome Coronavirus (MERS-CoV) Infection during Pregnancy: Report of Two Cases and Review of the Literature. *J. Microbiol. Immunol. Infect.* **2019**, *52*, 501–503. [CrossRef] [PubMed]
54. Ming-Zhu, Y.; Lijuan, Z.; Guangtong, D.; Chaofei, H.; Minxue, S.; Hongyin, S.; Furong, Z.; Wei, Z.; Lan, C.; Qingqing, L.; et al. Severe Acute Respiratory Syndrome Coronavirus 2 (SARS-CoV-2) Infection During Pregnancy in China: A Retrospective Cohort Study. *medRxiv* **2020**. [CrossRef]
55. Scheinost, D.; Sinha, R.; Cross, S.N.; Kwon, S.H.; Sze, G.; Constable, R.T.; Ment, L.R. Does Prenatal Stress Alter the Developing Connectome? *Pediatric Res.* **2017**, *81*, 214–226. [CrossRef]
56. Fatima, M.; Srivastav, S.; Mondal, A.C. Prenatal Stress and Depression Associated Neuronal Development in Neonates. *Int. J. Dev. Neurosci.* **2017**, *60*, 1–7. [CrossRef] [PubMed]

57. Abdoli, A.; Falahi, S.; Kenarkoohi, A.; Shams, M.; Mir, H.; Jahromi, M. The COVID-19 Pandemic, Psychological Stress during Pregnancy, and Risk of Neurodevelopmental Disorders in Offspring: A Neglected Consequence. *J. Psychosom. Obstet. Gynaecol.* **2020**, *41*, 247–248. [CrossRef] [PubMed]
58. Castro, P.; Narciso, C.; Matos, A.P.; Werner, H.; Araujo Júnior, E. Pregnant, Uninfected, Stressed, and Confined in the COVID-19 Period: What Can We Expect in the near Future? *Revista da Associacao Medica Brasileira* **2020**, *66*, 386–387. [CrossRef] [PubMed]
59. Shoib, S.; Arafat, S.; Ahmad, W. Perinatal Mental Health in Kashmir, India during the COVID-19 Pandemic. *Matern. Child Health J.* **2020**, *24*, 1365–1366. [CrossRef] [PubMed]
60. Ceulemans, M.; Verbakel, J.Y.; Van Calsteren, K.; Eerdekens, A.; Allegaert, K.; Foulon, V. SARS-CoV-2 Infections and Impact of the COVID-19 Pandemic in Pregnancy and Breastfeeding: Results from an Observational Study in Primary Care in Belgium. *Int. J. Environ. Res. Public Health* **2020**, *17*, 6766. [CrossRef] [PubMed]
61. Implementing Telehealth in Practice. ACOG Committee Opinion Summary, Number 798. *Obstet. Gynecol.* **2020**, *135*, 493–494. [CrossRef] [PubMed]
62. Rad, S.; Smith, D.; Malish, T.; Jain, V. SMFM Coding White Paper: Interim Coding Guidance: Coding for Telemedicine and Remote Patient Monitoring Services during the COVID-19 Pandemic. *Soc. Matern. Fetal Med.* **2020**. Available online: https://www.smfm.org/covid-19-white-paper (accessed on 19 January 2022).
63. Jakubowski, D.; Sys, D.; Kajdy, A.; Lewandowska, R.; Kwiatkowska, E.; Cymbaluk-Płoska, A.; Rabijewski, M.; Torbé, A.; Kwiatkowski, S. Application of Telehealth in Prenatal Care during the COVID-19 Pandemic—A Cross-Sectional Survey of Polish Women. *J. Clin. Med.* **2021**, *10*, 2570. [CrossRef] [PubMed]
64. Mazurkiewicz, D.W.; Piechocka, D.I.; Miela, R.; Koniecko, K.; Sawka, J.H.; Strzelecka, J. A New Challenge for Midwives and Medical Doctors in Time of the Threat of a Mass Terrorist Attack and a Life-Threatening Mass Disaster. *Prog. Health Sci.* **2018**, *8*, 181–193. [CrossRef]
65. Coelho, C.M.; Suttiwan, P.; Arato, N.; Zsido, A.N. On the Nature of Fear and Anxiety Triggered by COVID-19. *Front. Psychol.* **2020**, *11*, 581314. [CrossRef] [PubMed]
66. Janik, K.; Cwalina, U.; Iwanowicz-Palus, G.; Cybulski, M. An Assessment of the Level of COVID-19 Anxiety among Pregnant Women in Poland: A Cross-Sectional Study. *J. Clin. Med.* **2021**, *10*, 5869. [CrossRef]
67. Witteveen, D.; Velthorst, E. Economic Hardship and Mental Health Complaints during COVID-19. *Proc. Natl. Acad. Sci. USA* **2020**, *117*, 27277–27284. [CrossRef] [PubMed]
68. Takubo, Y.; Tsujino, N.; Aikawa, Y.; Fukiya, K.; Iwai, M.; Uchino, T.; Ito, M.; Akiba, Y.; Mizuno, M.; Nemoto, T. Psychological Impacts of the COVID-19 Pandemic on One-Month Postpartum Mothers in a Metropolitan Area of Japan. *BMC Pregnancy Childbirth* **2021**, *21*, 845. [CrossRef]
69. Choi, K.W.; Kim, H.H.; Basu, A.; Kwong, A.S.F.; Hernandez-Diaz, S.; Wyszynski, D.F.; Koenen, K.C. COVID-19 Perceived Impacts on Sleep, Fitness, and Diet and Associations with Mental Health during Pregnancy: A Cross-National Study. *J. Affect. Disord. Rep.* **2022**, *7*, 100288. [CrossRef] [PubMed]
70. Fryer, K.; Delgado, A.; Foti, T.; Reid, C.N.; Marshall, J. Implementation of Obstetric Telehealth During COVID-19 and beyond. *Matern. Child Health J.* **2020**, *24*, 1104–1110. [CrossRef] [PubMed]
71. Aryal, S.; Pant, S.B. Maternal Mental Health in Nepal and Its Prioritization during COVID-19 Pandemic: Missing the Obvious. *Asian J. Psychiatry* **2020**, *54*, 102281. [CrossRef] [PubMed]
72. Martins-Filho, P.R.; Tanajura, D.M.; Santos, H.P., Jr.; Santos, V.S. COVID-19 during Pregnancy: Potential Risk for Neurodevelopmental Disorders in Neonates? *Eur. J. Obstet. Gynecol. Reprod. Biol.* **2020**, *250*, 255–256. [CrossRef] [PubMed]
73. Shatri, H.; Faisal, E.; Putranto, R. Mass Panic Disaster Management in COVID-19 Pandemic. *Acta Medica Indones.* **2020**, *52*, 179–184.
74. Lehnig, F.; Nagl, M.; Stepan, H.; Wagner, B.; Kersting, A. Associations of Postpartum Mother-Infant Bonding with Maternal Childhood Maltreatment and Postpartum Mental Health: A Cross-Sectional Study. *BMC Pregnancy Childbirth* **2019**, *19*, 278. [CrossRef] [PubMed]
75. Zhang, C.; Okeke, J.C.; Levitan, R.D.; Murphy, K.E.; Foshay, K.; Lye, S.J.; Knight, J.A.; Matthews, S.G. Evaluating Depression and Anxiety throughout Pregnancy and after Birth: Impact of the COVID-19 Pandemic. *Am. J. Obstet. Gynecol. MFM* **2022**, *4*, 100605. [CrossRef]
76. Demissie, D.B.; Bitew, Z.W. Mental Health Effect of COVID-19 Pandemic among Women Who Are Pregnant and/or Lactating: A Systematic Review and Meta-Analysis. *SAGE Open Med.* **2021**, *9*, 20503121211026195. [CrossRef]
77. Serafini, G.; Parmigiani, B.; Amerio, A.; Aguglia, A.; Sher, L.; Amore, M. The Psychological Impact of COVID-19 on the Mental Health in the General Population. *QJM Mon. J. Assoc. Physicians* **2020**, *113*, 531–537. [CrossRef] [PubMed]

Journal of
Clinical Medicine

MDPI

Article

Impact of COVID-19 Related Maternal Stress on Fetal Brain Development: A Multimodal MRI Study

Vidya Rajagopalan [1,*], William T. Reynolds [2], Jeremy Zepeda [3], Jeraldine Lopez [4], Skorn Ponrartana [5], John Wood [6], Rafael Ceschin [7] and Ashok Panigrahy [8]

1 Department of Radiology, Children's Hospital Los Angeles, Keck School of Medicine University of Southern California, Los Angeles, CA 90033, USA
2 Department of Biomedical Informatics, University of Pittsburgh, Pittsburgh, PA 15206, USA
3 Department of Radiology, Children's Hospital Los Angeles, Los Angeles, CA 90027, USA
4 Neuropsychology Core, The Saban Research Institute, Children's Hospital Los Angeles, Los Angeles, CA 90027, USA
5 Department of Pediatric Radiology, Keck School of Medicine University of Southern California, Los Angeles, CA 90033, USA
6 Departments of Radiology and Pediatrics, Children's Hospital Los Angeles, Keck School of Medicine University of Southern California, Los Angeles, CA 90033, USA
7 Department of Radiology, University of Pittsburgh School of Medicine, Pittsburgh, PA 15206, USA
8 Department of Pediatric Radiology, Children's Hospital of Pittsburgh of UPMC, Pittsburgh, PA 15224, USA
* Correspondence: vrajagopalan@chla.usc.edu

Abstract: Background: Disruptions in perinatal care and support due to the COVID-19 pandemic was an unprecedented but significant stressor among pregnant women. Various neurostructural differences have been re-ported among fetuses and infants born during the pandemic compared to pre-pandemic counterparts. The relationship between maternal stress due to pandemic related disruptions and fetal brain is yet unexamined. Methods: Pregnant participants with healthy pregnancies were prospectively recruited in 2020–2022 in the greater Los Angeles Area. Participants completed multiple self-report assessments for experiences of pandemic related disruptions, perceived stress, and coping behaviors and underwent fetal MRI. Maternal perceived stress exposures were correlated with quantitative multimodal MRI measures of fetal brain development using multivariate models. Results: Increased maternal perception of pandemic related stress positively correlated with normalized fetal brainstem volume (suggesting accelerated brainstem maturation). In contrast, increased maternal perception of pandemic related stress correlated with reduced global fetal brain temporal functional variance (suggesting reduced functional connectivity). Conclusions: We report alterations in fetal brainstem structure and global functional fetal brain activity associated with increased maternal stress due to pandemic related disruptions, suggesting altered fetal programming. Long term follow-up studies are required to better understand the sequalae of these early multi-modal brain disruptions among infants born during the COVID-19 pandemic.

Keywords: fetal brain function; maternal stress; COVID-19 pandemic

Citation: Rajagopalan, V.; Reynolds, W.T.; Zepeda, J.; Lopez, J.; Ponrartana, S.; Wood, J.; Ceschin, R.; Panigrahy, A. Impact of COVID-19 Related Maternal Stress on Fetal Brain Development: A Multimodal MRI Study. *J. Clin. Med.* **2022**, *11*, 6635. https://doi.org/10.3390/jcm11226635

Academic Editor: Alfonso Troisi

Received: 10 October 2022
Accepted: 5 November 2022
Published: 9 November 2022

1. Introduction

The COVID-19 pandemic created many, unprecedented disruptions to everyday life particularly in 2020–2022 before vaccines were widespread. In addition to disruptions around employment, childcare, housing, and nutrition, pregnant women also suffered negative experiences related to support and care during pregnancy and childbirth. Social isolation, reduced access to child and elder care, COVID-19 infection risk, and changes to medical policies around pre and postpartum care were reported to be the most common stressors among pregnant women [1,2]. Pregnant women are particularly vulnerable to mood and anxiety related disorders [3] which are exacerbated during natural disasters or stressful events [4,5]. Unsurprisingly, pregnant women indicated elevated levels of stress during the COVID-19 pandemic [6]. In addition to health consequences for the mother, increased maternal stress has an intergenerational impact on fetal development [7,8]. Increased maternal stress during pregnancy is known to alter the fetal brain and adversely impact postnatal neurodevelopmental outcomes [9–12].

Studies of infants born during the COVID-19 pandemic have reported reduced cognitive, motor, and emotional development compared to those born pre-pandemic [7,8], with increased prenatal stress directly associated with adverse affect and temperament [13,14]. Simultaneously, changes to brain structure and function have also been reported in infants born during the pandemic [15]. Lu et al. [16] reported volumetric reductions in the brain among fetuses of women pregnant during the pandemic compared to a pre-pandemic cohort. Their findings showed a negative relationship between general maternal stress and fetal brain volumes. However, their cohort did not show an increase in maternal stress or anxiety during a pandemic, and they did not measure maternal stress or anxiety specifically linked to the pandemic. Additionally, there is no data on if or how emerging functional networks in the fetal brain, which are known to be sensitive to ma-ternal stress, were impacted by pandemic related maternal stress. Early aberrations to functional organization of the brain are well known to have deleterious downstream effects in brain and behavioral development. As such, a multimodal imaging study is important to better understand how prenatal maternal stress sets up the offspring's brain for a trajectory of compounding aberrant development.

Understanding the impact of pandemic related maternal stress on fetal development allows us to identify risk and resilience factors to mitigate maternal stress and consequently minimize the intergenerational effect of pandemic related stress. Coping behaviors, in response to stressful events, are known to be modifiable targets to mitigate maternal stress and anxiety [17,18]. Given the extraordinary nature of pandemic related stressors, there is little information on various coping behaviors that pregnant women have adopted during the pandemic [19–21]. Despite its observational nature, information on coping behaviors to pandemic related stressors allow clinical care teams to design and implement support programs aimed at improving maternal mental health during pregnancy and child outcomes.

In this work, we investigated the impact of maternal stress due to pandemic related disruptions in pregnancy support and care on structural and functional development of the human fetal brain. Our primary hypothesis is that increased maternal stress would predict quantitative alterations in structural and functional characteristics of the fetal brain. Secondarily, we compared coping behaviors between pregnant women reporting high vs. low levels of pandemic related stress.

2. Materials and Methods

2.1. Subject Demographics

Pregnant mothers, living in the greater Los Angeles area were recruited using flyers, social media ads, and referrals from community partner clinics at Children's Hospital Los Angeles (CHLA) from November 2020–November 2021. Enrollment eligibility included healthy, pregnant women between 18–45 years with singleton, uncomplicated pregnancies (confirmed by ultrasound) between 21–38 gestational weeks (GW). Exclusion criteria were multiple gestation, fetal or genetic anomalies, congenital infection, and maternal contraindication to MRI. Informed consent for the study was obtained under a protocol approved by the Institutional Review Board at CHLA. Demographics, perinatal health history, and self-assessment surveys of consented participants were gathered via online survey within 24 h prior to MRI.

2.2. Stress and Coping Behavioral Assessments

Participants were asked to complete the Coronavirus Perinatal Experiences-Impact Survey [22] (COPE-IS). This is a self-assessment questionnaire, available in multiple languages, to assess feelings and experiences of pregnant women and new mothers in relation to disruptions caused by the COVID-19 pandemic. Questions in this assessment were adapted from multiple validated questionnaires such as the Brief Symptom Inventory [23] PTSD checklist from DSM-5 [24], and the Johns Hopkins Mental Health Working Group. In this study, we only included questions pertinent to the prenatal period. Perceived maternal stress was computed as described here [21,22] and will be referred to as COPE-Stress going forward. Participants also completed the Brief COPE questionnaire [25], which is an abbreviated form of the COPE (Coping Orientation to Problems Exposed) questionnaire [26]. This is a self-assessment of a wide range of coping behaviors including both maladaptive coping (includes substance use, venting, behavioral disengagement, denial, self-blame, and self-distraction) [27] and adaptive coping (includes humor, planning and seeking social support, use of emotional and instrumental support, positive reframing, religion, and acceptance) [26,28]. This questionnaire has been validated in multiple languages and cultural contexts to be correlated to perceived stress and mental well-being.

2.3. *Child Opportunity Index (COI)*

Neighborhood socio-economic environment (SEE) is a known modifier of overall maternal stress during pregnancy [29], pandemic related stress [30], and offspring outcomes [31]. Family income is often used to measure SEE. However, the quality of life associated with absolute income number varies regionally based on cost of living, social policies, environmental factors, etc. To overcome these limitations, we chose to represent SEE using childhood opportunity index (COI). COI is a multi-dimensional, nationally normed measure of the quality of social, environmental, health, and educational resources available at each zip code [32]. We extracted maternal COI using self-reported zip code at the time of the MRI visit and will be referred to as COI-SEE going forward.

2.4. *Image Acquisition*

Pregnant mothers were prospectively recruited between 24–38 GW and imaged on 3.0 T Philips Ingenia scanner (Philips Healthcare, Best, The Netherlands). Multiplanar single-shot turbo spin echo imaging was per-formed (TE = 160 ms, TR = 9000–12,000 ms, 3 mm slice thickness, no interslice gap, 1×1 mm in plane resolution). Fetal brains were scanned in each of three planes for three times resulting in nine images per subject and images were repeated if excessive motion was present. Echo-planar imaging (EPI) BOLD images were also collected with the following parameters: FOV = 300 mm TR = 2000 ms, TE = 31–35 ms (set to shortest), flip angle = 80°, with an in-plane resolution of 3×3 mm^2, slice thickness of 3.0 mm and 0.0 mm intra-slice gap. 150 timepoints were recorded for each BOLD image and two images were collected for each subject.

2.5. *Image Processing*

2.5.1. Brain Structure

All structural brain images were verified as being typical for gestational age by a board certified neuroradiologist (SP). For each subject, various 2D stacks of the T2 images were visually assessed to identify and discard stacks with large, spontaneous fetal motion. In each stack, the fetal brain was localized from surrounding tissue. For each subject, multiple 2D stacks were motion corrected and reconstructed, using a slice-to-volume reconstruction [33] into a 3D volumetric T2 image with an isotropic resolution of 1 mm^3. Reconstructed fetal brains were processed through a bespoke, automated fetal segmentation pipeline. Each fetal brain was normalized (affine followed by non-rigid) to a probabilistic atlas [34] of equivalent gestational age using Advanced Normalization tools [35]. Segmentations were manually inspected for accuracy and subjects with failed segmentations were discarded. The resulting segmentation maps were subsequently refined. To ensure consistency across different gestational ages, transient structures only present in the tissue atlas from 21–30 weeks of gestation such as the subplate, intermediate zone, and ventricular zone were combined with the corpus collosum and labeled as developing WM (WM). Cerebrospinal fluid (CSF) segmentation was refined as intra-ventricular (within lateral ventricles) and extra-axial CSF.

Due to the small size and relative difficulty in segmenting the hippocampus and amygdala, both structures were combined into a hippocampus-amygdala complex. Deep grey tissue was defined as the combination of the caudate, putamen, thalamus, fornix, internal capsule, subthalamic nucleus, and hippocampal commissure. Right and left hemispheric labels were combined into a single volume for each structure. The final segmentation yielded volumes of the following structures: cortical plate, developing white matter, intra-ventricular CSF, extra-axial CSF, deep gray tis-sues, cerebellum, hippocampal-amygdala complex, and brainstem. A total brain volume (TBV) was generated for each subject as the sum of all tissues.

2.5.2. Brain Function

BOLD imaging of the fetal brain is prone to spontaneous fetal motion which is compounded by lower signal to noise ratio and spatial resolution. While modern motion correction algorithms effectively attenuate the effects of subject motion on the temporal data, they are limited in effect beyond small degrees of motion. Any robust voxel-wise approach to functional fetal imaging would yield a prohibitively low number of subjects with usable data. We therefore chose to implement a whole-brain temporal signal approach to fetal functional imaging. Resting state images were first motion corrected using FSL's MCFLIRT routine, using the first frame as the registration target, and a mean framewise displacement threshold >0.2 mm to eliminate frames with excessive motion. As the intent of this study was to use minimally processed data using framewise measures, as opposed to voxel wise measures, we made no prior assumptions on physiological or nuisance frequency thresholds in fetal functional imaging and did not apply any bandpass filtering. A mean brain signal image was then generated by averaging across every frame in the sequence. This mean signal image was used as the source image for brain extraction to generate a brain mask. Brain extraction was done by using an adaptive routine that iterated between using FSL's Brain Extraction Tool (BET) [36] and AFNI's Skullstrip, using decreasingly smaller thresholds for brain tissue [37]. This approach yielded a good approximation of the fetal brain, with a minimal manual correction step required for final brain masking. The brain mask was then propagated across each frame in the temporal sequence to extract only fetal brain voxels.

Using the mask generated above, we averaged the whole brain BOLD signal in each frame and generated statistical measures across time. The measures generated were temporal mean (average of the mean signal across frames), temporal variability (average of the standard deviation of the signal across frames), variance of the mean (variance of the mean signal in each frame), kurtosis of the mean (kurtosis of the mean signal in each frame). Finally, to assess for any signal or physiological drift, we calculated the autocorrelation of the mean signal in each frame, and the kurtosis and autocorrelation of the normalized signal across frames.

2.6. Statistical Analysis

2.6.1. Brain Structure

Regression analysis was performed in Python (3.7) using the Statsmodel.api v0.13.2. We used multiple, linear regression to model the relationship of COPE-Stress Score, COI-SEE, and their interaction on TBV after adjusting for gestational age at MRI. Nested models of the covariates without interaction were also evaluated. Models were deemed to be significant if one or more of the covariates were statistically significant, and models including the interaction term were only selected over the simpler counterpart if they had a higher explained variance (R-squared) and/or lower Bayes' Information Criteria (BIC). Using similar regression models, we individually assessed the relationship of COPE-Stress score and COI-SEE for each tissue volume listed in Section 2.5.1 (as a dependent variable). Secondarily, we also evaluated the relationship of COPE-Stress score and COI-SEE on tissue volumes normalized by TBV after adjusting for gestational age.

2.6.2. Brain Function

Statistical analysis for brain functional metrics was similar to Section 2.5.1. A separate regression model was evaluated for each, individual functional metric (Section 2.5.2) with COPE Stress, COI-SEE, and their interaction as predictor variables after accounting for GA at MRI.

2.6.3. Comparison of Coping Behaviors

Coping behaviors, both the Brief-COPE and COVID specific, were analyzed for differences between low and high stress mothers. Mothers were split into low, medium, and high stress categories based on tertiles of COVID Stress scores. Using Fischer Exact test, we compared if mothers reporting low and high stress used each coping behavior at significantly different amounts.

3. Results

3.1. Subject Demographics

Pregnant mothers were recruited prospectively for this study with a total of 45 mother-fetus dyads completed the MR imaging session. Three subjects had missing zip code information, and which resulted in missing COI-SEE data and was thus excluded from any analysis. After imaging, three subjects failed brain segmentation resulting in 39 subjects for structural regression results. A total of 43 subjects of the original 45 subjects had analyzable BOLD imaging and were used for the functional regression results (Table 1).

Table 1. Study participants' demographic information.

Characteristic	Total	Range/Percentage of Total
Total Participants	45	
Sex of fetus	18	
Female	18	40%
Male	20	44.5%
Unknown	7	15.5%
	45	
Total MRI's		
GA, median (range), wk.		
At MRI	31.57	(22.57 to 38.42)
At Birth	39.14	(33 to 41.86)
Maternal age at MRI, median, yr.	32	(18 to 43)
Maternal parity		
Primiparous	18	40%
Multiparous	22	49%
Unknown	5	11%
Infant Weight, median, kg	3.54	
Caucasian	8	18%
Hispanic or Latino	28	62%
Asian/Pacific Islander	7	16%
African American	1	2%
Middle Eastern	0	
Other or unknown	1	2%

3.2. Brain Structure

There were no significant associations between absolute volumes of the various brain structures and perceived maternal stress, COI-SEE, or their interaction (Table 2). However, there was a significant positive association between normalized brain stem volume and perceived maternal stress ($p = 0.03$) but not with COI-SEE and the interaction of COI-SEE and maternal stress (Table 3) There were no significant associations between normalized volumes of other structures with COPE-Stress or COI-SEE.

Table 2. Raw brain structure volumes relationship to COVID stress and COI-SEE.

Volume (cm^3)	COVID Stress Score		COI Nationally Normed Value		COI Stress Interaction	
	β (CI)	*p*-Value	β (CI)	*p*-Value	β (CI)	*p*-Value
Brainstem	3.89×10^0, (-7.62×10^1, 8.40×10^1)	0.97	-2.81×10^{-1}, (-1.41×10^1, 1.35×10^1)	0.99	4.06×10^{-1}, (-1.18×10^0, 1.99×10^0)	0.86
Cerebellum	1.54×10^2, (-4.84×10^1, 3.56×10^2)	0.61	3.28×10^1, (4.13×10^{-1}, 6.52×10^1)	0.49	-1.95×10^0, (-5.79×10^0, 1.89×10^0)	0.73
Cortical Plate	-7.33×10^2, (-1.35×10^3, -1.18×10^2)	0.42	-3.78×10^0, (-1.59×10^2, 1.52×10^2)	0.99	1.23×10^1, (-1.43×10^0, 2.60×10^1)	0.55
Deep Grey	1.93×10^1, (-1.83×10^2, 2.22×10^2)	0.95	2.76×10^0, (-3.17×10^1, 3.73×10^1)	0.96	1.65×10^0, (-2.28×10^0, 5.58×10^0)	0.78
Extra Axial CSF	-7.29×10^2, (-1.74×10^3, 2.81×10^2)	0.63	-9.28×10^1, (-3.06×10^2, 1.21×10^2)	0.77	1.76×10^1, (-5.28×10^0, 4.04×10^1)	0.60
Hippocampus amygdala complex	-1.31×10^0, (-2.72×10^1, 2.46×10^1)	0.97	-7.62×10^{-1}, (-6.21×10^0, 4.69×10^0)	0.92	2.17×10^{-1}, (-3.33×10^{-1}, 7.68×10^{-1})	0.79
Intra ventricular CSF	2.59×10^1, (-7.98×10^1, 1.32×10^2)	0.87	1.23×10^1, (-1.15×10^1, 3.60×10^1)	0.73	-5.07×10^{-1}, (-2.81×10^0, 1.79×10^0)	0.88
White Matter	-5.17×10^2, (-1.69×10^3, 6.58×10^2)	0.77	-8.47×10^1, (-2.99×10^2, 1.30×10^2)	0.79	1.19×10^1, (-1.25×10^1, 3.63×10^1)	0.74
Total Brain Volume	-2.51×10^3, (-6.81×10^3, 1.80×10^3)	0.69	-2.27×10^2, (-1.05×10^3, 5.96×10^2)	0.85	5.92×10^1, (-3.03×10^1, 1.49×10^2)	0.66

Table 3. Brain structure volumes', after normalization to total brain volume, relationship to COVID stress, COI-SEE, and their interaction. * denotes statistically significant relationships.

Volume Normalized by Total Brain Volume	COVID Stress		Overall COI by Zip Code		COVID Stress and COI Interaction	
	β (CI)	*p*-Value	β (CI)	*p*-Value	β (CI)	*p*-Value
Brainstem	1.30×10^{-4}, (9.00×10^{-5}, 1.70×10^{-4})	**0.03** *	1.00×10^{-5}, (0.00×10^0, 2.00×10^{-5})	0.65	0.00×10^0, (0.00×10^0, 0.00×10^0)	0.31
Cerebellum	3.40×10^{-4}, (1.50×10^{-4}, 5.40×10^{-4})	0.24	7.00×10^{-5}, (4.00×10^{-5}, 1.10×10^{-4})	0.12	-1.00×10^{-5}, (-1.00×10^{-5}, 0.00×10^0)	0.26

Table 3. *Cont.*

Volume Normalized by Total Brain Volume	COVID Stress		Overall COI by Zip Code		COVID Stress and COI Interaction	
	β (CI)	*p*-Value	β (CI)	*p*-Value	β (CI)	*p*-Value
Cortical Plate	-1.42×10^{-3}, $(-2.10 \times 10^{-3}$, $-7.40 \times 10^{-4})$	0.16	-1.00×10^{-5}, $(-2.20 \times 10^{-4}$, $2.00 \times 10^{-4})$	0.97	1.00×10^{-5}, $(-1.00 \times 10^{-5}$, $3.00 \times 10^{-5})$	0.64
Deep Grey	1.90×10^{-4}, $(3.00 \times 10^{-5}$, $3.60 \times 10^{-4})$	0.42	2.00×10^{-5}, $(-3.00 \times 10^{-5}$, $6.00 \times 10^{-5})$	0.82	0.00×10^{0}, $(0.00 \times 10^{0}$, $1.00 \times 10^{-5})$	0.90
Extra Axial CSF	1.10×10^{-4}, $(-7.00 \times 10^{-5}$, $2.80 \times 10^{-4})$	0.68	-5.00×10^{-5}, $(-1.20 \times 10^{-4}$, $2.00 \times 10^{-5})$	0.61	0.00×10^{0}, $(0.00 \times 10^{0}$, $1.00 \times 10^{-5})$	0.60
Hippocampus amygdala complex	4.00×10^{-5}, $(2.00 \times 10^{-5}$, $6.00 \times 10^{-5})$	0.22	0.00×10^{0}, $(-1.00 \times 10^{-5}$, $1.00 \times 10^{-5})$	0.94	0.00×10^{0}, $(0.00 \times 10^{0}$, $0.00 \times 10^{0})$	0.99
Intra ventricular CSF	1.20×10^{-4}, $(-4.00 \times 10^{-5}$, $2.80 \times 10^{-4})$	0.61	5.00×10^{-5}, $(-1.00 \times 10^{-5}$, $1.00 \times 10^{-4})$	0.55	0.00×10^{0}, $(-1.00 \times 10^{-5}$, $0.00 \times 10^{0})$	0.64
White Matter	3.80×10^{-4}, $(-1.60 \times 10^{-4}$, $9.20 \times 10^{-4})$	0.63	-3.00×10^{-5}, $(-1.80 \times 10^{-4}$, $1.20 \times 10^{-4})$	0.89	-1.00×10^{-5}, $(-3.00 \times 10^{-5}$, $0.00 \times 10^{0})$	0.62

3.3. Brain Function

Lack of significant relationship between autocorrelation metrics and the predictor variable confirmed the absence of any systematic signal or physiological drifts. We found a significant negative relationship between temporal variability and COPE Stress ($p < 0.028$) (Table 4). The temporal variability model including the interaction term between Cope Stress Score and COI SES had a slightly improved R-squared (0.267) but lower BIC and reduced statistical significance of the covariates, likely due to co-linearity. We there-fore report the original model without the interaction term. We found no other statistically significant relationships between fetal brain functional characteristics with COPE Stress or COI SEE.

Table 4. Brain functional metrics' relationship to COVID stress and COI-SEE using linear modeling. * denotes statistically significant relationships.

	COVID Stress		Overall COI by Zip Code	
	β (CI)	*p*-Value	β (CI)	*p*-Value
Temporal mean of BOLD Signal	135.369, (−509.52, 38.1)	0.09	316.9634, (−604.97, 1238.9)	0.49
Temporal variability of BOLD Signal	−113.94, (−215.18, −12. 71)	**0.03 ***	−19.5173, (−360.388, 321.354)	0.91
Variance of framewise mean BOLD signal	$-5336.81, (-2.87 \times 10^{4}, 1.81 \times 10^{4})$	0.65	$-5191.57, (-8.4 \times 10^{4}, 7.36 \times 10^{4})$	0.9
Kurtosis of framewise mean BOLD signal	0.329, (−0.144, 0.802)	0.17	0.457, (−1.135, 2.049)	0.57
Autocorrelation of framewise mean BOLD	$-6.828 \times 10^{6}, (-1.41 \times 10^{7}, 4.89 \times 10^{5})$	0.07	$1.005 \times 10^{7}, (-1.46 \times 10^{7}, 3.47 \times 10^{7})$	0.41

3.4. Comparison of Coping Behaviors

We compared coping behaviors between participants reporting high and low stress in our cohort. Figure 1 shows the prevalence of use of various coping behaviors, reported as percentage of total, among the participant in the study. Humor (p-value = 0.025) and venting (*p*-value = 0.048) were used more commonly by participants reporting low stress compared to those reporting high stress (Figure 1). We observed differential patterns of coping behavior use among mothers who reported high and low stress. Figure 2 shows, self-reported importance levels of potential resources for management of stress associated with COVID-19 related disruptions among pregnant women in the study. Access to a mental health provider (*p*-value = 0.038), and information about how to reduce stress (*p*-value = 0.038) were chosen as being 'Very Important' to women reporting low stress at a high amount than in women reporting high stress (Figure 2). No other behaviors were found to be significantly different between high and low stress mothers. A full summary of the results can be seen in Figures 1 and 2.

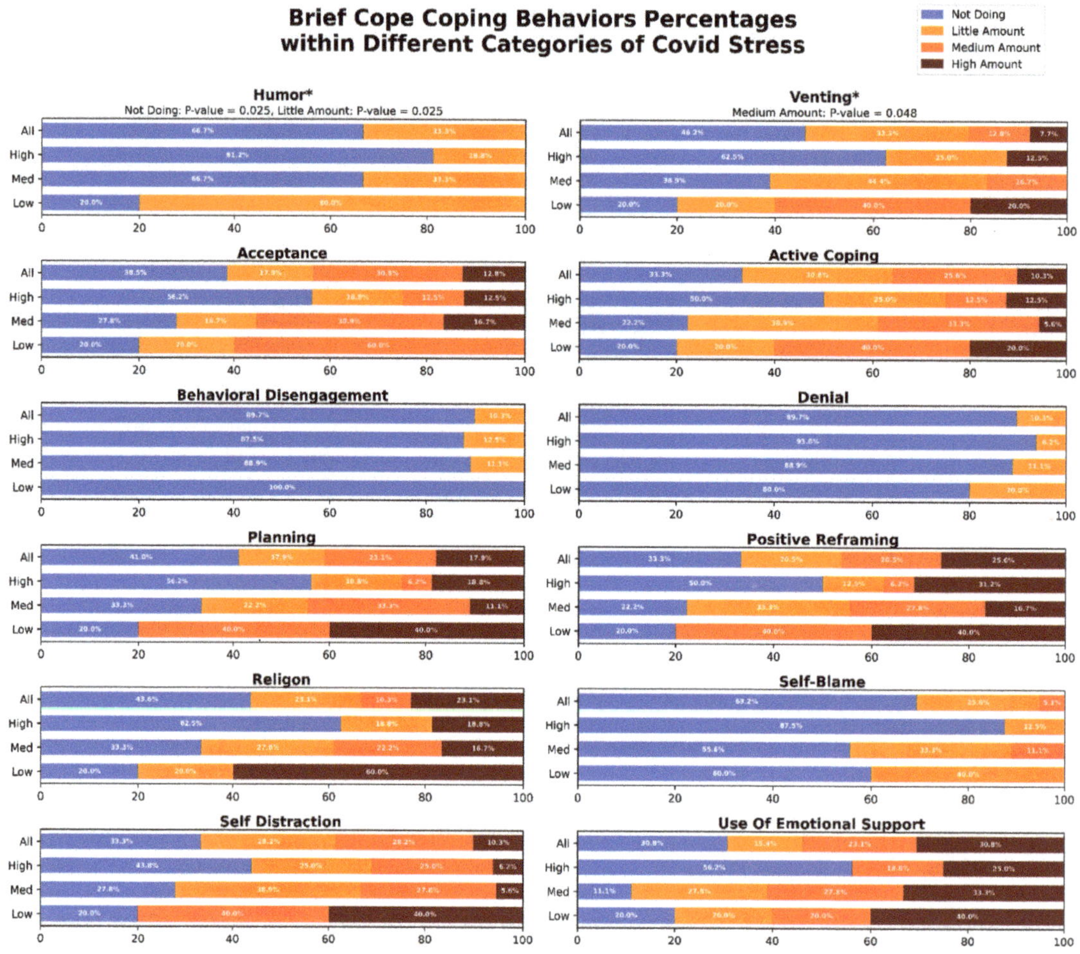

Figure 1. Prevalence of use of various subscales of coping behaviors within pregnant women in the study. The first row for each subscale represents the entire cohort. The second, third, and fourth rows correspond to prevalence of coping behaviors in participants reporting high, medium, and low COVID-19 related stress. * Denotes subscales with significantly different prevalence of use between mothers reporting high and low stress levels.

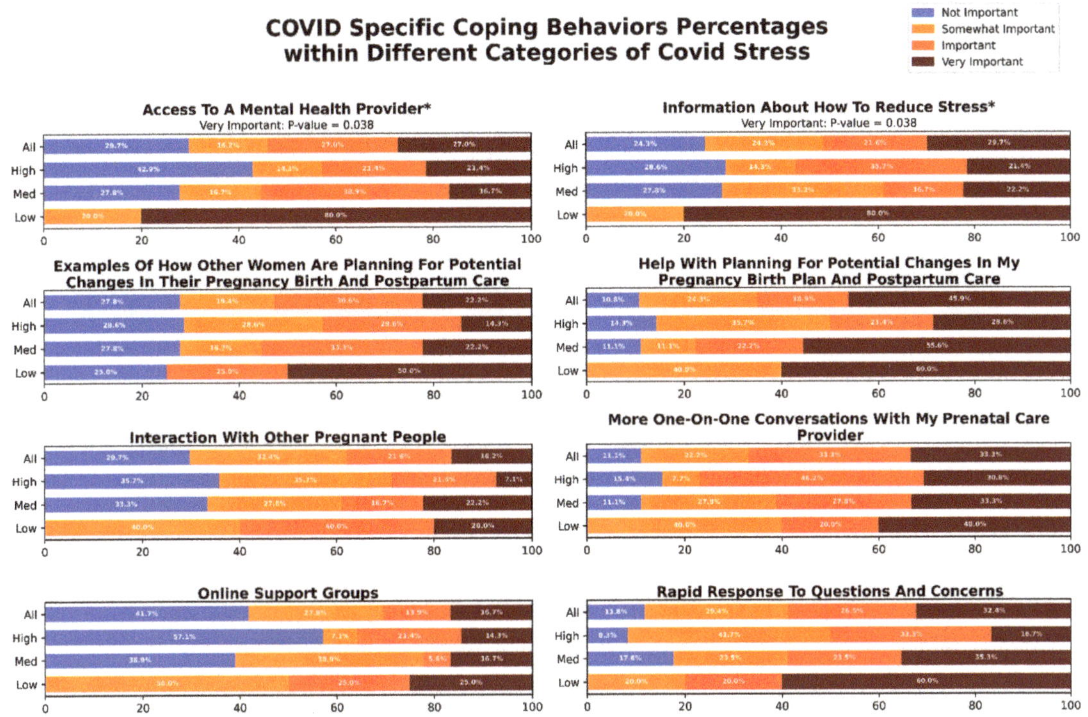

Figure 2. Self-reported importance of potential resources for management of stress associated with COVID-19 related disruptions among pregnant women in the study. The first row for each subscale represents the entire cohort. The second, third, and fourth rows correspond to prevalence of coping behaviors in participants reporting high, medium, and low COVID-19 related stress. * Denotes subscales with significantly different prevalence of use between mothers reporting high and low stress levels.

4. Discussion

Our findings show that perceived maternal stress, in the setting of COVID-19 related care disruptions, impacts with structural and functional developmental of the fetal brain. Higher maternal stress was associated with increased brainstem volume (suggesting accelerated brainstem maturation) and globally decreased temporal variability of function (suggesting reduced functional connectivity) in the fetal brain. Additionally, we also found differences in the prevalence of specific coping behaviors between pregnant women who reported high stress compared to those who reported low stress. Our study is novel in the following aspects: (1) use multi-modal imaging to characterize fetal brain developmental changes due to maternal stress during COVID, and (2) characterization of adaptive coping behaviors which may provide resilience during this period of increased maternal stress.

We found that increased levels of maternal stress correlated with increased normalized brainstem volume suggesting relatively increased acceleration of brainstem maturation relative to cortical/supratentorial cerebral regions. Importantly, these results are consistent with prior studies that have correlated prenatal maternal stress and neonatal brainstem auditory evoked potentials (the speed at which the brainstem auditory evoked potential is conducted through the auditory nerve serves as a proxy for greater neural maturation) [38,39]. These studies have found significant relations between higher maternal prenatal distress and faster conductance, suggesting that greater maternal prenatal stress is associated with accelerated subcortical/brainstem neural maturation in neonates [40]. Our results are also consistent with the recent study by De Asis-Cruz et al. [41] which found that altered functional connectivity between brainstem and sensorimotor regionals were associated with high maternal anxiety scores.

We found that higher perceived maternal stress was associated with lower temporal variability in the fetal brain suggesting aberrations to foundational characteristics of connectivity and organization of emerging brain networks [42]. It has been well-established that perturbations to early brain connectivity architecture, during the critical fetal period, has long-standing effects on behavioral and psychiatric development among these children [43–45]. Altered temporal variability of brain BOLD are known to associated with adverse neurocognitive functioning of the brain [46–48]. Our findings of altered brain connectivity agree with previous findings of altered brain connectivity in infants of mothers who reported higher stress during the pandemic [15]. Behavioral and functional deficits particularly in the motor, cognitive and temperamental domain have been widely reported in various studies investigating the impact of maternal stress during the pandemic on child outcomes [7,8,13,14]. Increased maternal stress and anxiety traits (outside the setting of the pandemic) have been shown to alter functional architecture of the fetal brain [49]. Collectively, our and prior findings suggest that in utero alterations to brain architecture, associated with maternal stress during the pandemic, could underlie developmental deficits reported in these children. Further meta studies are needed to investigate the trajectory of brain development in children conceived and born during the pandemic.

Our findings suggest key differences in coping behaviors between pregnant women who reported low and high stress. Increased use of adaptive coping behaviors (particularly humor and venting) was more common among pregnant women who reported lower stress compared to those who reported higher stress. This association between in-creased use of adaptive, active coping and lower stress perception was reported across multiple studies of mental health in peripartum women during COVID-19 pandemic [21,50,51]. Our findings are also in agreement with generalized findings of positive relationship between active coping behaviors and improved mental well-being in pregnant women [52]. In questions regarding COVID-19 specific coping behaviors, pregnant mothers reporting low stress endorsed access to mental health information and providers as being key to wellness. Routine screening for prenatal stress, provision of stress management information, and improved access to prenatal mental health care provide potential avenues for improving mental health and associated outcomes in pregnant women regardless of pandemic conditions.

This study's limitations include small sample size and recruitment limited to a single geographical area in the USA during the pandemic. Since the greater Los Angeles area was disproportionately affected by pandemic related disruptions, comparison to a multi-site cohort will provide greater statistical power thereby increasing the generalizability of our findings. The cross-sectional nature of prenatal stress assessment limits our ability to associate time-varying stress levels and fetal outcomes. However, all participating women became pregnant after pandemic-related restrictions were put in place. Lack of a pre-pandemic cohort limits our ability to pin-point if the differences in coping behaviors between pregnant women reporting low and high stress are specific adaptations to stress experienced during the pandemic. Consistent with the demographics of Los Angeles County, over 50% of the pregnant women in our study cohort identified as Hispanic. Cultural norms around coping behaviors, care and family support during pregnancy or postpartum periods should be factored into the interpretation of our findings. Future work could examine if disparities in healthcare utilization have been altered during the pandemic among pregnant women from diverse backgrounds [53,54].

5. Conclusions

Here, we reported the first multi-modal study of the impact of COVID-19 pandemic related maternal stress on fetal brain development. Our findings showed that increased maternal stress due to pandemic related disruptions was associated with structural and functional disruptions to fetal brain development and is suggestive of altered fetal programming. Comparing coping behaviors between pregnant women reporting higher and lower stress, our study provides insight into potential avenues for improved stress management and mental health outcomes among pregnant women.

Author Contributions: Conceptualization, V.R., R.C. and W.T.R.; methodology, V.R., R.C. and W.T.R.; validation, R.C., S.P. and W.T.R.; resources, V.R.; data curation, V.R., J.Z. and J.L.; writing—original draft preparation, V.R., R.C., W.T.R. and J.Z.; writing—review and editing, V.R., W.T.R., J.Z., J.W., R.C., S.P., J.W. and A.P.; visualization, V.R., R.C., W.T.R. and J.Z.; supervision, A.P. and V.R.; funding acquisition, V.R. and A.P. All authors have read and agreed to the published version of the manuscript.

Funding: This work was funded NIH/NHLBI K01HL153942 and The Saban Research Institute's Research Career Development Award to VR. Funding for WR was provided by the National Library of Medicine T15 Training program grant; award number 2T15LM007059-36. AP reported receiving grants from the Department of Defense (W81XWH-16-1-0613), the National Heart, Lung, and Blood Institute (R01 HL152740-1, R01 HL128818-05), and Additional Ventures.

Institutional Review Board Statement: The study was conducted in accordance with the Declaration of Helsinki and approved by the Institutional Review Board (or Ethics Committee) of Children's Hospital Los Angeles (protocol code CHLA-17-00292 and 9/14/2017).

Informed Consent Statement: Any research article describing a study involving humans Written informed consent to include deidentified data has been obtained from the patient(s) to publish this paper.

Data Availability Statement: Due to limitations of informed consent, data from the study cannot be shared. However, Methodologies and techniques from the study will be made available via direct email to the corresponding author.

Acknowledgments: We would like to acknowledge all the women and families who participated in the study during an unprecedented global pandemic. We would like to thank Rosa Rangel, Teddy Aguilar, and Veronica Gonzalez for their help with the study.

Conflicts of Interest: The authors declare no conflict of interest. The funders had no role in the design of the study; in the collection, analyses, or interpretation of data; in the writing of the manuscript; or in the decision to publish the results.

References

1. Zhou, J.; Havens, K.L.; Starnes, C.P.; Pickering, T.A.; Brito, N.H.; Hendrix, C.L.; Thomason, M.E.; Vatalaro, T.C.; Smith, B.A. Changes in Social Support of Pregnant and Postnatal Mothers during the COVID-19 Pandemic. *Midwifery* **2021**, *103*, 103162. [CrossRef] [PubMed]
2. Barbosa-Leiker, C.; Smith, C.L.; Crespi, E.J.; Brooks, O.; Burduli, E.; Ranjo, S.; Carty, C.L.; Hebert, L.E.; Waters, S.F.; Gartstein, M.A. Stressors, Coping, and Resources Needed during the COVID-19 Pandemic in a Sample of Perinatal Women. *BMC Pregnancy Childbirth* **2021**, *21*, 1–13. [CrossRef] [PubMed]
3. Shorey, S.; Chee, C.Y.I.; Ng, E.D.; Chan, Y.H.; Tam, W.W.S.; Chong, Y.S. Prevalence and Incidence of Postpartum Depression among Healthy Mothers: A Systematic Review and Meta-Analysis. *J. Psychiatr. Res.* **2018**, *104*, 235–248. [CrossRef] [PubMed]
4. King, S.; Dancause, K.; Turcotte-Tremblay, A.M.; Veru, F.; Laplante, D.P. Using Natural Disasters to Study the Effects of Prenatal Maternal Stress on Child Health and Development. *Birth Defects Res. C Embryo Today* **2012**, *96*, 273–288. [CrossRef] [PubMed]
5. Salm Ward, T.; Kanu, F.A.; Robb, S.W. Prevalence of Stressful Life Events during Pregnancy and Its Association with Postpartum Depressive Symptoms. *Arch. Womens Ment. Health* **2017**, *20*, 161–171. [CrossRef]
6. Motrico, E.; Domínguez-Salas, S.; Rodríguez-Domínguez, C.; Gómez-Gómez, I.; Rodríguez-Muñoz, M.F.; Gómez-Baya, D. The Impact of the COVID-19 Pandemic on Perinatal Depression and Anxiety: A Large Cross-Sectional Study in Spain. *Psicothema* **2022**, *34*, 200–208. [CrossRef]
7. Bianco, C.; Sania, A.; Kyle, M.H.; Beebe, B.; Barbosa, J.; Bence, M.; Coskun, L.; Fields, A.; Firestein, M.R.; Goldman, S.; et al. Pandemic beyond the Virus: Maternal COVID-Related Postnatal Stress Is Associated with Infant Temperament. *Pediatric Res.* **2022**, *2022*, 1–7. [CrossRef]
8. Shuffrey, L.C.; Firestein, M.R.; Kyle, M.H.; Fields, A.; Alcántara, C.; Amso, D.; Austin, J.; Bain, J.M.; Barbosa, J.; Bence, M.; et al. Association of Birth During the COVID-19 Pandemic With Neurodevelopmental Status at 6 Months in Infants with and without In Utero Exposure to Maternal SARS-CoV-2 Infection. *JAMA Pediatr.* **2022**, *176*, e215563. [CrossRef]
9. Schuurmans, C.; Kurrasch, D.M. Neurodevelopmental Consequences of Maternal Distress: What Do We Really Know? *Clin. Genet.* **2013**, *83*, 108–117. [CrossRef]
10. Talge, N.M.; Neal, C.; Glover, V. Antenatal Maternal Stress and Long-Term Effects on Child Neurodevelopment: How and Why? *J. Child Psychol. Psychiatry* **2007**, *48*, 245–261. [CrossRef]

11. Wu, Y.; Lu, Y.C.; Jacobs, M.; Pradhan, S.; Kapse, K.; Zhao, L.; Niforatos-Andescavage, N.; Vezina, G.; du Plessis, A.J.; Limperopoulos, C. Association of Prenatal Maternal Psychological Distress with Fetal Brain Growth, Metabolism, and Cortical Maturation. *JAMA Netw. Open* **2020**, *3*, e1919940. [CrossRef] [PubMed]
12. van den Heuvel, M.I.; Hect, J.L.; Smarr, B.L.; Qawasmeh, T.; Kriegsfeld, L.J.; Barcelona, J.; Hijazi, K.E.; Thomason, M.E. Maternal Stress during Pregnancy Alters Fetal Cortico-Cerebellar Connectivity in Utero and Increases Child Sleep Problems after Birth. *Sci. Rep.* **2021**, *11*, 2228. [CrossRef] [PubMed]
13. Griffin, M.; Ghassabian, A.; Majbri, A.; Brubaker, S.G.; Thomason, M. Evaluating the Association between Maternal Peripartum Care Interruptions and Infant Affect: A Longitudinal Study. *Am. J. Obstet. Gynecol.* **2022**, *226*, S310. [CrossRef]
14. Provenzi, L.; Grumi, S.; Altieri, L.; Bensi, G.; Bertazzoli, E.; Biasucci, G.; Cavallini, A.; Decembrino, L.; Falcone, R.; Freddi, A.; et al. Prenatal Maternal Stress during the COVID-19 Pandemic and Infant Regulatory Capacity at 3 Months: A Longitudinal Study. *Dev. Psychopathol.* **2021**, 1–9. [CrossRef] [PubMed]
15. Manning, K.Y.; Long, X.; Watts, D.; Tomfohr-Madsen, L.; Giesbrecht, G.F.; Lebel, C. Prenatal Maternal Distress During the COVID-19 Pandemic and Associations with Infant Brain Connectivity. *Biol. Psychiatry* **2022**, *92*, 701–708. [CrossRef] [PubMed]
16. Lu, Y.-C.; Andescavage, N.; Wu, Y.; Kapse, K.; Andersen, N.R.; Quistorff, J.; Saeed, H.; Lopez, C.; Henderson, D.; Barnett, S.D.; et al. Maternal Psychological Distress during the COVID-19 Pandemic and Structural Changes of the Human Fetal Brain. *Commun. Med.* **2022**, *2*, 47. [CrossRef]
17. Varescon, I.; Leignel, S.; Poulain, X.; Gerard, C. Coping Strategies and Perceived Stress in Pregnant Smokers Seeking Help for Cessation. *J. Smok. Cessat.* **2011**, *6*, 126–132. [CrossRef]
18. Razurel, C.; Kaiser, B.; Sellenet, C.; Epiney, M. Relation between Perceived Stress, Social Support, and Coping Strategies and Maternal Well-Being: A Review of the Literature. *Women Health* **2013**, *53*, 74–99. [CrossRef]
19. Rimal, S.P.; Thapa, K.; Shrestha, R. Psychological Distress and Coping among Pregnant Women during the COVID 19 Pandemic. *J. Nepal Health Res. Counc.* **2022**, *20*, 234–240. [CrossRef]
20. Kinser, P.A.; Jallo, N.; Amstadter, A.B.; Thacker, L.R.; Jones, E.; Moyer, S.; Rider, A.; Karjane, N.; Salisbury, A.L. Depression, Anxiety, Resilience, and Coping: The Experience of Pregnant and New Mothers during the First Few Months of the COVID-19 Pandemic. *J. Womens Health* **2021**, *30*, 654–664. [CrossRef]
21. Werchan, D.M.; Hendrix, C.L.; Ablow, J.C.; Amstadter, A.B.; Austin, A.C.; Babineau, V.; Anne Bogat, G.; Cioffredi, L.A.; Conradt, E.; Crowell, S.E.; et al. Behavioral Coping Phenotypes and Associated Psychosocial Outcomes of Pregnant and Postpartum Women during the COVID-19 Pandemic. *Sci. Rep.* **2022**, *12*, 1209. [CrossRef] [PubMed]
22. Thomason, M.; Graham, A.; Sullivan, E.; van den Heuvel, M.I. COVID-19 and Perinatal Experiences Study. Available online: https://osf.io/uqhcv/ (accessed on 28 August 2022).
23. Brief Symptom Inventory—PsycNET. Available online: https://psycnet.apa.org/doiLanding?doi=10.1037%2Ft00789-000 (accessed on 16 September 2022).
24. Blevins, C.A.; Weathers, F.W.; Davis, M.T.; Witte, T.K.; Domino, J.L. The Posttraumatic Stress Disorder Checklist for DSM-5 (PCL-5): Development and Initial Psychometric Evaluation. *J. Trauma. Stress* **2015**, *28*, 489–498. [CrossRef] [PubMed]
25. Carver, C.S. You Want to Measure Coping but Your Protocol's Too Long: Consider the Brief COPE. *Int. J. Behav. Med.* **1997**, *4*, 92–100. [CrossRef] [PubMed]
26. Carver, C.S.; Scheier, M.F.; Weintraub, J.K. Assessing Coping Strategies: A Theoretically Based Approach. *J. Pers. Soc. Psychol.* **1989**, *56*, 267–283. [CrossRef] [PubMed]
27. Connor-Smith, J.K.; Flachsbart, C. Relations between Personality and Coping: A Meta-Analysis. *J. Pers. Soc. Psychol.* **2007**, *93*, 1080–1107. [CrossRef]
28. García, F.E.; Barraza-Peña, C.G.; Wlodarczyk, A.; Alvear-Carrasco, M.; Reyes-Reyes, A. Psychometric Properties of the Brief-COPE for the Evaluation of Coping Strategies in the Chilean Population. *Psicol. Reflex. Crit.* **2018**, *31*, 1–11. [CrossRef]
29. Lefmann, T.; Combs-Orme, T. Prenatal Stress, Poverty, and Child Outcomes. *Child Adolesc. Soc. Work J.* **2014**, *31*, 577–590. [CrossRef]
30. Silverman, M.E.; Medeiros, C.; Burgos, L. Early Pregnancy Mood before and during COVID-19 Community Restrictions among Women of Low Socioeconomic Status in New York City: A Preliminary Study. *Arch. Womens Ment. Health* **2020**, *23*, 779. [CrossRef]
31. Sandel, M.; Faugno, E.; Mingo, A.; Cannon, J.; Byrd, K.; Garcia, D.A.; Collier, S.; McClure, E.; Jarrett, R.B. Neighborhood-Level Interventions to Improve Childhood Opportunity and Lift Children out of Poverty. *Acad. Pediatr.* **2016**, *16*, S128–S135. [CrossRef]
32. Acevedo-Garcia, D.; McArdle, N.; Hardy, E.F.; Crisan, U.I.; Romano, B.; Norris, D.; Baek, M.; Reece, J. The Child Opportunity Index: Improving Collaboration between Community Development and Public Health. *Health Aff.* **2014**, *33*, 1948–1957. [CrossRef]
33. Ebner, M.; Wang, G.; Li, W.; Aertsen, M.; Patel, P.A.; Aughwane, R.; Melbourne, A.; Doel, T.; Dymarkowski, S.; de Coppi, P.; et al. An Automated Framework for Localization, Segmentation and Super-Resolution Reconstruction of Fetal Brain MRI. *Neuroimage* **2020**, *206*, 116324. [CrossRef] [PubMed]
34. Gholipour, A.; Rollins, C.K.; Velasco-Annis, C.; Ouaalam, A.; Akhondi-Asl, A.; Afacan, O.; Ortinau, C.M.; Clancy, S.; Limperopoulos, C.; Yang, E.; et al. A Normative Spatiotemporal MRI Atlas of the Fetal Brain for Automatic Segmentation and Analysis of Early Brain Growth. *Sci. Rep.* **2017**, *7*, 476. [CrossRef] [PubMed]
35. Avants, B.B.; Tustison, N.J.; Song, G.; Cook, P.A.; Klein, A.; Gee, J.C. A Reproducible Evaluation of ANTs Similarity Metric Performance in Brain Image Registration. *Neuroimage* **2011**, *54*, 2033–2044. [CrossRef] [PubMed]
36. Smith, S.M. Fast Robust Automated Brain Extraction. *Hum. Brain Mapp.* **2002**, *17*, 143–155. [CrossRef]

37. Cox, R.W. AFNI: Software for Analysis and Visualization of Functional Magnetic Resonance Neuroimages. *Comput. Biomed. Res.* **1996**, *29*, 162–173. [CrossRef] [PubMed]
38. Amin, S.B.; Orlando, M.S.; Dalzell, L.E.; Merle, K.S.; Guillet, R. Morphological Changes in Serial Auditory Brain Stem Responses in 24 to 32 Weeks' Gestational Age Infants during the First Week of Life. *Ear Hear.* **1999**, *20*, 410–418. [CrossRef]
39. Jiang, Z.D.; Xiu, X.; Brosi, D.M.; Shao, X.M.; Wilkinson, A.R. Sub-Optimal Function of the Auditory Brainstem in Term Infants with Transient Low Apgar Scores. *Clin. Neurophysiol.* **2007**, *118*, 1088–1096. [CrossRef]
40. DiPietro, J.A.; Kivlighan, K.T.; Costigan, K.A.; Rubin, S.E.; Shiffler, D.E.; Henderson, J.L.; Pillion, J.P. Prenatal Antecedents of Newborn Neurological Maturation. *Child Dev.* **2010**, *81*, 115. [CrossRef]
41. de Asis-Cruz, J.; Krishnamurthy, D.; Zhao, L.; Kapse, K.; Vezina, G.; Andescavage, N.; Quistorff, J.; Lopez, C.; Limperopoulos, C. Association of Prenatal Maternal Anxiety with Fetal Regional Brain Connectivity. *JAMA Netw. Open* **2020**, *3*, e2022349. [CrossRef]
42. Garrett, D.D.; Kovacevic, N.; McIntosh, A.R.; Grady, C.L. The Importance of Being Variable. *J. Neurosci.* **2011**, *31*, 4496–4503. [CrossRef]
43. Rogers, C.E.; Lean, R.E.; Wheelock, M.D.; Smyser, C.D. Aberrant Structural and Functional Connectivity and Neurodevelopmental Impairment in Preterm Children. *J. Neurodev. Disord.* **2018**, *10*, 38. [CrossRef] [PubMed]
44. Evans, T.M.; Kochalka, J.; Ngoon, T.J.; Wu, S.S.; Qin, S.; Battista, C.; Menon, V. Brain Structural Integrity and Intrinsic Functional Connectivity Forecast 6 Year Longitudinal Growth in Children's Numerical Abilities. *J. Neurosci.* **2015**, *35*, 11743–11750. [CrossRef] [PubMed]
45. Barch, D.M.; Belden, A.C.; Tillman, R.; Whalen, D.; Luby, J.L. Early Childhood Adverse Experiences, Inferior Frontal Gyrus Connectivity, and the Trajectory of Externalizing Psychopathology. *J. Am. Acad. Child Adolesc. Psychiatry* **2018**, *57*, 183–190. [CrossRef] [PubMed]
46. Yang, S.; Zhao, Z.; Cui, H.; Zhang, T.; Zhao, L.; He, Z.; Liu, H.; Guo, L.; Liu, T.; Becker, B.; et al. Temporal Variability of Cortical Gyral-Sulcal Resting State Functional Activity Correlates with Fluid Intelligence. *Front. Neural Circuits* **2019**, *13*, 36. [CrossRef] [PubMed]
47. Stevens, W.D.; Spreng, R.N. Resting-State Functional Connectivity MRI Reveals Active Processes Central to Cognition. *Wiley Interdiscip. Rev. Cogn. Sci.* **2014**, *5*, 233–245. [CrossRef]
48. Vidaurre, D.; Llera, A.; Smith, S.M.; Woolrich, M.W. Behavioural Relevance of Spontaneous, Transient Brain Network Interactions in FMRI. *Neuroimage* **2021**, *229*, 117713. [CrossRef]
49. Thomason, M.E.; Hect, J.L.; Waller, R.; Curtin, P. Interactive Relations between Maternal Prenatal Stress, Fetal Brain Connectivity, and Gestational Age at Delivery. *Neuropsychopharmacology* **2021**, *46*, 1839–1847. [CrossRef]
50. Han, L.; Bai, H.; Lun, B.; Li, Y.; Wang, Y.; Ni, Q. The Prevalence of Fear of Childbirth and Its Association with Intolerance of Uncertainty and Coping Styles among Pregnant Chinese Women during the COVID-19 Pandemic. *Front. Psychiatry* **2022**, *13*, 935760. [CrossRef]
51. Anderson, M.R.; Salisbury, A.L.; Uebelacker, L.A.; Abrantes, A.M.; Battle, C.L. Stress, Coping and Silver Linings: How Depressed Perinatal Women Experienced the COVID-19 Pandemic. *J. Affect. Disord.* **2022**, *298*, 329–336. [CrossRef]
52. Giurgescu, C.; Penckofer, S.; Maurer, M.C.; Bryant, F.B. Impact of Uncertainty, Social Support, and Prenatal Coping on the Psychological Well-Being of High-Risk Pregnant Women. *Nurs. Res.* **2006**, *55*, 356–365. [CrossRef]
53. Yadav, A.K.; Jena, P.K. Explaining Changing Patterns and Inequalities in Maternal Healthcare Services Utilization in India. *J. Public Aff.* **2022**, *22*, e2570. [CrossRef]
54. Yadav, A.K.; Jena, P.K. Maternal Health Outcomes of Socially Marginalized Groups in India. *Int. J. Health Care Qual. Assur.* **2020**, *33*, 172–188. [CrossRef] [PubMed]

Journal of
Clinical Medicine

MDPI

Review

SARS-CoV-2 and the Brain: What Do We Know about the Causality of 'Cognitive COVID?

Hashir Ali Awan [1], Mufaddal Najmuddin Diwan [1], Alifiya Aamir [1], Muneeza Ali [1], Massimo Di Giannantonio [2], Irfan Ullah [3], Sheikh Shoib [4] and Domenico De Berardis [2,4,5,*]

[1] Department of Internal Medicine, Dow Medical College, Karachi 74200, Pakistan; hashiraliawan@gmail.com (H.A.A.); mufdiwan@gmail.com (M.N.D.); alifiya.aamir521@gmail.com (A.A.); muneeza1998@gmail.com (M.A.)
[2] Department of Neurosciences and Imaging, Chair of Psychiatry, University "G. D'Annunzio", 66100 Chieti, Italy; digiannantonio@unich.it
[3] Department of Internal Medicine, Kabir Medical College, Gandhara University, Peshawar 25000, Pakistan; irfanullahecp2@gmail.com
[4] Department of Internal Medicine, Jawahar Lal Nehru Memorial Hospital, Srinagar 190003, India; Sheikshoib22@gmail.com
[5] NHS, National Health Service, Department of Mental Health, Psychiatric Service for Diagnosis and Treatment, Hospital "G. Mazzini", ASL 4, 64100 Teramo, Italy
* Correspondence: domenico.deberardis@aslteramo.it; Tel.: +39-08-6142-0515

Abstract: The second year of the COVID-19 (coronavirus disease) pandemic has seen the need to identify and assess the long-term consequences of a SARS-CoV-2 infection on an individual's overall wellbeing, including adequate cognitive functioning. 'Cognitive COVID' is an informal term coined to interchangeably refer to acute changes in cognition during COVID-19 and/or cognitive sequelae with various deficits following the infection. These may manifest as altered levels of consciousness, encephalopathy-like symptoms, delirium, and loss of various memory domains. Dysexecutive syndrome is a peculiar manifestation of 'Cognitive COVID' as well. In the previous major outbreaks of viruses like SARS-CoV, MERS-CoV and Influenza. There have been attempts to understand the underlying mechanisms describing the causality of similar symptoms following SARS-CoV-2 infection. This review, therefore, is attempting to highlight the current understanding of the various direct and indirect mechanisms, focusing on the role of neurotropism of SARS-CoV-2, the general pro-inflammatory state, and the pandemic-associated psychosocial stressors in the causality of 'Cognitive COVID.' Neurotropism is associated with various mechanisms including retrograde neuronal transmission via olfactory pathway, a general hematogenous spread, and the virus using immune cells as vectors. The high amounts of inflammation caused by COVID-19, compounded with potential intubation, are associated with a deleterious effect on the cognition as well. Finally, the pandemic's unique psychosocial impact has raised alarm due to its possible effect on cognition. Furthermore, with surfacing reports of post-COVID-vaccination cognitive impairments after vaccines containing mRNA encoding for spike glycoprotein of SARS-CoV-2, we hypothesize their causality and ways to mitigate the risk. The potential impact on the quality of life of an individual and the fact that even a minor proportion of COVID-19 cases developing cognitive impairment could be a significant burden on already overwhelmed healthcare systems across the world make it vital to gather further evidence regarding the prevalence, presentation, correlations, and causality of these events and reevaluate our approach to accommodate early identification, management, and rehabilitation of patients exhibiting cognitive symptoms.

Keywords: COVID-19; SARS-CoV-2; brain; neurotropism; cognitive; prevention; diagnosis

Citation: Ali Awan, H.; Najmuddin Diwan, M.; Aamir, A.; Ali, M.; Di Giannantonio, M.; Ullah, I.; Shoib, S.; De Berardis, D. SARS-CoV-2 and the Brain: What Do We Know about the Causality of 'Cognitive COVID? *J. Clin. Med.* **2021**, *10*, 3441. https://doi.org/10.3390/jcm10153441

Academic Editor: Alfonso Troisi

Received: 17 June 2021
Accepted: 28 July 2021
Published: 2 August 2021

1. Introduction

Over one year since the first case surfaced in the Chinese city of Wuhan, COVID-19 has resulted in more than 3.7 million deaths globally [1]. Initially, focus was primarily on managing acute conditions, but the long-term consequences of SARS-CoV-2 infection are now being highlighted with time. An interesting example is the patient-coined term 'Long-COVID' [2], which denotes long-term outcomes or lasting symptoms of COVID-19 [3].

Apart from major respiratory symptoms, there are reports of acute and post-recovery cognitive deficits occurring in COVID-19 patients [4]. Some authors [5] have also coined a more generic term 'infectious disease-associated encephalopathy' to encompass neurological manifestations of both the classical and novel infections. While it is assumed to have a separate pathophysiology than encephalopathy of a non-infectious origin [5], and although evidence of central nervous system (CNS) involvement exists for the 1918 H1N1 Influenza Virus and 2002 SARS-CoV [6], there is a lack of academic evidence necessary to evaluate the causality of cognitive impairments accurately. Nevertheless, several mechanisms have been presented to explain SARS-CoV-2's acute and 'sequelae' effects [7–10] on the brain. These include viral neurotropism, widespread systemic inflammation, and psychological burden of the pandemic across the world.

These sequelae consist of cognitive impairment after COVID-19 and have also been associated with the medical interventions, especially mechanical ventilation, provided to alleviate conditions of those with severe forms of the infection, which mainly manifested as acute respiratory distress syndrome (ARDS) [11]. Moreover, the immense psychosocial strain due to the prevailing conditions, rising mortality, and government-mandated distancing mechanisms such as lockdowns [12] may also lead to psychological and cognitive consequences in the long run [6].

There has been a critical and time-sensitive [4] need to assess the cognitive impact of COVID-19 due to possible long-term implications it could have on the overall wellbeing of those surviving the infection. This review is attempting to collect the available clinical data, etiological models, and proposed recommendations currently available in the literature to highlight 'Cognitive COVID' and determine if it could change our approach in the second year of this global pandemic.

2. History of Cognitive Impairment in Previous Major Coronavirus Outbreaks and Other Classical Infectious Diseases

Before SARS-CoV-2, two coronaviruses caused significant outbreaks—the Severe Acute Respiratory Syndrome caused by SARS-CoV in 2002 [13], and the Middle Eastern Respiratory Syndrome caused by MERS-CoV in 2012 [14]. A rapid review published in 2020 highlighted the neurological manifestations of the previous coronaviruses to extrapolate the ratio and predict the number of COVID-19 patients that will potentially show neurological deficits [15].

Furthermore, the comparative pathophysiology of SARS and COVID-19 and a similar psychological strain caused by some of the disease processes and circumstances increase the likelihood that COVID-19 will present with cognitive impairments. SARS and COVID-19 both consist of extensive systemic inflammation, the level of which determines disease severity and outcomes [16]. Furthermore, a study on three MERS patients in Saudi Arabia revealed that they had altered levels of consciousness and confusion, which was correlated to new-onset changes on MRI imaging, indicating a neurological component of the viral infection [17]. Another study on 70 patients in Saudi Arabia found that a quarter of the patients (25.7%) developed confusion during the disease [18].

This link, however, expands beyond just coronaviruses. For example, multiple studies conducted on viral infections involving the Human Immunodeficiency Virus (HIV) and Zika Virus (ZIKV) have also underscored a cognitive aspect to the disease presentation with attention, memory, and learning defects [19,20]. The Influenza viruses have also been reported to affect cognition and result in a cognitive decline. Neurological manifestations of Influenza (NMI) have been reported for both global and seasonal outbreaks of the virus and have ranged from seizures to encephalopathies [21]. A study in Taiwan reported Influenza-associated encephalitis/encephalopathy (IAE) and noted that all 10 patients had different levels of consciousness disturbance on presentation [22]. The prevalence of NMI varies geographically [21] and depends on the dominant viral strain. Rao et al.

reported around 18% of all patients of Influenza A (H3N2) in Colorado (USA) had NMI during 2016–17 season [23]. On the other hand, a large national study in Malaysia showed prevalence of NMI to be 8.3% during the 2009 Influenza A (H1N1) pandemic [24]. While the risk of hospitalization is increased by NMI [23], most authors have considered a long-term sequela of such cognitive disturbances by Influenza rare [21,22].

3. Brief Review of Manifestation of Acute and Long-Term Cognitive Deficits

Cognitive deficits and impairments have a complex presentation with variable durations [15,25]. In addition, reports for both acute manifestations and long-term sequelae exist [6].

Acute decline in cognitive functions may result due to a combination of causes, including neurotropism of SARS-CoV-2 and sedation during mechanical ventilation. Encephalopathy is then cited as a general cause for the development of cognitive disturbances [26]. Early in the pandemic, a study involving 214 patients in Wuhan, China, noted CNS-related symptoms including dizziness, headache, and diminished consciousness in 24.8% of patients [27]. In April 2020, 'altered mental status' was listed as one of the 'clinical syndromes' associated with COVID-19 and defined as an 'acute alteration in personality, behavior, cognition, or consciousness' by a survey in the United Kingdom [28]. In the same survey, 31% of the patients recorded having an altered mental status following COVID-19, and nearly 5% of the total patients had dementia-like cognitive symptoms [28]. In addition, viral encephalitis has been identified in some COVID-19 patients, and it alone is possibly linked to the development of acute and lasting cognitive losses [6,29].

'Dysexecutive syndrome' is another peculiar concept that depicts cognitive defects in individuals, particularly of attention, control, and orientation loss [30]. Empirical evidence from a French study shows that loss of executive functions was reported in almost a quarter of COVID-19 patients presenting with ARDS [31]. Furthermore, there is promising evidence of even asymptomatic COVID-19 subjects scoring significantly lower in domains of visual perception, naming, and fluency when checked via the Montreal Cognitive Assessment (MoCA) test [32]. A review also noted symptoms more prevalent in older individuals and those with severe infections [6].

Apart from lasting psychiatric conditions, cognitive impairments may follow a SARS-CoV-2 infection, causing impaired memory, confusion, and attention deficits in the long term [6,33]. A study in Zhejiang, China administered multiple tests evaluating attention, memory, executive function, and information processing, checking for cognitive function of recovered COVID-19 patients against a control group, and finding the sustained attention domain significantly lesser in COVID-19 survivors [34]. Further exploring the link between hospitalization mostly with mechanical ventilation and cognitive deficits, a study using the BMET was conducted on 57 recovering patients with severe disease [4]. In total, 81% of the cohort exhibited some form of cognitive impairment; however, there was no significant correlation of such deficits with the length of intubation.

Further evidence of long-term deficits is available in two more studies [35,36]. First, Lu et al. [35] recorded data of 60 patients during acute SARS-CoV-2 infection and at a 3-month follow-up visit. The proportion of patients with memory loss more than doubled from 13.3% during the acute disease to 28.3% at the follow-up [35], demonstrating the long-term impact of COVID-19 on an individual's cognition. In addition, Woo et al. [36] investigated the cognitive status of 18 recovered patients using the Modified Telephone Interview for Cognitive Status (TICS-M). They contacted the patients at a median of 85 days following their recovery from mild or moderate COVID-19 without an ICU admission. Results showed 18 post-COVID-19 patients scoring appreciably lower than ten control patients on the cognitive assessment, with multiple other self-reported cognitive impairments, including attention deficits (50%), memory deficits (44.4%), and incoherent thoughts (5.6%) [36].

4. Causality

Owing to the nascency of the novel coronavirus causing the pandemic, the exact pathophysiology behind the cognitive sequelae has not been entirely understood. There is no clarity regarding SARS-CoV-2 *directly* affecting the brain or the symptoms resulting from the non-specific and indirect causes; for instance, systemic inflammation and medical interventions such as ventilation. Additionally, the piling psychosocial strain could also potentially act as the source of 'Cognitive COVID' [6,9].

The evidence so far is inconclusive of whether each aspect works solitarily or all elements are working together in causing symptoms. This section briefly outlines these mechanisms (also shown in Figure 1) with references to available evidence of SARS-CoV-2 and its predecessor coronaviruses.

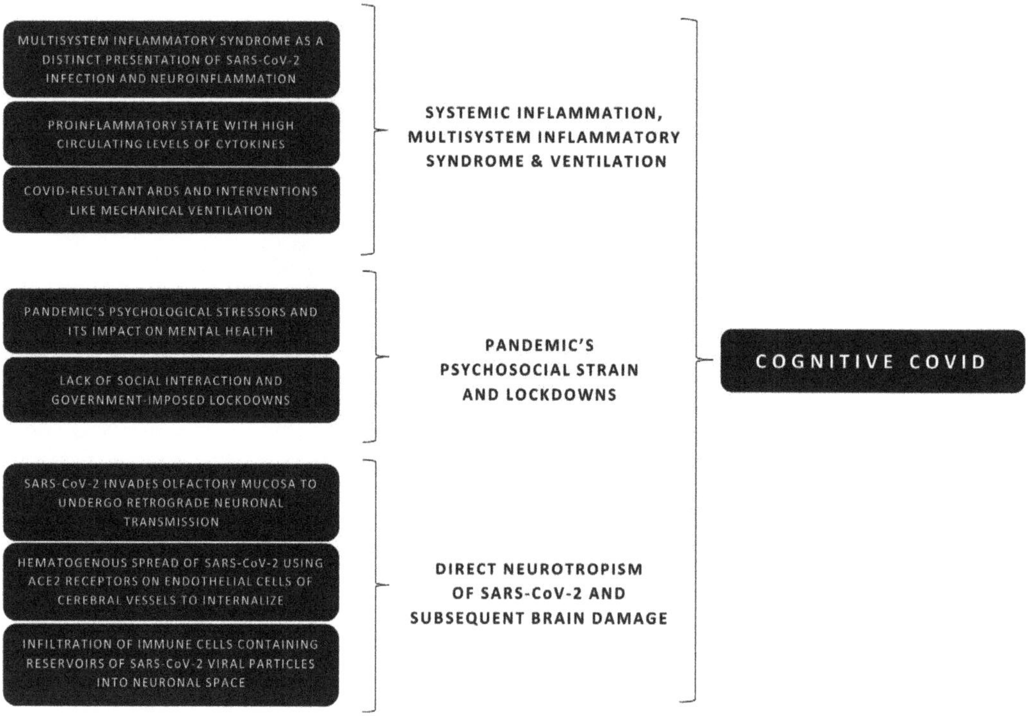

Figure 1. Summary of possible causal elements in the development of cognitive symptoms during and after a COVID-19 (coronavirus disease 2019) infection.

4.1. Neurotropism and the ACE2 Receptor

While still unclear, it is hypothesized that SARS-CoV-2, similarly to other coronaviruses, can infect and survive in nervous tissue [37,38]. Although rare, evidence of SARS-CoV-2's presence in cerebrospinal fluid (CSF) [29,39], as with other viruses [40], is available. There are numerous suggested pathways by which such neurotropism occurs. However, the exact mechanism is still uncertain. Retrograde neuronal access via peripheral nerves, hematogenous spread via directly infecting endothelial cells, and infiltration of infected cells are three main explanations [7,41–43] behind how respiratory viruses (such as SARS-CoV-2) enter the CNS.

i. Olfactory invasion: There is emerging evidence of SARS-CoV-2 affecting the olfactory and gustatory sensations, producing well-known symptoms of 'loss of taste and smell' in infected individuals [44–46]. With time, evidence has surfaced supporting the pathobiology of olfactory and gustatory dysfunction because of a direct invasion of the mucosal epithelium and olfactory bulb [47]. The invasion can potentially be attributed to their expression of the ACE2 surface receptor and Transmembrane Protease Serine 2 (TMPRSS2), cleaving the spike protein of SARS-CoV-2 and facilitating the fusion of SARS-CoV-2 with cellular membranes [48,49]. Furthermore, having a genome that is 79% similar to that of SARS-CoV, the spike glycoprotein of SARS-CoV-2 also binds to Angiotensin-Converting Enzyme 2 (ACE2) receptor on multiple organs, including the brain, acting as the viral functional receptor [50,51]. However, SARS-CoV-2 binds to ACE2 receptors with a considerably greater affinity than SARS-CoV [52]. Animal studies focusing on SARS-CoV have shown trans-neuronal spread from the olfactory bulb to certain 'connected' regions of the brain, providing key 'circumstantial evidence' in the potential neurotropic properties of SARS-CoV-2, as well [43,53]. The entorhinal cortex and the hippocampus are such 'connected' regions. They are involved in episodic memory and other domains, illustrating how damage directed at these areas may cause lasting cognitive dysfunction [54].

ii. Hematogenous spread: Some authors [8] claim hematogenous spread via the cerebral vasculature plays a more critical role in direct brain entry and damage-causing cognitive deficits in COVID-19. Evidence of SARS-CoV-2's presence in blood samples of some confirmed COVID-19 patients exists. As many as 41% [55] of the samples showed viremia [43], showcasing the ability of the virus to easily reach the brain once the blood-brain barrier (BBB) is damaged. The distribution of SARS-CoV-2's functional (ACE2) receptor is widespread in endothelial cells and pericytes throughout the body [56]. Analysis of available genomic databases confirms noteworthy expression of the receptor in neuronal and glial tissues of the CNS [56]. Consequently, the nervous tissue is potentially vulnerable if the virus comes in direct contact and interacts with the ACE2 receptors. In addition, SARS-CoV-2's potential neurotropic properties may allow it to assume latency inside neuronal tissue of patients even after recovery from COVID-19, putting them at greater risk of long-term or delayed cognitive deficits and neurological symptoms [6]. Notably, it is still unclear how abundantly ACE2 receptors are expressed in the cerebral vasculature. However, other docking receptors, importantly basigin (BSG) and neuropilin (NRP1), have been identified as facilitators of the viral entry or internalization—making the brain vulnerable to viral inflammation even with an intact BBB [7] In addition, SARS-CoV-2 and the accompanying inflammatory cytokines, including Interleukins (IL) and Tumor Necrosis Factor (TNF), may damage the BBB [57]. Moreover, evidence shows that SARS-CoV-2 affects vasculature integrity by direct viral infection, leading to endothelium damage and increased vascular permeability in peripheral vessels [58]; extrapolated from the cerebral endothelial cells, this could explain the disruption of the BBB. Therefore, immune-mediated action or direct inflammation may be responsible for endothelial dysfunction in the BBB, enabled by the recruitment of host immune cells. Additional factors that may aid in the hematogenous spread of SARS-CoV-2 to the brain include a pre-existing or underlying neurological pathology and entry via circumventricular organs such as the median eminence of the hypothalamus [7].

iii. Infiltration of infected cells: A 2005 study aimed at SARS-CoV found a sizeable proportion of immune cells (29.7% of monocytes and 51.5% of lymphocytes) in 6 out of 22 patients to contain viral particles [59], signaling their potential as a reservoir for the virus. If immune cells were to infiltrate the neuronal space by crossing the BBB, this would allow the viral particles in them to cause direct brain damage by binding to ACE2 receptors on neuronal and glial cells [7]. However, whether these findings can be accurately extrapolated to SARS-CoV-2 remains yet to be ascertained. In addition, autopsies and studies conducted on samples obtained from infected individuals have been inconclusive about direct immune cell infiltration during COVID-19 [60].

4.2. Non-Specific Systemic Inflammation, Multisystem Inflammatory Syndrome (MIS), and ARDS

i. Widespread systemic inflammation: A significant increase in inflammatory cytokines plays a role in SARS symptoms, with inflammation persisting even after the viral clearance, and a similar ramped up an innate immune response in the form of 'cytokine storm' is behind COVID-19 as well [16,34,61]. Highly circulating amounts of Interleukins and other mediators (including IL-6, IL-1β, and TNF, and others) resulting in a pro-inflammatory status are commonly found in COVID-19 patients [62,63]. This amplified immune response may cause increased vascular permeability and vasculopathy arising from disseminated intravascular coagulation (DIC). Subsequently, the BBB is compromised, allowing cytokines to activate a microglial inflammatory response [64]. This mechanism may potentially lead to delirium and seizures due to an immune-mediated encephalopathy [6]. There is a substantial risk of Cerebral Vascular Disease in infected individuals potentially due to this exact pathophysiology, with studies showing increased incidences of hypoxic-ischemic conditions [8]. A study in April 2020 investigated the histopathological changes during autopsy, and all 18 patients' brain specimens depicted hypoxic changes [60]. It also drew attention to how cerebral white matter is at high risk for damage due to ischemia, manifesting as loss of vital cognitive functions during and after COVID-19 [8]. Several studies investigating Alzheimer's Disease (AD) patients found a notable inflammation in patients showing cognitive deficits compared to the control group, indicating the link between the development of cognitive impairment and increased inflammatory molecules [65]. In addition, previous studies have highlighted the long-term detrimental effects of severe inflammation on the cognitive ability of a person, especially those already with or at high risk of developing a neurodegenerative disease [66–68]. A study investigated links between serum inflammatory markers and C-reactive protein (CRP) in COVID-19 patients with cognitive functions and found loss of some domains, such as sustained attention, to be significantly correlated to CRP levels in the blood [34]. In addition, previous longitudinal studies have confirmed a significant association between CRP levels and cognitive decline [69], affirming how underlying inflammation (using CRP as a marker) likely affects an individual's cognitive functioning in the long run. Some studies have claimed the role of NLRP3 inflammasome activity in exacerbating systemic inflammation and its outcomes [16]. In addition, some proteins of SARS-CoV have shown to induce NLRP4 inflammasome activity, making it likely that SARS-CoV-2 also utilizes similar pathways to cause extensive inflammation [70]. This pathway has further been suggested to explain cognitive deficits due to high IL-1β activity in the setting of hypercapnia caused by mechanical ventilation [71].

ii. Multisystem Inflammatory Syndrome (MIS): Demographically, COVID-19 has been shown to cause more severe disease in adults, but increasing reports of COVID-associated Multisystem Inflammatory Syndrome (MIS) have surfaced [72–74]. While more prevalent in children, as MIS in children (MIS-C), it can potentially occur in adults as well (MIS-A). A meta-analysis comparing MIS-C's clinical course to COVID-19 revealed how it can potentially lead to multi-organ failure [75]. MIS-C was also shown to have a relatively higher incidence of neurological manifestations compared to acute COVID-19 [75]. As a distinct manifestation of a SARS-CoV-2 infection even in adults [76], with a high risk of neurological symptoms, MIS warrants discussion as a potential causal factor in the development of Cognitive COVID. MIS-C is considered to cause a hyperinflammatory shock and resembles Kawasaki Disease (KD) [77] or Toxic Shock Syndrome (TSS) [78]. Several cases with serologic evidence of a SARS-CoV-2 infection reported symptoms of MIS-C such as shock, cardiac symptoms, gastrointestinal complains, and elevated markers of inflammation, particularly after it was recognized by the Centers for Disease Control and Prevention (CDC) in May 2020 [78]. The pathophysiology of MIS-C during and after a SARS-CoV-2 infection is largely unknown [78]. Generally, MIS-C is believed to cause a dysregulated immune response possibly by viral mimicry of the host and development of autoantibodies. This leads to widespread systemic inflammation that potentially has a damaging impact on multiple systems, including the neurological system [79–81]. Interestingly, some cases depicted a milder, 'overlapping' syndrome with acute COVID-19, while other cases reported MIS-C symptoms weeks after an acute infection. However, children with an active COVID-19 infection confirmed via a positive RT-PCR test form only one-third of the total MIS-C cases, with a majority showing evidence of a past infection confirmed via serological tests [80]. Jiang et al. uses epidemiological data from different countries to suggest that MIS-C is more likely caused by an acquired, albeit dysfunctional, immune response to SARS-CoV-2 instead of direct viral involvement [80]. The above discussion on widespread systemic inflammation in severe COVID-19 in adults is of value here when discussing MIS-C or MIS-A. The pathophysiology of MIS-C is also believed to involve a cytokine storm with elevated inflammatory mediators [80,82] which may ultimately lead to neurocognitive manifestations, as elucidated previously in this text.

iii. Acute respiratory distress syndrome (ARDS), mechanical ventilation, and associated cognitive decline: Although the exact ratio of COVID-19 patients developing severe disease and requiring hospitalization or intensive care unit (ICU) admission varies extensively, there is undoubtedly a noticeable proportion that progresses to life-threatening conditions [83]. Preliminary studies from China investigating data of more than 70 thousand patients suggested that around 19% of patients with COVID-19 develop severe or critical disease, most likely necessitating hospitalization [84]. A survey of 17 studies examining statistics of hospitalized COVID-19 patients from different regions found that one-third of all hospitalized and three-quarters of all ICU-admitted patients develop ARDS [83]. Cognitive impairment following ARDS of variable etiology is widely reported and reviewed [85]. Although severe inflammation, hemodynamic instability, and hypoxia have been indicted, the exact mechanism causing it is unknown. However, a review of studies has shown that cognitive impairment post-ARDS has a high incidence and ranges from 70–100% at hospital discharge, to 46–80% at one year after discharge, to 20% at five years after discharge [85]. In addition, an observational study in France described several ICU-admitted COVID-19 patients with complaints of ARDS developing encephalopathy manifesting as confusion and agitation [31]. According to Tzotzos et al., of the COVID-19 ICU-admitted patients who develop ARDS, more than 80% must receive mechanical ventilation [83]. Mechanical ventilation, regardless of ARDS, is associated with cognitive decline and reduced quality of life in the long run [86]. Since mechanical ventilation inextricably leads to the administration of sedatives, it is essential to note delirium and other cognitive consequences that may accompany, both in the short and long term [87]. The likelihood of a systemic inflammation playing a significant role in the development of cognitive loss compared to direct viral damage is underscored by the sparse evidence of the virus being found in the CSF [16]. Furthermore, instead of being two entirely independent processes, the neurotropism of SARS-CoV-2 and the widespread parallel inflammation may also operate in conjunction [7] and collectively lead to direct and indirect neuronal damage with cognitive deficits. Lastly, it is crucial to not trivialize non-specific but potentially key elements in developing cognitive sequelae, namely COVID-19 complications such as ARDS and subsequent mechanical ventilation [11].

4.3. The Psychosocial Strain of the Pandemic and Associated Lockdowns

i. Psychological stressors: While countries battle their second or third waves, confinement due to lockdowns and the fear of one or one's loved ones contracting

COVID-19 are just some of the reasons that continue to cause an unprecedented psychological burden on people across the world [12,88]. With psychological conditions such as anxiety and depression now being recorded globally, cognitive consequences can be reasonably expected as a unique symptomatic presentation [89]. A systematic review remarked that some studies had shown the prevalence of post-traumatic stress disorder (PTSD) ranging from 7% to as high as 53.8% during the pandemic [90]. Moreover, this psychological disorder has been correlated with diminishing cognitive function, especially in the elderly [91], showing how 'Cognitive COVID' is possibly related to an individual's psychological state.

ii. Social isolation and government-mandated lockdowns: An article published in late 2020 had reviewed the available evidence and stipulated that social distancing/isolation and lack of human interaction may have a detrimental effect on a person's cognition [92]. Echoing these findings, a study conducted in Italy during May 2020 investigated the effects of psychological stressors as a result of isolation in the form of national lockdown as a mitigation technique on the global cognitive function of the public [93]. Findings suggested cognitive function such as barring memory deteriorated during lockdowns. Furthermore, with a greater prevalence of anxiety, depression, and other mental health changes, a significant deleterious impact on cognitive function(s) was noted in those who had lesser social interactions [93].

Further research needs to correlate lockdowns and various psychosocial factors of the pandemic with cognitive ability to gather experimental evidence. Consequently, the findings may aid in ascertaining if this psychological burden is responsible for the reason why COVID-19 survivors may develop cognitive sequelae following their recovery. Likewise, any significant conclusions may also illustrate if psychosocial distress in the wake of lockdowns increases an individual's risk of being affected and the severity by which they are affected due to other causal factors outlined in this text earlier.

5. COVID-19 Vaccination, Autoimmunity, and Cognitive Impairment

The vaccine roll-out for COVID-19 began recently, but nearly 3.57 billion doses have been administered worldwide already [1]. Various vaccines were approved by the World Health Organization (WHO) for emergency use but all of them fall under three major subtypes: messenger RNA (mRNA), viral vector, and inactivated whole-virus [94]. As the pace of vaccine administration increases, more data is surfacing regarding post-vaccination adverse events. Neurocognitive symptoms following vaccinations COVID-19 vaccinations are rare but emerging case reports require due attention to accurately evaluate the pathophysiology and risk-factors carefully and accurately.

Two cases of encephalopathy within one week following inoculation via an mRNA vaccine were reported in patients with no prior neuropsychiatric history [95]. Furthermore, an 89-year-old patient developed delirium after a first dose of an mRNA vaccine [96]. The mRNA in the vaccines encodes antigen S-2B, which includes SARS-CoV-2 spike glycoprotein. The spike glycoprotein during a viral infection initiates a cascade of inflammatory reactions after attaching to ACE2 receptor, leading to COVID-19 encephalopathy [95]. Authors hypothesize that cells translating this vaccine mRNA may produce the same glycoprotein and in turn mimic the encephalopathy caused by an active viral infection [95]. Furthermore, acquired immunity via anti-spike antibodies linking to spike protein of SARS-CoV has been known to boost inflammation by activating macrophages [80]. A similar mechanism following development of anti-spike antibodies against SARS-CoV-2 after administration of mRNA vaccines may lead to widespread inflammation, macrophage activation, and development of neurological symptoms [80,95,96].

An interesting case is of an adult, who recovered from COVID-19 6 weeks ago, developing MIS following a second dose of an inactivated virus vaccine [97]. Features of shock and cardiac dysfunction were present in the patient along with elevated inflammatory markers, indicating MIS. The authors postulate that the vaccine may have accentuated their body's immune response which was 'already primed' following SARS-CoV-2 infection and therefore led to an uninhibited inflammatory condition in the body [97].

Some authors have warned against the use of certain immunogenic proteins of SARS-CoV-2 in vaccines that are homologous to the human immune system [98]. With most of SARS-CoV-2's immunogenic epitopes matching human proteins, there is a reasonable risk that vaccines containing these epitopes will lead to autoimmunity [98]. Excessive inflammation, creation of autoantibodies, and a series of biochemical processes due to autoimmunity may lead to neuroinflammation, damage to neuronal integrity and cognitive impairment [99]. Using Alzheimer's Disease as a parallel in mouse models, a temporal association between increasing autoimmunity and declining cognitive competence was found [100], highlighting the damaging effect accelerated autoimmunity may have on brain function.

6. Discussion

We have identified three major areas of discussion when debating on causality of cognitive symptoms occurring during and after a SARS-CoV-2 infection. The direct neurotropism of SARS-CoV-2 is largely based on information available for SARS-CoV. Several hypotheses on mechanisms of direct neurotropism have been outlined, such as infiltration of virus-laden immune cells, hematogenous spread through CVOs or breaks in BBB, and retrograde neuronal transmission through invasion of the olfactory system. Furthermore, non-specific systemic inflammation which also manifest as multisystemic inflammatory syndrome (MIS) due to a 'cytokine storm' reported in COVID patients predisposes them to vascular injuries, leading to neuroinflammation. As mentioned earlier, treatment methods such as intubation to treat ARDS can also lead to cognitive symptoms. Lastly, a neuropsychiatric vantage point allows us to underscore the importance of prevailing psychological stressors and their effect on a person's cognitive ability.

For the first time, to our knowledge, in this text we have also reviewed case studies of cognitive impairment and adverse-events following COVID-19 vaccinations, especially the mRNA subtype. We have discussed the occurrence of a heightened immune response to spike glycoprotein encoded by the mRNA in the vaccine which leads to a condition similar to COVID-19 encephalopathy. By discussing the potential occurrence of autoimmunity following inoculation, we have identified the risk of using viral epitopes that are homologous to proteins in the human immune system.

Furthermore, despite the varying prevalence and presentations of cognitive deficits, due to the sheer scale of the pandemic, with global cases crossing 173 million [1], any proportion will result in substantial implications on health systems and a massive influx of patients with cognitive complaints. Therefore, with more significant evidence through research, greater awareness regarding the probable emergence of 'Cognitive COVID' in some patients is required—both for the public, early seeking medical care, and healthcare workers, for readiness and early detection.

As described above, the varying levels of cognitive impairment will require a thorough evaluation, planned follow-ups, and in-patient management if required. Consequently, facilities and institutions should allocate adequate resources and enable their healthcare workers via training to effectively respond to those COVID-19 survivors at high risk for developing cognitive sequelae [6].

Additionally, the therapeutic significance of understanding and ascertaining the etiology of 'Cognitive COVID', particularly on a cellular level, is manifold. There are available interventions that may mitigate the negative impact of high inflammation levels with a potential cytokine storm, including cytokine antagonists and other anti-inflammatory modulators [64]. Importantly, due to the requirement of physical distancing to avoid transmission of SARS-CoV-2, telemedicine for diagnosis and cognitive rehabilitation is an exciting and promising avenue to be utilized [101]. Moreover, as a psychosocial burden and mental health disorders are possible causal elements, telepsychiatry services can play a crucial role in preventing cognitive impairments [102].

7. Conclusions, Limitations and Way Forward

Cognitive COVID is an oft-ignored aspect of the pandemic, but with greater attention now being paid to the non-respiratory and long-term cognitive consequences of COVID, it is vital to collect further evidence regarding the prevalence, presentation, correlations, and causality of these events. Furthermore, the potentially long-term nature of these deficits and their devastating effect on quality of life, especially the elderly, makes it more pressing to review our current approach in early identification, management, and rehabilitation of patients exhibiting cognitive symptoms [6]. In this article, we have highlighted the probable causality of Cognitive COVID by reviewing the available hypotheses, case reports, and clinical data that has been published after the pandemic started and used previous coronaviruses as a basis to form a parallel to the novel coronavirus 2019.

Due to the relative recency of the pandemic and unavailability of coherent data, it is extremely challenging to reach a plausible conclusion regarding the intricate interplay of causal factors. Criteria to determine causality such as the Bradford-Hill criteria [103] are difficult to apply on the causal factors. The lack of consistent data available from different regions across the world and various methods of measuring inflammation or cognitive deficits disallow direct comparison. The biological plausibility criterion of Bradford-Hill criteria, however, has been discussed at depth in the text to decipher neurological and inflammatory mechanisms that lead to clinical symptoms. Another criterion of analogy can be extrapolated to use of available data from SARS-CoV and MERS-CoV to predict SARS-CoV-2's effect on the brain. We are also limited by a lack of research conducted into different variants of SARS-CoV-2 and their effect on cognition.

The way forward is to develop a standardized protocol for neurocognitive assessment of COVID-19 patients, especially at times of discharge from hospitalization and end of medical interventions such as intubation. These steps will mitigate the threat posed by 'Cognitive COVID' and will undoubtedly decrease the burden on already overwhelmed healthcare systems.

Moving forward, greater attention should be paid to cognitive impairment during and after COVID-19 and vaccination. With the emergence of new strains of COVID-19, such as the Delta and the Lambda variant [104], the variation in prevalence of cognitive manifestations of the viral infection needs to be ascertained. Therefore, it is imperative to collect empirical data from multiple demographics in order to attain uniform clinical and biochemical information regarding causality and risk-factors in developing cognitive impairments.

Author Contributions: Conceptualization, I.U.; methodology, H.A.A. and A.A.; formal analysis, H.A.A.; data curation, M.N.D. and M.A.; writing—original draft preparation, H.A.A., M.D.G., A.A. and M.A.; writing—review and editing, S.S. and D.D.B.; visualization, I.U. and D.D.B.; supervision, I.U. and D.D.B.; project administration, I.U. All authors have read and agreed to the published version of the manuscript.

Funding: This research received no external funding.

Institutional Review Board Statement: Not applicable.

Informed Consent Statement: Not applicable.

Data Availability Statement: No new data were created or analyzed in this study. Data sharing does not apply to this article.

Conflicts of Interest: The authors declare no conflict of interest.

References

1. Dong, E.; Du, H.; Gardner, L. An interactive web-based dashboard to track COVID-19 in real time. *Lancet Infect. Dis.* **2020**, *20*, 533–534. [CrossRef]
2. Nabavi, N. Long covid: How to define it and how to manage it. *BMJ* **2020**, *370*, m3489. [CrossRef] [PubMed]
3. Mahase, E. Covid-19: What do we know about "long covid"? *BMJ* **2020**, *370*, m2815. [CrossRef]
4. Jaywant, A.; Vanderlind, W.M.; Alexopoulos, G.S.; Fridman, C.B.; Perlis, R.H.; Gunning, F.M. Frequency and profile of objective cognitive deficits in hospitalized patients recovering from COVID-19. *Neuropsychopharmacology* **2021**, *15*, 1–6. [CrossRef]

5. Barbosa-Silva, M.C.; Lima, M.N.; Battaglini, D.; Robba, C.; Pelosi, P.; Rocco, P.R.M.; Maron-Gutierrez, T. Infectious disease-associated encephalopathies. *Crit. Care* **2021**, *25*, 236. [CrossRef]
6. Kumar, S.; Veldhuis, A.; Malhotra, T. Neuropsychiatric and cognitive sequelae of COVID-19. *Front. Psychol.* **2021**, *12*, 577529. [CrossRef] [PubMed]
7. Iadecola, C.; Anrather, J.; Kamel, H. Effects of COVID-19 on the nervous system. *Cell* **2020**, *183*, 16–27.e1. [CrossRef]
8. Miners, S.; Kehoe, P.G.; Love, S. Cognitive impact of COVID-19: Looking beyond the short term. *Alzheimers Res. Ther.* **2020**, *12*, 170. [CrossRef] [PubMed]
9. Pereira, A. Long-term neurological threats of COVID-19: A call to update the thinking about the outcomes of the coronavirus pandemic. *Front. Neurol.* **2020**, *11*, 308. [CrossRef]
10. Uversky, V.N.; Elrashdy, F.; Aljadawi, A.; Ali, S.M.; Khan, R.H.; Redwan, E.M. Severe acute respiratory syndrome coronavirus 2 infection reaches the human nervous system: How? *J. Neurosci. Res.* **2020**, *99*, 750–777. [CrossRef] [PubMed]
11. Rabinovitz, B.; Jaywant, A.; Fridman, C.B. Neuropsychological functioning in severe acute respiratory disorders caused by the coronavirus: Implications for the current COVID-19 pandemic. *Clin. Neuropsychol.* **2020**, *34*, 1453–1479. [CrossRef]
12. Dubey, S.; Biswas, P.; Ghosh, R.; Chatterjee, S.; Dubey, M.J.; Chatterjee, S.; Lahiri, D.; Lavie, C.J. Psychosocial impact of COVID-19. *Diabetes Metab. Syndr. Clin. Res. Rev.* **2020**, *14*, 779–788. [CrossRef]
13. Ksiazek, T.G.; Erdman, D.; Goldsmith, C.S.; Zaki, S.R.; Peret, T.; Emery, S.; Tong, S.; Urbani, C.; Comer, J.A.; Lim, W.; et al. A novel coronavirus associated with severe acute respiratory syndrome. *N. Engl. J. Med.* **2003**, *348*, 1953–1966. [CrossRef]
14. Al-Osail, A.M.; Al-Wazzah, M.J. The history and epidemiology of Middle East respiratory syndrome corona virus. *Multidiscip. Respir. Med.* **2017**, *12*, 20. [CrossRef]
15. Ellul, M.A.; Benjamin, L.; Singh, B.; Lant, S.; Michael, B.D.; Easton, A.; Kneen, R.; Defres, S.; Sejvar, J.; Solomon, T. Neurological associations of COVID-19. *Lancet Neurol.* **2020**, *19*, 767–783. [CrossRef]
16. Heneka, M.T.; Golenbock, D.; Latz, E.; Morgan, D.; Brown, R. Immediate and long-term consequences of COVID-19 infections for the development of neurological disease. *Alzheimers Res. Ther.* **2020**, *12*, 69. [CrossRef]
17. Arabi, Y.M.; Harthi, A.; Hussein, J.; Bouchama, A.; Johani, S.; Hajeer, A.H.; Saeed, B.T.; Wahbi, A.; Saedy, A.; Aldabbagh, T.; et al. Severe neurologic syndrome associated with Middle East respiratory syndrome corona virus (MERS-CoV). *Infection* **2015**, *43*, 495–501. [CrossRef]
18. Saad, M.; Omrani, A.; Baig, K.; Bahloul, A.; Elzein, F.; Matin, M.A.; Selim, M.A.; Al Mutairi, M.; Al Nakhli, D.; Al Aidaroos, A.Y.; et al. Clinical aspects and outcomes of 70 patients with Middle East respiratory syndrome coronavirus infection: A single-center experience in Saudi Arabia. *Int. J. Infect. Dis.* **2014**, *29*, 301–306. [CrossRef]
19. Kanmogne, G.D.; Fonsah, J.Y.; Umlauf, A.; Moul, J.; Doh, R.F.; Kengne, A.M.; Tang, B.; Tagny, C.T.; Nchindap, E.; Kenmogne, L.; et al. Attention/Working memory, learning and memory in adult cameroonians: Normative data, effects of HIV infection and viral genotype. *J. Int. Neuropsychol. Soc.* **2020**, *26*, 607–623. [CrossRef] [PubMed]
20. Raper, J.; Kovacs-Balint, Z.; Mavigner, M.; Gumber, S.; Burke, M.W.; Habib, J.; Mattingly, C.; Fair, D.; Earl, E.; Feczko, E.; et al. Long-term alterations in brain and behavior after postnatal Zika virus infection in infant macaques. *Nat. Commun.* **2020**, *11*, 2534. [CrossRef] [PubMed]
21. Ekstrand, J.J. Neurologic Complications of Influenza. *Semin. Pediatr. Neurol.* **2012**, *19*, 96–100. [CrossRef] [PubMed]
22. Chen, L.-W.; Teng, C.-K.; Tsai, Y.-S.; Wang, J.-N.; Tu, Y.-F.; Shen, C.-F.; Liu, C.-C. Influenza-associated neurological complications during 2014–2017 in Taiwan. *Brain Dev.* **2018**, *40*, 799–806. [CrossRef] [PubMed]
23. Rao, S.; Martin, J.; Ahearn, M.A.; Osborne, C.; Moss, A.; Dempsey, A.; Dominguez, S.R.; Weinberg, A.; Messacar, K.B. Neurologic manifestations of influenza A(H3N2) infection in children during the 2016–2017 season. *J. Pediatr. Infect. Dis. Soc.* **2018**, *9*, 71–74. [CrossRef] [PubMed]
24. Ismail, H.I.M.; Teh, C.M.; Lee, Y.L. Neurologic manifestations and complications of pandemic influenza A H1N1 in Malaysian children: What have we learnt from the ordeal? *Brain Dev.* **2015**, *37*, 120–129. [CrossRef]
25. Rogers, J.P.; Chesney, E.; Oliver, D.; Pollak, T.V.; McGuire, P.; Fusar-Poli, P.; Zandi, M.; Lewis, G.; David, A. Psychiatric and neuropsychiatric presentations associated with severe coronavirus infections: A systematic review and meta-analysis with comparison to the COVID-19 pandemic. *Lancet Psychiatry* **2020**, *7*, 611–627. [CrossRef]
26. Filatov, A.; Sharma, P.; Hindi, F.; Espinosa, P.S. Neurological complications of coronavirus disease (COVID-19): Encephalopathy. *Cureus* **2020**, *12*, e7352. [CrossRef]
27. Mao, L.; Jin, H.; Wang, M.; Hu, Y.; Chen, S.; He, Q.; Chang, J.; Hong, C.; Zhou, Y.; Wang, D.; et al. Neurologic manifestations of hospitalized patients with coronavirus disease 2019 in Wuhan, China. *JAMA Neurol.* **2020**, *77*, 683. [CrossRef]
28. Varatharaj, A.; Thomas, N.; Ellul, M.A.; Davies, N.W.S.; Pollak, T.A.; Tenorio, E.L.; Sultan, M.; Easton, A.; Breen, G.; Zandi, M.; et al. Neurological and neuropsychiatric complications of COVID-19 in 153 patients: A UK-wide surveillance study. *Lancet Psychiatry* **2020**, *7*, 875–882. [CrossRef]
29. Moriguchi, T.; Harii, N.; Goto, J.; Harada, D.; Sugawara, H.; Takamino, J.; Ueno, M.; Sakata, H.; Kondo, K.; Myose, N.; et al. A first case of meningitis/encephalitis associated with SARS-Coronavirus-2. *Int. J. Infect. Dis.* **2020**, *94*, 55–58. [CrossRef]
30. Ardila, A.; Lahiri, D. Executive dysfunction in COVID-19 patients. *Diabetes Metab. Syndr. Clin. Res. Rev.* **2020**, *14*, 1377–1378. [CrossRef]
31. Helms, J.; Kremer, S.; Merdji, H.; Clere-Jehl, R.; Schenck, M.; Kummerlen, C.; Collange, O.; Boulay, C.; Fafi-Kremer, S.; Ohana, M.; et al. Neurologic Features in Severe SARS-CoV-2 Infection. *N. Engl. J. Med.* **2020**, *382*, 2268–2270. [CrossRef]

32. Amalakanti, S.; Arepalli, K.V.R.; Jillella, J.P. Cognitive assessment in asymptomatic COVID-19 subjects. *Virusdisease* **2021**, *32*, 146–149. [CrossRef]
33. Wang, F.; Kream, R.M.; Stefano, G.B. Long-term respiratory and neurological sequelae of COVID-19. *Med. Sci. Monit.* **2020**, *26*, e928996. [CrossRef]
34. Zhou, H.; Lu, S.; Chen, J.; Wei, N.; Wang, D.; Lyu, H.; Shi, C.; Hu, S. The landscape of cognitive function in recovered COVID-19 patients. *J. Psychiatr. Res.* **2020**, *129*, 98–102. [CrossRef]
35. Lu, Y.; Li, X.; Geng, D.; Mei, N.; Wu, P.-Y.; Huang, C.-C.; Jia, T.; Zhao, Y.; Wang, D.; Xiao, A.; et al. Cerebral micro-structural changes in COVID-19 patients–An MRI-based 3-month follow-up study. *EClinicalMedicine* **2020**, *25*, 100484. [CrossRef]
36. Woo, M.S.; Malsy, J.; Pöttgen, J.; Zai, S.S.; Ufer, F.; Hadjilaou, A.; Schmiedel, S.; Addo, M.M.; Gerloff, C.; Heesen, C.; et al. Frequent neurocognitive deficits after recovery from mild COVID-19. *Brain Commun.* **2020**, *2*, fcaa205. [CrossRef]
37. Kwong, K.C.N.K.; Mehta, P.R.; Shukla, G.; Mehta, A.R. COVID-19, SARS and MERS: A neurological perspective. *J. Clin. Neurosci.* **2020**, *77*, 13–16. [CrossRef]
38. Valiuddin, H.M.; Kalajdzic, A.; Rosati, J.; Boehm, K.; Hill, D. Update on neurological manifestations of SARS-CoV-2. *West. J. Emerg. Med.* **2020**, *21*, 45–51. [CrossRef] [PubMed]
39. Lewis, A.; Frontera, J.; Placantonakis, D.G.; Lighter, J.; Galetta, S.; Balcer, L.; Melmed, K. Cerebrospinal fluid in COVID-19: A systematic review of the literature. *J. Neurol. Sci.* **2021**, *421*, 117316. [CrossRef] [PubMed]
40. Bohmwald, K.; Gálvez, N.M.S.; Ríos, M.; Kalergis, A.M. Neurologic alterations due to respiratory virus infections. *Front. Cell. Neurosci.* **2018**, *12*, 386. [CrossRef]
41. Desforges, M.; Le Coupanec, A.; Dubeau, P.; Bourgouin, A.; Lajoie, L.; Dube, M.; Talbot, P.J. Human coronaviruses and other respiratory viruses: Underestimated opportunistic pathogens of the central nervous system? *Viruses* **2019**, *12*, 14. [CrossRef] [PubMed]
42. Wu, Y.; Xu, X.; Chen, Z.; Duan, J.; Hashimoto, K.; Yang, L.; Liu, C.; Yang, C. Nervous system involvement after infection with COVID-19 and other coronaviruses. *Brain Behav. Immun.* **2020**, *87*, 18–22. [CrossRef]
43. Zhou, Z.; Kang, H.; Li, S.; Zhao, X. Understanding the neurotropic characteristics of SARS-CoV-2: From neurological manifestations of COVID-19 to potential neurotropic mechanisms. *J. Neurol.* **2020**, *267*, 2179–2184. [CrossRef] [PubMed]
44. Hornuss, D.; Lange, B.; Schröter, N.; Rieg, S.; Kern, W.; Wagner, D. Anosmia in COVID-19 patients. *Clin. Microbiol. Infect.* **2020**, *26*, 1426–1427. [CrossRef]
45. Dawson, P.; Rabold, E.M.; Laws, R.L.; Conners, E.E.; Gharpure, R.; Yin, S.; Buono, S.A.; Dasu, T.; Bhattacharyya, S.; Westergaard, R.P.; et al. Loss of taste and smell as distinguishing symptoms of coronavirus disease 2019. *Clin. Infect. Dis.* **2020**, *72*, 682–685. [CrossRef]
46. Mullol, J.; Alobid, I.; Mariño-Sánchez, F.; Izquierdo-Domínguez, A.; Marin, C.; Klimek, L.; Wang, D.-Y.; Liu, Z. The loss of smell and taste in the COVID-19 outbreak: A tale of many countries. *Curr. Allergy Asthma Rep.* **2020**, *20*, 61. [CrossRef]
47. Mehraeen, E.; Behnezhad, F.; Salehi, M.A.; Noori, T.; Harandi, H.; SeyedAlinaghi, S. Olfactory and gustatory dysfunctions due to the coronavirus disease (COVID-19): A review of current evidence. *Eur. Arch. Oto-Rhino-Laryngol.* **2020**, *278*, 307–312. [CrossRef] [PubMed]
48. Brann, D.H.; Tsukahara, T.; Weinreb, C.; Lipovsek, M.; Berge, K.V.D.; Gong, B.; Chance, R.; Macaulay, I.C.; Chou, H.-J.; Fletcher, R.B.; et al. Non-neuronal expression of SARS-CoV-2 entry genes in the olfactory system suggests mechanisms underlying COVID-19-associated anosmia. *Sci. Adv.* **2020**, *6*, eabc5801. [CrossRef]
49. Dong, M.; Zhang, J.; Ma, X.; Tan, J.; Chen, L.; Liu, S.; Xin, Y.; Zhuang, L. ACE2, TMPRSS2 distribution and extrapulmonary organ injury in patients with COVID-19. *Biomed. Pharmacother.* **2020**, *131*, 110678. [CrossRef]
50. Lu, R.; Zhao, X.; Li, J.; Niu, P.; Yang, B.; Wu, H.; Wang, W.; Song, H.; Huang, B.; Zhu, N.; et al. Genomic characterisation and epidemiology of 2019 novel coronavirus: Implications for virus origins and receptor binding. *Lancet* **2020**, *395*, 565–574. [CrossRef]
51. Zhou, P.; Yang, X.-L.; Wang, X.-G.; Hu, B.; Zhang, L.; Zhang, W.; Si, H.-R.; Zhu, Y.; Li, B.; Huang, C.-L.; et al. Addendum: A pneumonia outbreak associated with a new coronavirus of probable bat origin. *Nat. Cell Biol.* **2020**, *588*, E6. [CrossRef]
52. Wrapp, D.; Wang, N.; Corbett, K.S.; Goldsmith, J.A.; Hsieh, C.-L.; Abiona, O.; Graham, B.S.; McLellan, J.S. Cryo-EM structure of the 2019-nCoV spike in the prefusion conformation. *Science* **2020**, *367*, 1260–1263. [CrossRef]
53. Netland, J.; Meyerholz, D.K.; Moore, S.; Cassell, M.; Perlman, S. Severe acute respiratory syndrome coronavirus infection causes neuronal death in the absence of encephalitis in mice transgenic for human ACE2. *J. Virol.* **2008**, *82*, 7264–7275. [CrossRef]
54. Ritchie, K.; Chan, D. The emergence of cognitive COVID. *World Psychiatr.* **2021**, *20*, 52–53. [CrossRef]
55. Zheng, S.; Fan, J.; Yu, F.; Feng, B.; Lou, B.; Zou, Q.; Xie, G.; Lin, S.; Wang, R.; Yang, X.; et al. Viral load dynamics and disease severity in patients infected with SARS-CoV-2 in Zhejiang province, China, January-March 2020: Retrospective cohort study. *BMJ* **2020**, *369*, m1443. [CrossRef]
56. Baig, A.M.; Khaleeq, A.; Ali, U.; Syeda, H. Evidence of the COVID-19 virus targeting the CNS: Tissue distribution, host–virus interaction, and proposed neurotropic mechanisms. *ACS Chem. Neurosci.* **2020**, *11*, 995–998. [CrossRef] [PubMed]
57. Teuwen, L.-A.; Geldhof, V.; Pasut, A.; Carmeliet, P. COVID-19: The vasculature unleashed. *Nat. Rev. Immunol.* **2020**, *20*, 389–391. [CrossRef]
58. Varga, Z.; Flammer, A.J.; Steiger, P.; Haberecker, M.; Andermatt, R.; Zinkernagel, A.S.; Mehra, M.R.; Schuepbach, R.; Ruschitzka, F.; Moch, H. Endothelial cell infection and endotheliitis in COVID-19. *Lancet* **2020**, *395*, 1417–1418. [CrossRef]

59. Gu, J.; Gong, E.; Zhang, B.; Zheng, J.; Gao, Z.; Zhong, Y.; Zou, W.; Zhan, J.; Wang, S.; Xie, Z.; et al. Multiple organ infection and the pathogenesis of SARS. *J. Exp. Med.* **2005**, *202*, 415–424. [CrossRef]
60. Solomon, I.H.; Normandin, E.; Bhattacharyya, S.; Mukerji, S.S.; Keller, K.; Ali, A.S.; Adams, G.; Hornick, J.L.; Padera, R.F.; Sabeti, P. Neuropathological features of Covid-19. *N. Engl. J. Med.* **2020**, *383*, 989–992. [CrossRef]
61. Hu, B.; Huang, S.; Yin, L. The cytokine storm and COVID-19. *J. Med. Virol.* **2020**, *93*, 250–256. [CrossRef] [PubMed]
62. Wang, J.; Jiang, M.; Chen, X.; Montaner, L.J. Cytokine storm and leukocyte changes in mild versus severe SARS-CoV-2 infection: Review of 3939 COVID-19 patients in China and emerging pathogenesis and therapy concepts. *J. Leukoc. Biol.* **2020**, *108*, 17–41. [CrossRef]
63. Anderberg, S.B.; Luther, T.; Berglund, M.; Larsson, R.; Rubertsson, S.; Lipcsey, M.; Larsson, A.; Frithiof, R.; Hultström, M. Increased levels of plasma cytokines and correlations to organ failure and 30-day mortality in critically ill Covid-19 patients. *Cytokine* **2021**, *138*, 155389. [CrossRef]
64. Boldrini, M.; Canoll, P.D.; Klein, R.S. How COVID-19 affects the brain. *JAMA Psychiatry* **2021**, *78*, 682–683. [CrossRef] [PubMed]
65. Shen, X.-N.; Niu, L.-D.; Wang, Y.-J.; Cao, X.-P.; Liu, Q.; Tan, L.; Zhang, C.; Yu, J.-T. Inflammatory markers in Alzheimer's disease and mild cognitive impairment: A meta-analysis and systematic review of 170 studies. *J. Neurol. Neurosurg. Psychiatry* **2019**, *90*, 590–598. [CrossRef]
66. Iwashyna, T.J.; Ely, E.W.; Smith, D.M.; Langa, K. Long-term cognitive impairment and functional disability among survivors of severe sepsis. *JAMA* **2010**, *304*, 1787–1794. [CrossRef] [PubMed]
67. Widmann, C.N.; Heneka, M.T. Long-term cerebral consequences of sepsis. *Lancet Neurol.* **2014**, *13*, 630–636. [CrossRef]
68. Chakrabarty, T.; Torres, I.J.; Bond, D.J.; Yatham, L.N. Inflammatory cytokines and cognitive functioning in early-stage bipolar I disorder. *J. Affect. Disord.* **2019**, *245*, 679–685. [CrossRef]
69. Zheng, F.; Xie, W. High-sensitivity C-reactive protein and cognitive decline: The english longitudinal study of ageing. *Psychol. Med.* **2017**, *48*, 1381–1389. [CrossRef]
70. Siu, K.; Yuen, K.; Castano-Rodriguez, C.; Ye, Z.; Yeung, M.; Fung, S.; Yuan, S.; Chan, C.P.; Yuen, K.-Y.; Enjuanes, L.; et al. Severe acute respiratory syndrome Coronavirus ORF3a protein activates the NLRP3 inflammasome by promoting TRAF3-dependent ubiquitination of ASC. *FASEB J.* **2019**, *33*, 8865–8877. [CrossRef]
71. Ding, H.-G.; Deng, Y.-Y.; Yang, R.-Q.; Wang, Q.-S.; Jiang, W.-Q.; Han, Y.-L.; Huang, L.-Q.; Wen, M.-Y.; Zhong, W.-H.; Li, X.-S.; et al. Hypercapnia induces IL-1β overproduction via activation of NLRP3 inflammasome: Implication in cognitive impairment in hypoxemic adult rats. *J. Neuroinflamm.* **2018**, *15*, 4. [CrossRef] [PubMed]
72. Leon, M.P.D.; Redzepi, A.; McGrath, E.; Abdel-Haq, N.; Shawaqfeh, A.; Sethuraman, U.; Tilford, B.; Chopra, T.; Arora, H.; Ang, J.; et al. COVID-19–Associated pediatric multisystem inflammatory syndrome. *J. Pediatr. Infect. Dis. Soc.* **2020**, *9*, 407–408. [CrossRef]
73. Cheung, E.W.; Zachariah, P.; Gorelik, M.; Boneparth, A.; Kernie, S.; Orange, J.S.; Milner, J.D. Multisystem inflammatory syndrome related to COVID-19 in previously healthy children and adolescents in New York City. *JAMA* **2020**, *324*, 294–296. [CrossRef] [PubMed]
74. Sadiq, M.; Aziz, O.A.; Kazmi, U.; Hyder, N.; Sarwar, M.; Sultana, N.; Bari, A.; Rashid, J. Multisystem inflammatory syndrome associated with COVID-19 in children in Pakistan. *Lancet Child. Adolesc. Health* **2020**, *4*, e36–e37. [CrossRef]
75. Yasuhara, J.; Watanabe, K.; Takagi, H.; Sumitomo, N.; Kuno, T. COVID-19 and multisystem inflammatory syndrome in children: A systematic review and meta-analysis. *Pediatr. Pulmonol.* **2021**, *56*, 837–848. [CrossRef] [PubMed]
76. Morris, S.B.; Schwartz, N.G.; Patel, P.; Abbo, L.; Beauchamps, L.; Balan, S.; Lee, E.H.; Paneth-Pollak, R.; Geevarughese, A.; Lash, M.K.; et al. Case series of multisystem inflammatory syndrome in adults associated with SARS-CoV-2 infection—United Kingdom and United States, March–August 2020. *MMWR. Morb. Mortal. Wkly. Rep.* **2020**, *69*, 1450–1456. [CrossRef]
77. Ebina-Shibuya, R.; Namkoong, H.; Shibuya, Y.; Horita, N. Multisystem inflammatory syndrome in children (MIS-C) with COVID-19: Insights from simultaneous familial Kawasaki disease cases. *Int. J. Infect. Dis.* **2020**, *97*, 371–373. [CrossRef]
78. Godfred-Cato, S.; Bryant, B.; Leung, J.; Oster, M.E.; Conklin, L.; Abrams, J.; Roguski, K.; Wallace, B.; Prezzato, E.; Koumans, E.H.; et al. COVID-19–Associated multisystem inflammatory syndrome in children—United States, March–July 2020. *MMWR. Morb. Mortal. Wkly. Rep.* **2020**, *69*, 1074–1080. [CrossRef]
79. Diorio, C.; Henrickson, S.E.; Vella, L.A.; McNerney, K.O.; Chase, J.M.; Burudpakdee, C.; Lee, J.H.; Jasen, C.; Balamuth, F.; Barrett, D.M.; et al. Multisystem inflammatory syndrome in children and COVID-19 are distinct presentations of SARS–CoV-2. *J. Clin. Investig.* **2020**, *130*, 5967–5975. [CrossRef]
80. Jiang, L.; Tang, K.; Levin, M.; Irfan, O.; Morris, S.K.; Wilson, K.; Klein, J.D.; A Bhutta, Z. COVID-19 and multisystem inflammatory syndrome in children and adolescents. *Lancet Infect. Dis.* **2020**, *20*, e276–e288. [CrossRef]
81. Maltezou, H.; Pavli, A.; Tsakris, A. Post-COVID syndrome: An insight on its pathogenesis. *Vaccines* **2021**, *9*, 497. [CrossRef]
82. Rowley, A.H.; Shulman, S.T.; Arditi, M. Immune pathogenesis of COVID-19–related multisystem inflammatory syndrome in children. *J. Clin. Investig.* **2020**, *130*, 5619–5621. [CrossRef]
83. Tzotzos, S.J.; Fischer, B.; Fischer, H.; Zeitlinger, M. Incidence of ARDS and outcomes in hospitalized patients with COVID-19: A global literature survey. *Crit. Care* **2020**, *24*, 516. [CrossRef]
84. Wu, Z.; McGoogan, J.M. Characteristics of and important lessons from the Coronavirus disease 2019 (COVID-19) outbreak in China. *JAMA* **2020**, *323*, 1239. [CrossRef]

85. Sasannejad, C.; Ely, E.W.; Lahiri, S. Long-term cognitive impairment after acute respiratory distress syndrome: A review of clinical impact and pathophysiological mechanisms. *Crit. Care* **2019**, *23*, 352. [CrossRef]
86. Jackson, J.C.; Hart, R.P.; Gordon, S.M.; Shintani, A.; Truman, B.; May, L.; Ely, E.W. Six-month neuropsychological outcome of medical intensive care unit patients. *Crit. Care Med.* **2003**, *31*, 1226–1234. [CrossRef]
87. Girard, T.D.; Thompson, J.L.; Pandharipande, P.; Brummel, N.E.; Jackson, J.C.; Patel, M.B.; Hughes, C.G.; Chandrasekhar, R.; Pun, B.T.; Boehm, L.M.; et al. Clinical phenotypes of delirium during critical illness and severity of subsequent long-term cognitive impairment: A prospective cohort study. *Lancet Respir. Med.* **2018**, *6*, 213–222. [CrossRef]
88. Ammar, A.; Mueller, P.; Trabelsi, K.; Chtourou, H.; Boukhris, O.; Masmoudi, L.; Bouaziz, B.; Brach, M.; Schmicker, M.; Bentlage, E.; et al. Psychological consequences of COVID-19 home confinement: The ECLB-COVID19 multicenter study. *PLoS ONE* **2020**, *15*, e0240204. [CrossRef]
89. Ritchie, K.; Chan, D.; Watermeyer, T. The cognitive consequences of the COVID-19 epidemic: Collateral damage? *Brain Commun.* **2020**, *2*, fcaa069. [CrossRef]
90. Xiong, J.; Lipsitz, O.; Nasri, F.; Lui, L.M.; Gill, H.; Phan, L.; Chen-Li, D.; Iacobucci, M.; Ho, R.; Majeed, A.; et al. Impact of COVID-19 pandemic on mental health in the general population: A systematic review. *J. Affect. Disord.* **2020**, *277*, 55–64. [CrossRef]
91. Qureshi, S.U.; Long, M.E.; Bradshaw, M.R.; Pyne, J.M.; Magruder, K.M.; Kimbrell, T.; Hudson, T.J.; Jawaid, A.; E Schulz, P.; E Kunik, M. Does PTSD impair cognition beyond the effect of trauma? *J. Neuropsychiatry Clin. Neurosci.* **2011**, *23*. [CrossRef] [PubMed]
92. Bzdok, D.; Dunbar, R.I. The neurobiology of social distance. *Trends Cogn. Sci.* **2020**, *24*, 717–733. [CrossRef]
93. Fiorenzato, E.; Zabberoni, S.; Costa, A.; Cona, G. Cognitive and mental health changes and their vulnerability factors related to COVID-19 lockdown in Italy. *PLoS ONE* **2021**, *16*, e0246204. [CrossRef]
94. *Drugs and Lactation Database(LactMed)*; National Library of Medicine(US): Bethesda, MD, USA, 2006; COVID-19 Vaccines. Available online: https://www.ncbi.nlm.nih.gov/books/NBK565969/ (accessed on 19 July 2021).
95. Liu, B.D.; Ugolini, C.; Jha, P. Two Cases of Post-Moderna COVID-19 Vaccine Encephalopathy Associated With Nonconvulsive Status Epilepticus. *Cureus* **2021**, *13*, e16172. [CrossRef]
96. Zavala-Jonguitud, L.F.; Pérez-García, C.C. Delirium triggered by COVID -19 vaccine in an elderly patient. *Geriatr. Gerontol. Int.* **2021**, *21*, 540. [CrossRef] [PubMed]
97. Uwaydah, A.K.; Hassan, N.M.M.; Abu Ghoush, M.S.; Shahin, K.M.M. Adult multisystem inflammatory syndrome in a patient who recovered from COVID-19 postvaccination. *BMJ Case Rep.* **2021**, *14*, e242060. [CrossRef]
98. Lyons-Weiler, J. Pathogenic priming likely contributes to serious and critical illness and mortality in COVID-19 via autoimmunity. *J. Transl. Autoimmun.* **2020**, *3*, 100051. [CrossRef]
99. Terrando, N.; Pavlov, V.A. Editorial: Neuro-immune interactions in inflammation and autoimmunity. *Front. Immunol.* **2018**, *9*, 772. [CrossRef]
100. Lal, H.; Forster, M.J. Autoimmunity and age-associated cognitive decline. *Neurobiol. Aging* **1988**, *9*, 733–742. [CrossRef]
101. Mantovani, E.; Zucchella, C.; Bottiroli, S.; Federico, A.; Giugno, R.; Sandrini, G.; Chiamulera, C.; Tamburin, S. Telemedicine and virtual reality for cognitive rehabilitation: A roadmap for the COVID-19 pandemic. *Front. Neurol.* **2020**, *11*, 926. [CrossRef]
102. O'Brien, M.; McNicholas, F. The use of telepsychiatry during COVID-19 and beyond. *Ir. J. Psychol. Med.* **2020**, *37*, 250–255. [CrossRef] [PubMed]
103. Fedak, K.M.; Bernal, A.; Capshaw, Z.A.; Gross, S. Applying the Bradford Hill criteria in the 21st century: How data integration has changed causal inference in molecular epidemiology. *Emerg. Themes Epidemiol.* **2015**, *12*, 14. [CrossRef]
104. Callaway, E. Delta coronavirus variant: Scientists brace for impact. *Nat. Cell Biol.* **2021**, *595*, 17–18. [CrossRef]

Journal of
Clinical Medicine

MDPI

Review

Impact of COVID-19 on Neuropsychiatric Disorders

Niloufar Zia [1], Parsa Ravanfar [2], Sepideh Allahdadian [3] and Mehdi Ghasemi [4,*]

1 Department of Psychology, Lesley University, Cambridge, MA 02138, USA
2 Department of Psychiatry, University of Texas Southwestern, Dallas, TX 75390, USA
3 Department of Neurology, Penn State Milton S. Hershey Medical Center, Hershey, PA 17033, USA
4 Department of Neurology, University of Massachusetts Chan Medical School, Worcester, MA 01655, USA
* Correspondence: mehdi.ghasemi@umassmemorial.org or m82.ghasemi@gmail.com

Abstract: Since the Coronavirus disease 2019 (COVID-19) pandemic, caused by severe acute respiratory syndrome coronavirus 2 (SARS-CoV-2), many studies have shown that besides common COVID-19 symptoms, patients may develop various neuropsychiatric conditions including anxiety, mood disorders, psychosis, neurodegenerative diseases (e.g., dementia), insomnia, and even substance abuse disorders. COVID-19 can also worsen the patients underlying neuropsychiatric and neurodevelopmental conditions during or after the system phase of disease. In this review, we discuss the impact of SARS-CoV-2 infection on development or status of neuropsychiatric conditions during or following COVID-19.

Keywords: coronavirus disease 2019 (COVID-19); severe acute respiratory syndrome coronavirus 2 (SARS-CoV-2); neuropsychiatry; neurodegenerative diseases; neurodevelopmental diseases

1. Introduction

In December 2019, a novel Coronavirus named Severe Acute Respiratory Syndrome Coronavirus 2 (SARS-CoV-2) was identified in Wuhan, China. Soon after it became an epidemic throughout the world. SARS-CoV-2 has some spikes on its surface which are the membrane-anchored tiners consisting of receptor binding s1 and membrane-fusion s2 segment. The Cov name originated from these spikes. S1 segment consists of the receptor binding domain (RBD) that causes pathogenicity and infects the host cell via binding to the angiotensin-converting receptor-2 (ACE-2) on all tissues [1,2]. RBD has greater affinity for ACE-2 on cells of the ileum, kidney, heart, brain, lung, and vasculatures. It is responsible for the different manifestations it has, including respiratory disease and mild pneumonia; its usual symptoms include fever, shortness of breath, cough, and fatigue [3]. Besides systemic manifestation, accumulating reports indicate that patients with COVID-19 may develop a variety of neuropsychiatric conditions during or after COVID-19 (Figure 1) [4–7]. SARS-CoV-2 infection may also affect the patients' current neuropsychiatric conditions in various ways. Given the high burden of neuropsychiatric conditions on society besides COVID-19 itself, in this review, we will discuss the impact of SARS-CoV-2 infection on new-onset and current neuropsychiatric conditions in patients with COVID-19.

Citation: Zia, N.; Ravanfar, P.; Allahdadian, S.; Ghasemi, M. Impact of COVID-19 on Neuropsychiatric Disorders. *J. Clin. Med.* **2022**, *11*, 5213. https://doi.org/10.3390/jcm11175213

Academic Editor: Alfonso Troisi

Received: 6 August 2022
Accepted: 2 September 2022
Published: 3 September 2022

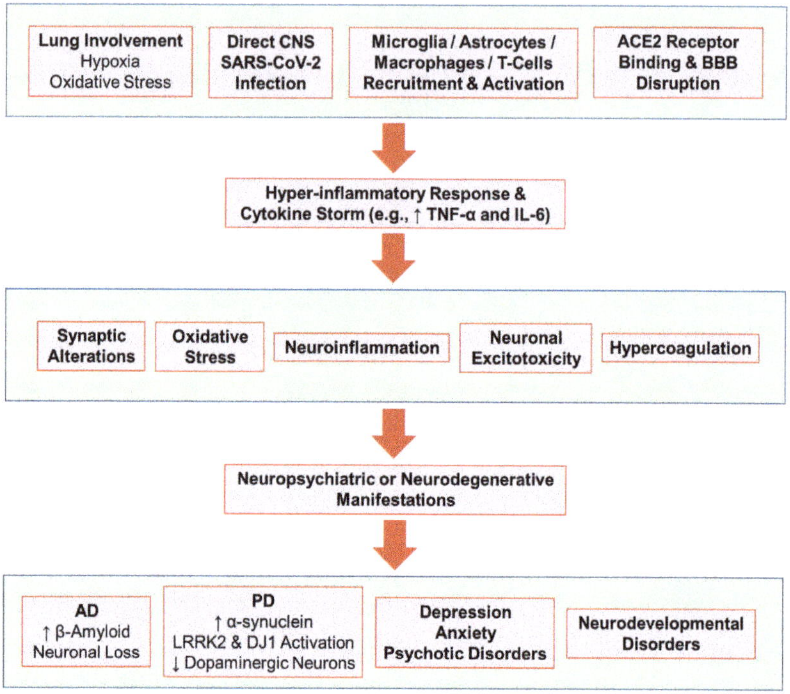

Figure 1. Neuropsychiatric manifestations and possible underlying mechanisms after SARS-CoV-2 infection. ACE2, angiotensin-converting enzyme 2; AD, Alzheimer's disease; BBB, blood-brain barrier; IL-6, interleukin-6; LRRK2, leucine-rich repeat kinase 2; PD, Parkinson's disease; TNF-α, tumor necrosis factor-α.

2. Neuropsychiatric Complications of COVID-19

Acute neuropsychiatric presentations and potentially long-term complications have been reported in people infected with COVID-19 as well as those who recovered from it [5]. In a large study using the TriNetX Analytics Network (a federated network recording anonymized data from electronic health records in 62 healthcare organizations, primarily in the United States [US]) and including 62,354 patients with confirmed diagnosis of COVID-19 [8], it was shown that COVID-19 was associated with increased incidence of a first psychiatric diagnosis in the following 14 to 90 days compared with six other health events (i.e., influenza, other respiratory tract infections, skin infection, cholelithiasis, urolithiasis, and a large bone fracture). The hazard ratios were greatest for anxiety disorders, insomnia, and dementia. The incidence of any psychiatric diagnosis in the 14 to 90 days after COVID-19 diagnosis was 18.1%, with 5.8% having a first diagnosis (e.g., first diagnosis of dementia 1.6% in patients older than 65 years) [8,9]. There is a wide range of underlying etiologic factors both within and beyond the CNS that lead to neuropsychiatric sequelae (Figure 1) [7].

In two large sample retrospective studies of 40,469 patients who recovered from COVID-19 in the TriNetX database, diagnosis of anxiety (and related disorders) and mood disorders was established in 4.6% and 3.8%, respectively, on or within one month after diagnosis of COVID-19 [6] (Table 1). Another retrospective study on 44,779 COVID-19 patients without previous psychiatric illness in the TriNetX Analytics Network revealed that the rate of all diagnoses of psychiatric disorders (i.e., including relapses) was higher within 14 to 90 days after COVID-19 diagnosis than after control health events (i.e., influenza, other respiratory tract infections, skin infection, cholelithiasis, urolithiasis, and a large bone fracture) [9]. The most common psychiatric diagnosis after COVID-19 diagnosis was anxiety disorder (12.8%, 95% confidence interval [CI] 12.4–13.3), followed by mood disorders (9.9%, 9.5–10.3). The probability of a first diagnosis of mood disorder within 14 to 90 days after COVID-19 diagnosis was 2% (95% CI 1.7–2.4), with depressive episode as the most common first diagnosis of mood disorder (1.7%, 95% CI 1.4–2.1) [9]. In another retrospective cohort study on 236,379 survivors of COVID-19 in the TriNetX Analytics Network, estimated incidences for first-time anxiety disorders in the following 6 months in the whole cohort and those admitted to intensive care unit (ICU) were 17.39% (95% CI 17.04–17.74) and 19.15% (95% CI 17.90–20.48), respectively [8]. Moreover, the estimated incidences for first-time mood disorders in the following 6 months in this study were 4.22% (95% CI 3.99–4.47) and 5.82% (95% CI 4.86–6.97) [8]. The prevalence of self-reported symptoms of depression and anxiety was much higher. Studies using self-report tools have suggested a markedly greater frequency of depressed mood (29.2%), anxiety, and post-traumatic anxiety symptoms (20.8–96.2%) in different countries including China and Italy [10–13] (Table 1).

Table 1. Incidence of anxiety and depressive psychiatric conditions in patients with COVID-19.

Population (Country)	Assessment	Psychiatric Conditions	Incidence	Ref.
126 (China)	Self-report questionnaire	Anxiety PTSD Depression	22.2% 31% 38.1%	[11]
402 (one month after hospital treatment) (Italy)	Self-report questionnaire	PTSD Depression Anxiety Obsessive Compulsive Symptoms Insomnia	28% 31% 42% 20% 40%	[12]
Prospective study in 44 hospitalized patients (USA)	HAD-A HAS-D	Depressive symptoms Anxiety Acute stress disorder syndrome	29% (20% after 2 weeks) 36% (9% after 2 weeks) 25% mild-moderate (after two weeks)	[14]
44,779 (the TriNetX Analytics Network)	Clinical diagnosis at 14–90 days (all first diagnoses)	Psychotic disorder Any mood disorder Depressive episode Insomnia Dementia	0.1% 2% 1.7% 1.9% 1.6%	[9]
236,379 (the TriNetX Analytics Network)	Clinical diagnosis at 6 months (all first diagnosis):	First dementia Mood disorder Anxiety Psychotic features Insomnia	0.67% 4.22% 7.11% 0.42% 2.56%	[8]
100 (UK)	Clinical evaluation	Any PTSD symptoms Thoughts of self-harm	41% 2%	[15]
714 clinically stable patients (China)	Online PTSD questionnaire (PCL-C)	Significant post-traumatic stress symptoms	96.2%	[10]
57 (China)	Chinese version 9-item Patient Health Questionnaire (PHQ-9) and 7-item Generalized Anxiety Disorder (GAD-7) scale	Depression Anxiety	29.2% 20.8%	[13]
153 (UK)	Clinical diagnosis	Affective disorder	2.6%	[16]

Table 1. *Cont.*

Population (Country)	Assessment	Psychiatric Conditions	Incidence	Ref.
40,469 (the TriNetX Analytics Network)	Clinical diagnosis	Anxiety Mood disorders Suicidal ideation	4.6% 3.8% 0.2%	[6]
2150 hospital admitted patients (Spain)	Clinical diagnosis	Mood disorder Anxiety-stress-adjustment disorder	1.4% 11.9%	[17]

There are multiple factors that contribute to the development of mood and anxiety disorders associated with COVID-19. These factors can be categorized into three domains: contextual factors and life stressors, disease-related reduction in quality of life such as fatigue and breathlessness, and biological factors impacting the brain such as neuro-immunological phenomena. Based on the evidence provided by Taquet et al., this higher occurrence of first-time mood and anxiety disorders cannot be solely attributed to the contextual factors such as economic and social adversities/challenges/stressors associated with COVID-19. Here, we focus on the disease-related pathophysiological mechanisms that may account for the occurrence of these psychiatric manifestations. The association between COVID-19 and depression and anxiety can be due to neurotropism of the virus, or the immunological reactions of the body such as cytokine storm [18]. In a study by Mazza et al. in Italy, there was a significant association between systemic immune-inflammation index (SII) with measures of anxiety and depression [12]. COVID-19 has been characterized by an exaggerated inflammatory response known as a "cytokine storm", and inflammatory cytokines have been associated with depression [19]. Conversely, the presence of a previous diagnosis of mood disorder is associated with higher mortality rates after prolonged hospitalization [20].

First-time psychosis may also occur among patients with COVID-19 as assessed in the TriNetX Analytics Network as well as systematic reviews of case reports and case series from different regions worldwide [8,9,21]. Although there has been shown a low probability of being newly diagnosed with a psychotic disorder in the 14 to 90 days after COVID-19 diagnosis (0.1%, 95% CI 0.08–0.2), broadly similar to the probability after control health events [9], the estimated incidences of psychotic disorders within 6 months after COVID-19 was higher by 1.40% (95% CI 1.30–1.51). It was even more increased in those patients initially admitted to the ICU due to COVID-19 (2.77%, 95% CI 2.31–3.33) [8]. A more recent systematic review of case reports and case series of 57 patients with COVID-19 (collected from six electronic databases including PubMed, Scopus, Web of Science, PsycInfo, PsycArticles, and CINAHL) also reported that the mean age for onset of psychotic symptoms (predominantly delusions and hallucinations) was the early 40s (men: 43.4 and women: 40.3), more than two thirds (~69%) of patients did not have any prior psychiatric disorders [21]. Only 26.3% of patients presented with moderate-severe COVID-19-related disease and complications. Overall, psychotic symptoms resolved markedly in 63.2% of cases after treatment with antipsychotics, benzodiazepines, valproic acid, and electroconvulsive treatment [21]. COVID-19-related new-onset psychosis and mania have been also reported in children and adolescents, even in those with asymptomatic COVID-19 infections as described in some case reports in the U.S. [22].

New onset dementia and cognitive dysfunction can occur in relation with COVID-19 [8,9,16,23]. A retrospective analysis of 50 patients with COVID-19 in the U.S. found cognitive impairment in 26% of cases [23]. Another study on 153 COVID-19 cases in the United Kingdom (UK) also showed that overall, 23 (15.3%) patients developed neuropsychiatric disorders related to COVID-19, among which 10 (43%) patients had new-onset psychosis, 6 (26%) had a neurocognitive (dementia-like) syndrome, and 4 (17%) had an affective disorder [16]. Further larger cohort studies showed that the estimated incidence of dementia during the first 14 to 90 days after a diagnosis of COVID-19 is 0.44% (95% CI 0.33–0.60); which was higher in those patients older than 65 years (1.6%,

95% CI 1.2–2.1), with a hazard ratio (HR) between 1.89 and 3.18 [9]. The estimated incidence of new dementia in the following 6 months was even higher by 0.67% (95% CI 0.59–0.75) and again with an increased rate in those patients initially admitted to ICU due to COVID-19 (1.74%, 95% CI 1.31–2.30) or in those who had encephalopathy by 4.72% (3.80–5.85) [8].

Both short-term (i.e., within 14 to 90 days) and 6-month onset of other neuropsychiatric conditions, such as insomnia and substance use disorder, may rise in the COVID-19 population as assessed in the TriNetX Analytics Network [8,9]. A post-discharge evaluation of 120 COVID-19 patients in France after an average of 110.9 days following admission showed that the most frequently reported persistent symptoms were fatigue (55%), dyspnea (42%), loss of memory (34%), difficulty in concentration (28%), and sleep disorders (30.8%) [24]. The probability of a first diagnosis of insomnia in the 14 to 90 days after COVID-19 diagnosis was further shown to be 1.9% (95% CI 1.6–2.2), more common than after controlled health events (HRs 1.85–3.29), in agreement with predictions that circadian disturbances will follow COVID-19 infection [9,25]. Close to 60% of the insomnia diagnoses were not accompanied by a concurrent diagnosis of an anxiety disorder [9]. The estimated incidence of first insomnia within 6 months post-COVID-19 was 2.53% (95% CI 2.37–2.71) [8]. The estimated incidence of new substance use disorder within 6 months following COVID-19 was 1.92% (95% CI 1.77–2.07) [8]. Overall, the above data indicate that COVID-19 is followed by remarkable rates of long-term neuropsychiatric diagnoses.

3. Impact of COVID-19 on Neuropsychiatric Disorders

The COVID-19 virus infection and the impact of the virus on society causes several different sequels and comorbidities in physical and mental health [26]. Infection with COVID-19 may cause the worsening of neuropsychiatric disorders and/or the development of neuropsychiatric disorders [26,27]. In addition, the societal consequences of the pandemic (i.e., isolation and quarantine) have caused the worsening and development of neuropsychiatric disorders [26]. Examples of relevant neuropsychiatric disorders in the context of COVID-19 include depression, anxiety, delirium, mood compulsivity, cognitive impairment, and obsessive-compulsive symptoms [26,28]. There are a variety of mechanisms that likely cause the worsening of the development of neuropsychiatric disorders in the context of COVID-19 infection and the ongoing pandemic [26].

Recent research examining the impact of COVID-19 infection on mental health functioning suggests that the virus causes an inflammation of the CNS which, in turn, may stress mental health processes and functioning through cytokine secretion [26]. Other research suggests that COVID-19 increases the risk of or exacerbates neuropsychiatric disorders via hypoxemia, which is common among individuals infected with COVID-19 [29,30]. Moreover, other research identifies additional ways by which COVID-19 infection and the pandemic negatively impact mental health (e.g., isolation, changes in social support, economic stressors) [26].

Individuals with pre-existing neuropsychiatric disorders and symptoms are likely at greater risk of poor mental health outcomes in the context of COVID-19 [26,31]. Indeed, the worldwide virus appears to affect people differently based on their baseline psychiatric functioning. As such, individuals with mood disorders, anxiety disorders, and psychotic disorders, may have a different baseline of psychiatric functioning and could be at higher risk of developing neuropsychiatric disorders or experiencing a worsening of neuropsychiatric symptoms following COVID-19 infection, as assessed in different studies and regions including the U.S. and Brazil [8,9,26,31,32].

Individuals with neuropsychiatric disorders demonstrate different and worse symptoms and functioning as compared to their counterparts in the context of the ongoing COVID-19 pandemic [26,33]. Specifically, individuals with pre-existing mood and anxiety disorders report increased stress and fear of pollution in the current pandemic [31]. In addition, these symptoms reached clinically significant or concerning levels. Among individuals with a pre-existing neuropsychiatric disorder who contracted COVID-19, many experienced an exacerbation of mental health symptoms [26,31,34,35]. Specifically, individuals may have experienced serious neuropsychiatric complications, including delirium, cognitive impairment, significant mood alterations, or even psychosis [26,31,32]. Indeed, even among people without pre-existing neuropsychiatric disorders, delirium occurs in most individuals who contract COVID-19 [26,36].

3.1. Anxiety Disorders

Individuals with anxiety disorders are at risk of poorer outcomes in the context of the COVID-19 pandemic [34]. Using an online subject pool from the U.S. and Canada, researchers found that individuals with anxiety-related disorders experienced higher stress as well as greater fear, socioeconomic consequences, xenophobia, and traumatic stress as compared to individuals with mood disorders and individuals without clinically significant mental health concerns in the context of the COVID-19 pandemic [34]. As such, individuals with anxiety disorders are at greater risk of certain poor outcomes even as compared to individuals with mood disorders in the context of the ongoing COVID-19 pandemic [34]. Regarding mechanisms behind the relationship between anxiety disorders and poor outcomes, individuals with anxiety disorders were more likely to engage in effortful isolation and ineffective coping strategies [34]. Perhaps these behaviors, in combination with other associated behaviors, increased the risk of certain poor outcomes for individuals with anxiety disorders as opposed to their counterparts [34]. The increased risk of poor outcomes across several domains (i.e., psychological or economic) among individuals with anxiety disorders in the context of the COVID-19 pandemic cannot be ignored. There is a need for research, intervention, and policy to address the increased risk and poor outcomes among this population.

3.2. Mood Disorders

Based on a recent meta-analysis, individuals with a pre-existing mood disorder have a significantly higher chance of hospitalization and death as compared to those without a pre-existing mood disorder following COVID-19 infection [37]. These meta-analytic results highlight the vulnerability of individuals with pre-existing mood disorders for poor health outcomes in the context of contracting COVID-19. As such, researchers and policymakers should consider those with pre-existing mood disorders when creating policy regarding vaccinations and other relevant public health decisions [37]. Mood disorders may confer a greater risk of susceptibility to COVID-19 for a variety of reasons. Individuals with pre-existing mood disorders experience increased psychological stress during the COVID-19 pandemic, which was further associated with maladaptive life and behavioral changes [34,38]. Certain mood disorders are associated with a greater risk of poor outcomes. For instance, a study in Australia demonstrated that specifically men with bipolar disorder are the most at-risk group among individuals with mood disorders regarding risk of depression and financial concerns [38]. As such, it is important to consider how individuals with pre-existing mood disorders may be at risk of certain poor health and psychological outcomes in the context of the ongoing COVID-19 pandemic.

3.3. Neurodevelopmental Disorders

Neurodevelopmental disorders typically emerge during early-to-middle childhood and may result in functional impairment and/or limitations regarding neuropsychological, cognitive, and adaptive development. Examples of neurodevelopmental disorders include autism spectrum disorder (ASD), attention-deficit/hyperactivity disorder (ADHD), intellectual disabilities, and specific learning disabilities [39].

Unfortunately, children with neurodevelopmental disorders (e.g., ASD and ADHD) are at higher risk of poor mental health and difficulties with functioning than their counterparts in the context of the COVID-19 pandemic, as evidenced by a cross-sectional parent-reported study in the UK [40]. Indeed, children with neurodevelopmental disorders experienced an increase in emotional difficulties and conduct problems as well as a decrease in prosocial behaviors during the pandemic [40]. Depression and anxiety among children and their parents with ASD have increased as reported by studies in different countries such as the US and Switzerland [41,42]. Among children with neurodevelopmental disorders studied in the UK, female children with ASD experienced the highest emotional symptoms [40]. The severity of neurodevelopmental symptoms increased during the course of the pandemic among children and adolescents in the U.S. [43]. In addition, a recent study on 238 adolescents (ages 15–17 years) from two sites in the Southeastern and Midwestern U.S. showed that associated behavioral considerations, including opposition/defiance and impulsivity, also increased during the pandemic [44]. The stressors and increased symptomatology of children with neurodevelopmental disorders also impacted parents; indeed, parents of children with neurodevelopmental disorders reported worse mental health than their counterparts during the pandemic in the UK [40].

Research has provided potential mechanisms or avenues by which individuals with neurodevelopmental disorders experienced worse outcomes in the context of the pandemic. Specifically, individuals with neurodevelopmental disorders experienced closures in or abrupt disruption of their health services [45], which likely caused decreases in physical and mental health [46,47]. The lack of access to physical exercise during lockdown and quarantine(s) may have been particularly detrimental to individuals with neurodevelopmental disorders as exercise may be used to regulate several symptoms of neurodevelopmental disorders [46]. Researchers have also postulated that boredom and associated decreases in motivation have engendered rises in depression and poor outcomes among children and young people with neurodevelopmental disorders [48]. In addition, changes in remote and hybrid schools were associated with increased dropout rates from school among children and young adults with ADHD in the U.S. [43].

Certain aspects of the ongoing pandemic may have increased risk of poor outcomes among children with ASD specifically. Indeed, individuals with ASD may have certain vulnerabilities that were exacerbated by the pandemic [48]. Quarantine and isolation policies in response to the pandemic caused severe disruption to the routines and services typically accessed by people with ASD [49]. In some cases, individuals with ASD lost complete access to services partially because individuals with ASD were not considered a marginalized population [20]. In addition, the evaluation of individuals with suspected ASD was also interrupted and services and diagnoses were delayed [20]. As such, individuals with ASD and individuals yet to be diagnosed with ASD experienced specific stressors that likely impeded effective intervention and support services. As a result, the research described above regarding poor outcomes among individuals with ASD and their families is not surprising.

Although initial research indicates that the negative impact of quarantine and lockdown on mental and physical health does not appear to be long-lasting among children and young people with neurodevelopmental disorders, longitudinal research has not yet been conducted to examine the long-lasting impact of COVID-19 on individuals with neurodevelopmental disorders [44].

3.4. *Psychotic Disorders*

Psychotic disorders are characterized by cognitive and perceptual dysfunction, usually hallucinations or delusions [50]. Psychotic disorders may be accompanied by mood disturbances and can be caused by [50]. In the U.S., between 0.25% and 0.64% of the population is diagnosed with a psychotic disorder [51]. However, over the course of the pandemic, the incidence of psychotic disorders and symptoms has risen [51]. Moreover, the risk of psychosis among individuals with COVID-19 is higher than the average population, with between 0.9% and 4% of individuals with COVID-19 experiencing psychosis [51].

As among individuals with neurodevelopmental disorders, services and supports for individuals with psychotic disorders were severely disrupted over the course of the pandemic. In addition, because of the symptoms and vulnerabilities associated with psychotic disorders, this population is highly vulnerable to the changes in routine and access to care caused by the COVID-19 pandemic [51]. Individuals with psychotic disorders may have experienced disruptions in their access to medication and face-to-face services [51–54]. These changes and barriers to services caused significant decompensation among many individuals with psychotic disorders and were also associated with increased paranoia and anxiety [51,52]. Decompensation refers to a significant deterioration in psychological functioning and an increase in severity of symptoms that is not typical [51]. Because of the transition to telehealth and phone services, providers may not have been able to accurately track and identify patients' decompensation over the course of the pandemic [51]. As such, individuals with psychotic disorders may have been uniquely at risk for experiencing worsening symptoms without proper support or intervention [51].

A single-center retrospective and observational study in Spain found that SARS-CoV-2 infection has also increased risk of and severity of psychosis symptoms [55]. Indeed, psychosis (e.g., delusions) has emerged among individuals with no history of these symptoms following infection with the virus [55]. However, it is unclear to what extent psychosis following infection with COVID-19 is caused by the virus itself versus the medications used by health providers to treat the virus [55]. Certain researchers posit that COVID-19 causes inflammation in the central nervous system, which then causes individuals to experience psychosis [55]. Regardless of the exact cause, individuals with COVID-19 are at increased risk of experiencing psychosis, even those without a prior history [55]. More research studies are needed to understand the cause of psychosis among individuals with COVID-19 as well as assessment and intervention strategies.

3.5. *Cognitive Disorders*

Cognitive disorders are overall characterized by executive function impairment and are associated with difficulties with organization, regulation, and perception [56]. Individuals with cognitive disorders may experience difficulties with processing speed, reasoning, decision-making, awareness, attention, learning, impulsivity, memory, or language [56]. More than 16 million individuals in the United States are currently diagnosed with a cognitive disorder [57].

Individuals with cognitive disorders are at significantly higher risk of contracting the virus given baseline difficulties with executive functioning [54]. Indeed, because individuals with cognitive disorders may struggle to care for themselves, it may be harder for them to adhere to safety standards regarding isolation, social distancing, and quarantine [58]. As part of this concern, individuals with cognitive disorders may live in collective housing or treatment units and the functioning of these structures has been severely impacted by the pandemic. As such, it is highly likely the functioning of individuals within these communities has also been severely affected. In addition, such facilities for individuals with cognitive disorders may allow the virus to spread easily across patients and staff putting individuals with cognitive disorders at even higher risk of contracting the virus [59]. If infected with COVID-19, individuals with cognitive disorders may also have worse outcomes, especially if their access to caregivers or supervision is limited in the context of ongoing social distancing and quarantine policy [58,60]. Research is needed to identify and develop standards for communal living facilities for individuals with cognitive disorders that prioritizes the delivery of services and the safety of patients.

Intellectual disabilities are a subset of cognitive disorders. Unfortunately, the health and well-being of individuals with cognitive disorders has been negatively impacted by the ongoing pandemic. Specifically, research indicates that mental health and physical activity have significantly decreased among children and young adults with both physical and intellectual disabilities [47]. Decreases in physical activity were due to quarantine and isolation policies as well as the closing of community centers and exercise facilities [47]. Among parents of children with intellectual disabilities, 90% reported worsening mood and increased behavioral problems among their children [47]. Although this study identified the potential for the development of solutions to the problems and barriers experienced by individuals with intellectual disabilities, no such solutions have been systematically implemented [47]. Thus, both research and advocacy are needed to address the problems and outcomes among individuals with intellectual disabilities over the course of the ongoing pandemic.

3.6. Neurodegenerative Disorders

Studies have revealed that ACE-2 is also expressed on neurons, glial cells, epithelial cells of blood-brain barrier (BBB), as well as oligodendrocytes. Interestingly a high concentration of substantia nigra may help the virus to enter, which itself may be the cause of reported neuropsychiatric sequelae of the infection [61]. Varieties of neurological symptoms including headache, ageusia, anosmia, and different forms of neurodegenerative disorders have been reported as consequences of SARS-CoV-2 infection [62]. Inflammation as a consequence of viral entry to the brain can cause oxidative damage and apoptosis of the cells in the brain, which has been reported as a cause of neurodegeneration and neurodegenerative disease [63]. Alzheimer's disease (AD) and Parkinson's disease (PD) are two neurodegenerative disorders reported to be caused by prolonged inflammation in patients infected by SARS-CoV-2 as a possible postinfectious manifestation. Inflammatory processes are also involved in other neurodegenerative disorders such as progressive supranuclear palsy syndrome (PSPS) [64], corticobasal syndrome (CBS) [64], and multiple system atrophy-parkinsonian type (MSA-P) [65]. COVID-19 has been reported to affect the international classification of functioning, disability, and health functioning in patients with MSA [66]. Accumulating evidence also suggests that SARS-CoV-2 infection can induce neurodegenerative disorders [67].

In view of the above, SARS-CoV-2-induced reactive oxygen species (ROS) caused by oxidative damage has been reported to cause accumulation of the amyloid beta (Aβ) proteins which itself is involved in the pathogenesis of AD. In addition, increased tau level as a result of neuroinflammation followed by viral entry to the brain has been reported as another possible cause of cognitive impairment within patients of SARS-CoV-2 [67,68]. COVID-19 incidence and complications are increased in patients with AD and related dementia. Patients with AD or related dementias have a cognitive impairment which causes difficulty understanding and remembering the recommendations. This disease is also more associated with other comorbidities such as cardiovascular disease, which may be another reason for high mortality of COVID-19 in these patients (90%) [69,70]. It has been also reported that APOE4 isoform of AD which causes a decreased amount of APO has increased the risk for COVID-19 infection and progression [71].

Several possible pathogeneses have been reported as a cause of PD in COVID-19 patients. Vulnerability of the basal ganglia and dopamine-rich region as well as the neuroinflammation caused by SARS-CoV-2 has been reported as a possible cause of failure of dopamine synthesis in COVID-19 patients [67]. Moreover, DJ1 and Leucine-rich repeat kinase 2 (LRRK2), key proteins in dopamine regulation and oxidative reaction, can be affected by SARS-CoV-2, resulting in dopamine dysregulation and inflammation in substantia nigra and α-synuclein aggregation [67,72].

Apart from the effect of COVID-19 on patients' access to different medical and psychological care, decreased physical activity and family support [73] and different neuropsychiatric outcomes have been reported that may be due to dopamine depletion in PD patients as a neurotransmitter to help with adoption to different changes in healthy individuals, which is lacking in PD patients. Anxiety and stress may remain and become chronic due to lack of adaptation as a result of dopamine depletion [74]. There are three different hypotheses about the effect of COVID-19-induced stress in PD patients. Stress can interfere with the levodopa effect and reduce it [75]. In addition, chronic stress has been revealed to decrease the dopamine activity within the rodent's ventral tegmentum compared to healthy controls and has been reported as a cause of neurodegeneration in PD and AD [76]. Emotional stress as a trigger for freezing gait has been reported as well [77]. One important aspect of COVID-19 infection is dehydration, diarrhea, fever and decrease in water intake which may be another important aspect to consider when adjusting the medication dosage. However, COVID-19 infection has been reported as a trigger for worsening of PD motor and nonmotor symptoms. Although, the patients with higher age and duration of illness had been reported to have more mortality risk compared to the participants with younger age and shorter disease duration [73,78], worsening of motor and non-motor symptoms, such as rigidity, tremor, fatigue, pain, and concentration, has not been related to disease duration or severity [79]. In view of the above, it can be concluded that COVID-19 can cause different effects on PD via decreasing dopamine secretion, neurodegeneration, and can be a trigger for the developing or worsening of symptoms in PD and AD.

4. Conclusions

Since the COVID-19 pandemic, accumulating lines of evidence have revealed that besides common clinical manifestations, SARS-CoV-2 infection is associated with development or worsening of a variety of neuropsychiatric conditions. These can occur during or shortly after the onset of COVID-19. However, more recent longitudinal studies have revealed that COVID-19 increases the estimated risk of developing or worsening of neuropsychiatric conditions, such as mood, anxiety, psychotic disorders, dementia, insomnia, or even substance abuse disorders, after 6 months following COVID-19. These data indicate that close and long-term neuropsychiatric and cognitive monitoring of patients with COVID-19 are critical in order to diagnose these sequels and take appropriate therapeutic approaches as early as possible, and eventually improve patients' and their families quality of life.

Although SARS-CoV-2 infection itself can be associated with the above-mentioned neuropsychiatric sequela, one should not overlook the multiple factors that contribute to the development or worsening of neuropsychiatric conditions during the COVID-19 pandemic. Overall, we can categorize these into three major domains: (i) the pandemic's burden on the society acting as psycho-socio-economic stressors (e.g., deterioration of economic state, lockdown or quarantine, disruption of health care provision, and loss of job or family members due to COVID-19), (ii) disease-related reduction in quality of life (e.g., fatigue and breathlessness), and (iii) the impact of infection itself on brain function. These factors separately or in combination with each other may play critical roles in development or exacerbation of neuropsychiatric conditions during the pandemic. For instance, a population-based longitudinal study on 16,910 participants in the UK revealed an independent association between COVID-19 and increased risk of economic vulnerability among participants, measured by both household income sufficiency and sickness absence from work [80]. The economic recession resulting from the COVID-19 pandemic has adversely affected many people's mental health and created new barriers for people already suffering from mental illness [81]. This is not only limited to COVID-19 pandemic, as such negative impacts on mental health and neuropsychiatric conditions have been seen in other global or regional shocks including wars [82–84], natural disasters [85,86], or other disease outbreaks, e.g., with Ebola [87,88], Zika virus [89], Middle East respiratory syndrome coronavirus (MERS) [90,91], and severe acute respiratory syndrome coronavirus (SARS-CoV) [90]. Social isolation due to lockdown or quarantine may have been particularly detrimental to individuals with neuropsychiatric and neurodevelopmental disorders, as social interaction and exercise may be used to regulate several symptoms of these disorders [46,92]. Data from an online questionnaire from 55,589 participants from 40 countries during the COVID-19 pandemic have revealed that lockdown significantly increases anxiety and depression at every degree of lockdown intensity, especially in combination with the presence of prior mental health issue [92]. This emphasizes the need for a proactive intervention to protect mental health of the general population but more specifically of vulnerable groups [92].

Almost over 2.5 years have passed since the COVID-19 pandemic; and as our knowledge about different neuropsychiatric manifestations directly or indirectly related to COVID-19 is improving, it overall highlights the critical need for global preparedness in the mental health sector during outbreaks of such infectious diseases. Important steps and innovations have been taken over the last 2 years to enable better service delivery to the affected populations. For instance, use of telemedicine and electronic prescriptions have become pivotal tools to be implemented globally [93]. This could be an essential element of continuity of care, especially during the lockdown or quarantine period. The promotion and empowerment of community-based mental health services especially in low-and-middle-income countries can also decrease the present treatment gap even during infectious disease outbreaks [94]. The development of global or local guidelines or consensus recommendations for such neuropsychiatric issues during or after the outbreak seems to be another effective way in reducing such psychiatric and mental health complications [94].

In the end, with an improvement of our knowledge about the pathophysiology of SARS-CoV-2 in brain dysfunction and neuropsychiatric conditions as well as the development of mediations targeting the infection itself or its related pathologic molecular signaling pathways, we may improve or even prevent the development of such neuropsychiatric manifestations. For instance, due to the presence of immune dysfunction and cytokine storm in COVID-19 patients, anti-inflammatory, immunomodulatory, or immunosuppressive medications have been tested or even in animal models of SARS-CoV-2 infections with variable benefits [95,96]. Vaccination has also created a new epoch in improving survival rate and acute critical illness related to COVID-19 [97]. Notably, a large retrospective cohort of 9479 individuals who developed COVID-19 despite SARS-CoV-2 vaccination, well-matched to controls, found that vaccination protected against severe acute illness, stroke, seizures, and psychotic disorders after breakthrough COVID-19 as assessed within 6 months post-vaccination. However, it may not protect from fatigue and other post-COVID-19 behavioral and cognitive symptoms [98]. Overall, research in this area is advancing. For instance, some studies have found an association between low neurotrophic factors and COVID-19-related neuropsychiatric complications [99]; thus, neurotrophic drugs such as cerebrolysin may serve as a potential therapeutic approach to improve neuropsychiatric manifestations of COVID-19 [100]. Clearly, more research studies and clinical trials are needed in this regard.

Author Contributions: N.Z., P.R., S.A. and M.G. conceived and designed the review, outlined the performed rigorous literature search, designed the table and figure, and wrote the manuscript. All authors have read and agreed to the published version of the manuscript.

Funding: M.G. is supported by a clinical research training scholarship in ALS funded by The ALS Association and The American Brain Foundation, in collaboration with the American Academy of Neurology as well as NIH-funded Wellstone fellowship training grant (NIH 5P50HD060848-15) for research on FSHD.

Institutional Review Board Statement: Not applicable.

Informed Consent Statement: Not applicable.

Data Availability Statement: Not applicable.

Conflicts of Interest: The authors declare no conflict of interest.

References

1. Ghasemi, M.; Umeton, R.P.; Keyhanian, K.; Mohit, B.; Rahimian, N.; Eshaghhosseiny, N.; Davoudi, V. SARS-CoV-2 and Acute Cerebrovascular Events: An Overview. *J. Clin. Med.* **2021**, *10*, 3349. [CrossRef] [PubMed]
2. Keyhanian, K.; Umeton, R.P.; Mohit, B.; Davoudi, V.; Hajighasemi, F.; Ghasemi, M. SARS-CoV-2 and nervous system: From pathogenesis to clinical manifestation. *J. Neuroimmunol.* **2020**, *350*, 577436. [CrossRef]
3. Ghosh, A.; Kar, P.K.; Gautam, A.; Gupta, R.; Singh, R.; Chakravarti, R.; Ravichandiran, V.; Ghosh Dastidar, S.; Ghosh, D.; Roy, S. An insight into SARS-CoV-2 structure, pathogenesis, target hunting for drug development and vaccine initiatives. *RSC Med. Chem.* **2022**, *13*, 647–675. [CrossRef] [PubMed]
4. Ferrando, S.J.; Klepacz, L.; Lynch, S.; Tavakkoli, M.; Dornbush, R.; Baharani, R.; Smolin, Y.; Bartell, A. COVID-19 Psychosis: A Potential New Neuropsychiatric Condition Triggered by Novel Coronavirus Infection and the Inflammatory Response? *Psychosomatics* **2020**, *61*, 551–555. [CrossRef] [PubMed]
5. Kumar, S.; Veldhuis, A.; Malhotra, T. Neuropsychiatric and Cognitive Sequelae of COVID-19. *Front. Psychol.* **2021**, *12*, 577529. [CrossRef]
6. Nalleballe, K.; Reddy Onteddu, S.; Sharma, R.; Dandu, V.; Brown, A.; Jasti, M.; Yadala, S.; Veerapaneni, K.; Siddamreddy, S.; Avula, A.; et al. Spectrum of neuropsychiatric manifestations in COVID-19. *Brain Behav. Immun.* **2020**, *88*, 71–74. [CrossRef]

7. Pantelis, C.; Jayaram, M.; Hannan, A.J.; Wesselingh, R.; Nithianantharajah, J.; Wannan, C.M.J.; Syeda, W.T.; Choy, K.H.C.; Zantomio, D.; Christopoulos, A.; et al. Neurological, neuropsychiatric and neurodevelopmental complications of COVID-19. *Aust. N. Z. J. Psychiatry* **2020**, *55*, 750–762. [CrossRef]
8. Taquet, M.; Geddes, J.R.; Husain, M.; Luciano, S.; Harrison, P.J. 6-month neurological and psychiatric outcomes in 236 379 survivors of COVID-19: A retrospective cohort study using electronic health records. *Lancet. Psychiatry* **2021**, *8*, 416–427. [CrossRef]
9. Taquet, M.; Luciano, S.; Geddes, J.R.; Harrison, P.J. Bidirectional associations between COVID-19 and psychiatric disorder: Retrospective cohort studies of 62354 COVID-19 cases in the USA. *Lancet Psychiatry* **2021**, *8*, 130–140. [CrossRef]
10. Bo, H.X.; Li, W.; Yang, Y.; Wang, Y.; Zhang, Q.; Cheung, T.; Wu, X.; Xiang, Y.T. Posttraumatic stress symptoms and attitude toward crisis mental health services among clinically stable patients with COVID-19 in China. *Psychol. Med.* **2021**, *51*, 1052–1053. [CrossRef]
11. Cai, X.; Hu, X.; Ekumi, I.O.; Wang, J.; An, Y.; Li, Z.; Yuan, B. Psychological Distress and Its Correlates Among COVID-19 Survivors During Early Convalescence Across Age Groups. *Am. J. Geriatr. Psychiatry* **2020**, *28*, 1030–1039. [CrossRef] [PubMed]
12. Mazza, M.G.; De Lorenzo, R.; Conte, C.; Poletti, S.; Vai, B.; Bollettini, I.; Melloni, E.M.T.; Furlan, R.; Ciceri, F.; Rovere-Querini, P.; et al. Anxiety and depression in COVID-19 survivors: Role of inflammatory and clinical predictors. *Brain Behav. Immun.* **2020**, *89*, 594–600. [CrossRef]
13. Zhang, J.; Lu, H.; Zeng, H.; Zhang, S.; Du, Q.; Jiang, T.; Du, B. The differential psychological distress of populations affected by the COVID-19 pandemic. *Brain Behav. Immun.* **2020**, *87*, 49–50. [CrossRef] [PubMed]
14. Parker, C.; Slan, A.; Shalev, D.; Critchfield, A. Abrupt Late-onset Psychosis as a Presentation of Coronavirus 2019 Disease (COVID-19): A Longitudinal Case Report. *J. Psychiatr. Pract.* **2021**, *27*, 131–136. [CrossRef] [PubMed]
15. Halpin, S.J.; McIvor, C.; Whyatt, G.; Adams, A.; Harvey, O.; McLean, L.; Walshaw, C.; Kemp, S.; Corrado, J.; Singh, R.; et al. Postdischarge symptoms and rehabilitation needs in survivors of COVID-19 infection: A cross-sectional evaluation. *J. Med. Virol.* **2021**, *93*, 1013–1022. [CrossRef]
16. Varatharaj, A.; Thomas, N.; Ellul, M.A.; Davies, N.W.S.; Pollak, T.A.; Tenorio, E.L.; Sultan, M.; Easton, A.; Breen, G.; Zandi, M.; et al. Neurological and neuropsychiatric complications of COVID-19 in 153 patients: A UK-wide surveillance study. *Lancet Psychiatry* **2020**, *7*, 875–882. [CrossRef]
17. Diez-Quevedo, C.; Iglesias-González, M.; Giralt-López, M.; Rangil, T.; Sanagustin, D.; Moreira, M.; López-Ramentol, M.; Ibáñez-Caparrós, A.; Lorán, M.E.; Bustos-Cardona, T.; et al. Mental disorders, psychopharmacological treatments, and mortality in 2150 COVID-19 Spanish inpatients. *Acta Psychiatr. Scand.* **2021**, *143*, 526–534. [CrossRef]
18. Ragab, D.; Salah Eldin, H.; Taeimah, M.; Khattab, R.; Salem, R. The COVID-19 Cytokine Storm; What We Know So Far. *Front. Immunol.* **2020**, *11*, 1446. [CrossRef]
19. Perlmutter, A. Immunological Interfaces: The COVID-19 Pandemic and Depression. *Front. Neurol.* **2021**, *12*, 657004. [CrossRef]
20. Castro, V.M.; Gunning, F.M.; McCoy, T.H.; Perlis, R.H. Mood Disorders and Outcomes of COVID-19 Hospitalizations. *Am. J. Psychiatry* **2021**, *178*, 541–547. [CrossRef]
21. Chaudhary, A.M.D.; Musavi, N.B.; Saboor, S.; Javed, S.; Khan, S.; Naveed, S. Psychosis during the COVID-19 pandemic: A systematic review of case reports and case series. *J. Psychiatr. Res.* **2022**, *153*, 37–55. [CrossRef] [PubMed]
22. Meeder, R.; Adhikari, S.; Sierra-Cintron, K.; Aedma, K. New-Onset Mania and Psychosis in Adolescents in the Context of COVID-19 Infection. *Cureus* **2022**, *14*, e24322. [CrossRef] [PubMed]
23. Pinna, P.; Grewal, P.; Hall, J.P.; Tavarez, T.; Dafer, R.M.; Garg, R.; Osteraas, N.D.; Pellack, D.R.; Asthana, A.; Fegan, K.; et al. Neurological manifestations and COVID-19: Experiences from a tertiary care center at the Frontline. *J. Neurol. Sci.* **2020**, *415*, 116969. [CrossRef] [PubMed]
24. Garrigues, E.; Janvier, P.; Kherabi, Y.; Le Bot, A.; Hamon, A.; Gouze, H.; Doucet, L.; Berkani, S.; Oliosi, E.; Mallart, E.; et al. Post-discharge persistent symptoms and health-related quality of life after hospitalization for COVID-19. *J. Infect.* **2020**, *81*, e4–e6. [CrossRef] [PubMed]
25. McCarthy, M.J. Circadian rhythm disruption in Myalgic Encephalomyelitis/Chronic Fatigue Syndrome: Implications for the post-acute sequelae of COVID-19. *Brain Behav Immun Health* **2022**, *20*, 100412. [CrossRef]
26. Robinson-Agramonte, M.A.; Gonçalves, C.A.; Noris-García, E.; Préndes Rivero, N.; Brigida, A.L.; Schultz, S.; Siniscalco, D.; García García, R.J. Impact of SARS-CoV-2 on neuropsychiatric disorders. *World J. Psychiatry* **2021**, *11*, 347–354. [CrossRef]
27. Idehen, J.B.; Kazi, U.; Quainoo-Acquah, J.A.; Sperry, B.; Zaman, I.; Goodarzi, A.; Chida, S.; Nalbandyan, L.; Hernandez, E.W.; Sharma, V.; et al. On Patterns of Neuropsychiatric Symptoms in Patients With COVID-19: A Systematic Review of Case Reports. *Cureus* **2022**, *14*, e25004. [CrossRef]
28. Pacitti, F.; Socci, V.; D'Aurizio, G.; Jannini, T.B.; Rossi, A.; Siracusano, A.; Rossi, R.; Di Lorenzo, G. Obsessive-compulsive symptoms among the general population during the first COVID-19 epidemic wave in Italy. *J. Psychiatr. Res.* **2022**, *153*, 18–24. [CrossRef]
29. Chippa, V.; Aleem, A.; Anjum, F. Post Acute Coronavirus (COVID-19) Syndrome. In *StatPearls*; StatPearls Publishing Copyright © 2022, StatPearls Publishing LLC.: Treasure Island, FL, USA, 2022.
30. Xiang, Y.T.; Yang, Y.; Li, W.; Zhang, L.; Zhang, Q.; Cheung, T.; Ng, C.H. Timely mental health care for the 2019 novel coronavirus outbreak is urgently needed. *Lancet Psychiatry* **2020**, *7*, 228–229. [CrossRef]

31. Carvalho, P.M.M.; Moreira, M.M.; de Oliveira, M.N.A.; Landim, J.M.M.; Neto, M.L.R. The psychiatric impact of the novel coronavirus outbreak. *Psychiatry Res.* **2020**, *286*, 112902. [CrossRef]
32. Goularte, J.F.; Serafim, S.D.; Colombo, R.; Hogg, B.; Caldieraro, M.A.; Rosa, A.R. COVID-19 and mental health in Brazil: Psychiatric symptoms in the general population. *J. Psychiatr. Res.* **2021**, *132*, 32–37. [CrossRef] [PubMed]
33. O'Connor, K.; Wrigley, M.; Jennings, R.; Hill, M.; Niazi, A. Mental health impacts of COVID-19 in Ireland and the need for a secondary care mental health service response. *Ir. J. Psychol. Med.* **2021**, *38*, 99–107. [CrossRef] [PubMed]
34. Asmundson, G.J.G.; Paluszek, M.M.; Landry, C.A.; Rachor, G.S.; McKay, D.; Taylor, S. Do pre-existing anxiety-related and mood disorders differentially impact COVID-19 stress responses and coping? *J. Anxiety Disord.* **2020**, *74*, 102271. [CrossRef] [PubMed]
35. Zarei, M.; Bose, D.; Nouri-Vaskeh, M.; Tajiknia, V.; Zand, R.; Ghasemi, M. Long-term side effects and lingering symptoms post COVID-19 recovery. *Rev. Med. Virol.* **2022**, *32*, e2289. [CrossRef] [PubMed]
36. González-Pinto, T.; Luna-Rodríguez, A.; Moreno-Estébanez, A.; Agirre-Beitia, G.; Rodríguez-Antigüedad, A.; Ruiz-Lopez, M. Emergency room neurology in times of COVID-19: Malignant ischaemic stroke and SARS-CoV-2 infection. *Eur. J. Neurol.* **2020**, *27*, e35–e36. [CrossRef]
37. Ceban, F.; Nogo, D.; Carvalho, I.P.; Lee, Y.; Nasri, F.; Xiong, J.; Lui, L.M.W.; Subramaniapillai, M.; Gill, H.; Liu, R.N.; et al. Association Between Mood Disorders and Risk of COVID-19 Infection, Hospitalization, and Death: A Systematic Review and Meta-analysis. *JAMA Psychiatry* **2021**, *78*, 1079–1091. [CrossRef]
38. Van Rheenen, T.E.; Meyer, D.; Neill, E.; Phillipou, A.; Tan, E.J.; Toh, W.L.; Rossell, S.L. Mental health status of individuals with a mood-disorder during the COVID-19 pandemic in Australia: Initial results from the COLLATE project. *J. Affect. Disord.* **2020**, *275*, 69–77. [CrossRef]
39. Termine, C.; Dui, L.G.; Borzaga, L.; Galli, V.; Lipari, R.; Vergani, M.; Berlusconi, V.; Agosti, M.; Lunardini, F.; Ferrante, S. Investigating the effects of COVID-19 lockdown on Italian children and adolescents with and without neurodevelopmental disorders: A cross-sectional study. *Curr. Psychol.* 2021, 1–17, *Online ahead of print*. [CrossRef]
40. Nonweiler, J.; Rattray, F.; Baulcomb, J.; Happé, F.; Absoud, M. Prevalence and Associated Factors of Emotional and Behavioural Difficulties during COVID-19 Pandemic in Children with Neurodevelopmental Disorders. *Children* **2020**, *7*, 128. [CrossRef]
41. Rezendes, D.L.; Scarpa, A. Associations between Parental Anxiety/Depression and Child Behavior Problems Related to Autism Spectrum Disorders: The Roles of Parenting Stress and Parenting Self-Efficacy. *Autism Res. Treat.* **2011**, *2011*, 395190. [CrossRef]
42. Werling, A.M.; Walitza, S.; Eliez, S.; Drechsler, R. Impact of the COVID-19 pandemic on mental health and family situation of clinically referred children and adolescents in Switzerland: Results of a survey among mental health care professionals after 1 year of COVID-19. *J. Neural Transm. (Vienna Austria 1996)* **2022**, *129*, 675–688. [CrossRef] [PubMed]
43. Sibley, M.H.; Ortiz, M.; Gaias, L.M.; Reyes, R.; Joshi, M.; Alexander, D.; Graziano, P. Top problems of adolescents and young adults with ADHD during the COVID-19 pandemic. *J. Psychiatr. Res.* **2021**, *136*, 190–197. [CrossRef] [PubMed]
44. Breaux, R.; Dvorsky, M.R.; Marsh, N.P.; Green, C.D.; Cash, A.R.; Shroff, D.M.; Buchen, N.; Langberg, J.M.; Becker, S.P. Prospective impact of COVID-19 on mental health functioning in adolescents with and without ADHD: Protective role of emotion regulation abilities. *J. Child Psychol. Psychiatry Allied Discip.* **2021**, *62*, 1132–1139. [CrossRef]
45. Morris-Rosendahl, D.J.; Crocq, M.A. Neurodevelopmental disorders-the history and future of a diagnostic concept. *Dialogues Clin. Neurosci.* **2020**, *22*, 65–72. [CrossRef]
46. Shuai, L.; He, S.; Zheng, H.; Wang, Z.; Qiu, M.; Xia, W.; Cao, X.; Lu, L.; Zhang, J. Influences of digital media use on children and adolescents with ADHD during COVID-19 pandemic. *Glob. Health* **2021**, *17*, 48. [CrossRef]
47. Theis, N.; Campbell, N.; De Leeuw, J.; Owen, M.; Schenke, K.C. The effects of COVID-19 restrictions on physical activity and mental health of children and young adults with physical and/or intellectual disabilities. *Disabil. Health J.* **2021**, *14*, 101064. [CrossRef]
48. Bellomo, T.R.; Prasad, S.; Munzer, T.; Laventhal, N. The impact of the COVID-19 pandemic on children with autism spectrum disorders. *J. Pediatric Rehabil. Med.* **2020**, *13*, 349–354. [CrossRef]
49. Amaral, D.G.; de Vries, P.J. COVID-19 and Autism Research: Perspectives from Around the Globe. *Autism Res. Off. J. Int. Soc. Autism Res.* **2020**, *13*, 844–869. [CrossRef]
50. Lieberman, J.A.; First, M.B. Psychotic Disorders. *N. Engl. J. Med.* **2018**, *379*, 270–280. [CrossRef]
51. Jay, J.; Garrels, E.; Korenis, P. Effects of the COVID-19 Pandemic on Patients with Psychotic Disorders: Review of the Literature and Case Series. *J. Sci. Innov. Med.* **2021**, *4*, 27.
52. Mongan, D.; Cannon, M.; Cotter, D.R. COVID-19, hypercoagulation and what it could mean for patients with psychotic disorders. *Brain Behav. Immun.* **2020**, *88*, 9–10. [CrossRef] [PubMed]
53. Valdés-Florido, M.J.; López-Díaz, Á.; Palermo-Zeballos, F.J.; Garrido-Torres, N.; Álvarez-Gil, P.; Martínez-Molina, I.; Martín-Gil, V.E.; Ruiz-Ruiz, E.; Mota-Molina, M.; Algarín-Moriana, M.P.; et al. Clinical characterization of brief psychotic disorders triggered by the COVID-19 pandemic: A multicenter observational study. *Eur. Arch. Psychiatry Clin. Neurosci.* **2022**, *272*, 5–15. [CrossRef]
54. Valdés-Florido, M.J.; López-Díaz, Á.; Palermo-Zeballos, F.J.; Martínez-Molina, I.; Martín-Gil, V.E.; Crespo-Facorro, B.; Ruiz-Veguilla, M. Reactive psychoses in the context of the COVID-19 pandemic: Clinical perspectives from a case series. *Rev. De Psiquiatr. Y Salud Ment.* **2020**, *13*, 90–94. [CrossRef]
55. Parra, A.; Juanes, A.; Losada, C.P.; Álvarez-Sesmero, S.; Santana, V.D.; Martí, I.; Urricelqui, J.; Rentero, D. Psychotic symptoms in COVID-19 patients. A retrospective descriptive study. *Psychiatry Res.* **2020**, *291*, 113254. [CrossRef] [PubMed]

56. Berryhill, M.E.; Peterson, D.; Jones, K.; Tanoue, R. Cognitive Disorders. In *Encyclopedia of Human Behavior*, 2nd ed.; Ramachandran, V.S., Ed.; Academic Press: San Diego, CA, USA, 2012; pp. 536–542. [CrossRef]
57. Small, G.W. What we need to know about age related memory loss. *BMJ (Clin. Res. Ed.)* **2002**, *324*, 1502–1505. [CrossRef]
58. Kozloff, N.; Mulsant, B.H.; Stergiopoulos, V.; Voineskos, A.N. The COVID-19 Global Pandemic: Implications for People with Schizophrenia and Related Disorders. *Schizophr. Bull.* **2020**, *46*, 752–757. [CrossRef]
59. Chen, Y.; Chen, C. How to support the quality of life of people living with cognitive disorders: A (k)new challenge in the post-COVID-19 world. *Eur. J. Neurol.* **2020**, *27*, 1742–1743. [CrossRef] [PubMed]
60. Akiyama, M.J.; Spaulding, A.C.; Rich, J.D. Flattening the Curve for Incarcerated Populations—COVID-19 in Jails and Prisons. *N. Engl. J. Med.* **2020**, *382*, 2075–2077. [CrossRef]
61. Zubair, A.S.; McAlpine, L.S.; Gardin, T.; Farhadian, S.; Kuruvilla, D.E.; Spudich, S. Neuropathogenesis and Neurologic Manifestations of the Coronaviruses in the Age of Coronavirus Disease 2019: A Review. *JAMA Neurol.* **2020**, *77*, 1018–1027. [CrossRef]
62. Acharya, A.; Kevadiya, B.D.; Gendelman, H.E.; Byrareddy, S.N. SARS-CoV-2 Infection Leads to Neurological Dysfunction. *J. Neuroimmune Pharmacol. Off. J. Soc. NeuroImmune Pharmacol.* **2020**, *15*, 167–173. [CrossRef]
63. Obulesu, M.; Lakshmi, M.J. Apoptosis in Alzheimer's disease: An understanding of the physiology, pathology and therapeutic avenues. *Neurochem. Res.* **2014**, *39*, 2301–2312. [CrossRef] [PubMed]
64. Alster, P.; Madetko, N.; Friedman, A. Neutrophil-to-lymphocyte ratio (NLR) at boundaries of Progressive Supranuclear Palsy Syndrome (PSPS) and Corticobasal Syndrome (CBS). *Neurol. I Neurochir. Pol.* **2021**, *55*, 97–101. [CrossRef] [PubMed]
65. Madetko, N.; Migda, B.; Alster, P.; Turski, P.; Koziorowski, D.; Friedman, A. Platelet-to-lymphocyte ratio and neutrophil-tolymphocyte ratio may reflect differences in PD and MSA-P neuroinflammation patterns. *Neurol. I Neurochir. Pol.* **2022**, *56*, 148–155. [CrossRef] [PubMed]
66. Haruyama, K.; Kawakami, M.; Miyai, I.; Nojiri, S.; Fujiwara, T. COVID-19 pandemic and the international classification of functioning in multiple system atrophy: A cross-sectional, nationwide survey in Japan. *Sci. Rep.* **2022**, *12*, 14163. [CrossRef]
67. ElBini Dhouib, I. Does coronaviruses induce neurodegenerative diseases? A systematic review on the neurotropism and neuroinvasion of SARS-CoV-2. *Drug Discov. Ther.* **2021**, *14*, 262–272. [CrossRef]
68. Sy, M.; Kitazawa, M.; Medeiros, R.; Whitman, L.; Cheng, D.; Lane, T.E.; Laferla, F.M. Inflammation induced by infection potentiates tau pathological features in transgenic mice. *Am. J. Pathol.* **2011**, *178*, 2811–2822. [CrossRef]
69. Brown, E.E.; Kumar, S.; Rajji, T.K.; Pollock, B.G.; Mulsant, B.H. Anticipating and Mitigating the Impact of the COVID-19 Pandemic on Alzheimer's Disease and Related Dementias. *Am. J. Geriatr Psychiatry* **2020**, *28*, 712–721. [CrossRef]
70. Xia, X.; Wang, Y.; Zheng, J. COVID-19 and Alzheimer's disease: How one crisis worsens the other. *Transl. Neurodegener.* **2021**, *10*, 15. [CrossRef]
71. Xiong, N.; Schiller, M.R.; Li, J.; Chen, X.; Lin, Z. Severe COVID-19 in Alzheimer's disease: APOE4's fault again? *Alzheimer's Res. Ther.* **2021**, *13*, 111. [CrossRef]
72. Limphaibool, N.; Iwanowski, P.; Holstad, M.J.V.; Kobylarek, D.; Kozubski, W. Infectious Etiologies of Parkinsonism: Pathomechanisms and Clinical Implications. *Front. Neurol.* **2019**, *10*, 652. [CrossRef]
73. van der Heide, A.; Meinders, M.J.; Bloem, B.R.; Helmich, R.C. The Impact of the COVID-19 Pandemic on Psychological Distress, Physical Activity, and Symptom Severity in Parkinson's Disease. *J. Parkinson's Dis.* **2020**, *10*, 1355–1364. [CrossRef] [PubMed]
74. Helmich, R.C.; Bloem, B.R. The Impact of the COVID-19 Pandemic on Parkinson's Disease: Hidden Sorrows and Emerging Opportunities. *J. Parkinson's Dis.* **2020**, *10*, 351–354. [CrossRef] [PubMed]
75. Zach, H.; Dirkx, M.F.; Pasman, J.W.; Bloem, B.R.; Helmich, R.C. Cognitive Stress Reduces the Effect of Levodopa on Parkinson's Resting Tremor. *CNS Neurosci. Ther.* **2017**, *23*, 209–215. [CrossRef]
76. Djamshidian, A.; Lees, A.J. Can stress trigger Parkinson's disease? *J. Neurol. Neurosurg. Psychiatry* **2014**, *85*, 878–881. [CrossRef] [PubMed]
77. Ehgoetz Martens, K.A.; Hall, J.M.; Georgiades, M.J.; Gilat, M.; Walton, C.C.; Matar, E.; Lewis, S.J.G.; Shine, J.M. The functional network signature of heterogeneity in freezing of gait. *Brain A J. Neurol.* **2018**, *141*, 1145–1160. [CrossRef] [PubMed]
78. Antonini, A.; Leta, V.; Teo, J.; Chaudhuri, K.R. Outcome of Parkinson's Disease Patients Affected by COVID-19. *Mov. Disord. Off. J. Mov. Disord. Soc.* **2020**, *35*, 905–908. [CrossRef] [PubMed]
79. Cilia, R.; Bonvegna, S.; Straccia, G.; Andreasi, N.G.; Elia, A.E.; Romito, L.M.; Devigili, G.; Cereda, E.; Eleopra, R. Effects of COVID-19 on Parkinson's Disease Clinical Features: A Community-Based Case-Control Study. *Mov. Disord. Off. J. Mov. Disord. Soc.* **2020**, *35*, 1287–1292. [CrossRef]
80. Williamson, A.E.; Tydeman, F.; Miners, A.; Pyper, K.; Martineau, A.R. Short-term and long-term impacts of COVID-19 on economic vulnerability: A population-based longitudinal study (COVIDENCE UK). *BMJ Open* **2022**, *12*, e065083. [CrossRef]
81. Panchal, N.; Kamal, R.; Cox, C.; Garfield, R. The Implications of COVID-19 for Mental Health and Substance Use. Available online: https://www.kff.org/coronavirus-covid-19/issue-brief/the-implications-of-covid-19-for-mental-health-and-substance-use/ (accessed on 24 August 2022).
82. Shoib, S.; Zharkova, A.; Pal, A.; Jain, N.; Saleem, S.M.; Kolesnyk, P. Refugees and Mental health crisis in Ukraine. *Asian J. Psychiatry* **2022**, *74*, 103169. [CrossRef]
83. Mohammadsadeghi, H.; Bazrafshan, S.; Seify-Moghadam, N.; Mazaheri Nejad Fard, G.; Rasoulian, M.; Eftekhar Ardebili, M. War, immigration and COVID-19: The experience of Afghan immigrants to Iran Amid the pandemic. *Front. Psychiatry* **2022**, *13*, 908321. [CrossRef]

84. Dangmann, C.; Solberg, Ø.; Myhrene Steffenak, A.K.; Høye, S.; Andersen, P.N. Syrian Refugee Youth Resettled in Norway: Mechanisms of Resilience Influencing Health-Related Quality of Life and Mental Distress. *Front. Public Health* **2021**, *9*, 711451. [CrossRef] [PubMed]
85. Evans, J.; Bansal, A.; Schoenaker, D.; Cherbuin, N.; Peek, M.J.; Davis, D.L. Birth Outcomes, Health, and Health Care Needs of Childbearing Women following Wildfire Disasters: An Integrative, State-of-the-Science Review. *Environ. Health Perspect.* **2022**, *130*, 86001. [CrossRef] [PubMed]
86. Lafarga Previdi, I.; Welton, M.; Díaz Rivera, J.; Watkins, D.J.; Díaz, Z.; Torres, H.R.; Galán, C.; Guilloty, N.I.; Agosto, L.D.; Cordero, J.F.; et al. The Impact of Natural Disasters on Maternal Health: Hurricanes Irma and María in Puerto Rico. *Children* **2022**, *9*, 940. [CrossRef]
87. Vivalya, B.M.N.; Vagheni, M.M.; Kitoko, G.M.B.; Vutegha, J.M.; Kalume, A.K.; Piripiri, A.L.; Masika, Y.D.; Mbeva, J.K. Developing mental health services during and in the aftermath of the Ebola virus disease outbreak in armed conflict settings: A scoping review. *Glob. Health* **2022**, *18*, 71. [CrossRef]
88. Mohammed, A.; Sheikh, T.L.; Poggensee, G.; Nguku, P.; Olayinka, A.; Ohuabunwo, C.; Eaton, J. Mental health in emergency response: Lessons from Ebola. *Lancet. Psychiatry* **2015**, *2*, 955–957. [CrossRef]
89. Kotzky, K.; Allen, J.E.; Robinson, L.R.; Satterfield-Nash, A.; Bertolli, J.; Smith, C.; Ornelas Pereira, I.; Faria, E.S.S.A.C.; Peacock, G. Depressive Symptoms and Care Demands Among Primary Caregivers of Young Children with Evidence of Congenital Zika Virus Infection in Brazil. *J. Dev. Behav. Pediatr. JDBP* **2019**, *40*, 344–353. [CrossRef]
90. Delanerolle, G.; Zeng, Y.; Shi, J.Q.; Yeng, X.; Goodison, W.; Shetty, A.; Shetty, S.; Haque, N.; Elliot, K.; Ranaweera, S.; et al. Mental health impact of the Middle East respiratory syndrome, SARS, and COVID-19: A comparative systematic review and meta-analysis. *World J. Psychiatry* **2022**, *12*, 739–765. [CrossRef]
91. Jeong, H.; Yim, H.W.; Song, Y.J.; Ki, M.; Min, J.A.; Cho, J.; Chae, J.H. Mental health status of people isolated due to Middle East Respiratory Syndrome. *Epidemiol. Health* **2016**, *38*, e2016048. [CrossRef]
92. Fountoulakis, K.N.; Karakatsoulis, G.N.; Abraham, S.; Adorjan, K.; Ahmed, H.U.; Alarcón, R.D.; Arai, K.; Auwal, S.S.; Berk, M.; Bjedov, S.; et al. The effect of different degrees of lockdown and self-identified gender on anxiety, depression and suicidality during the COVID-19 pandemic: Data from the international COMET-G study. *Psychiatry Res.* **2022**, *315*, 114702. [CrossRef]
93. Zangani, C.; Ostinelli, E.G.; Smith, K.A.; Hong, J.S.W.; Macdonald, O.; Reen, G.; Reid, K.; Vincent, C.; Syed Sheriff, R.; Harrison, P.J.; et al. Impact of the COVID-19 Pandemic on the Global Delivery of Mental Health Services and Telemental Health: Systematic Review. *JMIR Ment. Health* **2022**, *9*, e38600. [CrossRef]
94. Ojeahere, M.I.; de Filippis, R.; Ransing, R.; Karaliuniene, R.; Ullah, I.; Bytyçi, D.G.; Abbass, Z.; Kilic, O.; Nahidi, M.; Hayatudeen, N.; et al. Management of psychiatric conditions and delirium during the COVID-19 pandemic across continents: Lessons learned and recommendations. *Brain Behav. Immun. Health* **2020**, *9*, 100147. [CrossRef] [PubMed]
95. Mehta, P.; McAuley, D.F.; Brown, M.; Sanchez, E.; Tattersall, R.S.; Manson, J.J. COVID-19: Consider cytokine storm syndromes and immunosuppression. *Lancet* **2020**, *395*, 1033–1034. [CrossRef]
96. Han, Y.; Yuan, K.; Wang, Z.; Liu, W.J.; Lu, Z.A.; Liu, L.; Shi, L.; Yan, W.; Yuan, J.L.; Li, J.L.; et al. Neuropsychiatric manifestations of COVID-19, potential neurotropic mechanisms, and therapeutic interventions. *Transl. Psychiatry* **2021**, *11*, 499. [CrossRef] [PubMed]
97. Rogers, J.P.; Rooney, A.G. Neuropsychiatric sequelae of COVID-19 after vaccination: A gathering storm? *Brain Behav. Immun.* **2022**, *106*, 30–31. [CrossRef] [PubMed]
98. Taquet, M.; Dercon, Q.; Harrison, P.J. Six-month sequelae of post-vaccination SARS-CoV-2 infection: A retrospective cohort study of 10,024 breakthrough infections. *Brain Behav. Immun.* **2022**, *103*, 154–162. [CrossRef]
99. Asgarzadeh, A.; Fouladi, N.; Asghariazar, V.; Sarabi, S.F.; Khiavi, H.A.; Mahmoudi, M.; Safarzadeh, E. Serum Brain-Derived Neurotrophic Factor (BDNF) in COVID-19 Patients and its Association with the COVID-19 Manifestations. *J. Mol. Neurosci. MN* **2022**, *72*, 1820–1830. [CrossRef]
100. Putilina, M.V.; Teplova, N.V.; Poryadin, G.V. Prospects for pharmacological adaptation of neurovascular unit in conditions of neurotropic viral infection. *Zhurnal Nevrol. I Psikhiatrii Im. S.S. Korsakova* **2021**, *121*, 144–150. [CrossRef]

MDPI
St. Alban-Anlage 66
4052 Basel
Switzerland
Tel. +41 61 683 77 34
Fax +41 61 302 89 18
www.mdpi.com

Journal of Clinical Medicine Editorial Office
E-mail: jcm@mdpi.com
www.mdpi.com/journal/jcm

www.ingramcontent.com/pod-product-compliance
Lightning Source LLC
LaVergne TN
LVHW070441100526
838202LV00014B/1640